The Healthy and Sick Newborn

Editor

DAVID A. CLARK

PEDIATRIC CLINICS
OF NORTH AMERICA

www.pediatric.theclinics.com

Consulting Editor
BONITA F. STANTON

April 2015 • Volume 62 • Number 2

ELSEVIER

1600 John F. Kennedy Boulevard ● Suite 1800 ● Philadelphia, Pennsylvania, 19103-2899

http://www.theclinics.com

THE PEDIATRIC CLINICS OF NORTH AMERICA Volume 62, Number 2
April 2015 ISSN 0031-3955, ISBN-13: 978-0-323-35981-8

Editor: Kerry Holland
Developmental Editor: Casey Jackson

The Pediatric Clinics of North America (ISSN 0031-3955) is published bimonthly by Elsevier Inc., 360 Park Avenue South, New York, New York 10010-1710. Months of issue are February, April, June, August, October, and December. Periodicals postage paid at New York, NY and additional mailing offices. Subscription prices are $200.00 per year (US individuals), $493.00 per year (US institutions), $270.00 per year (Canadian individuals), $657.00 per year (Canadian institutions), $325.00 per year (international individuals), $657.00 per year (international institutions), $100.00 per year (US students and residents), and $165.00 per year (international and Canadian residents and students). To receive students/resident rare, orders must be accompanied by name of affiliated institution, date of term, and the signature of program/residency coordinator on institution letterhead. Orders will be billed at individual rate until proof of status is received. Foreign air speed delivery is included in all Clinics subscription prices. All prices are subject to change without notice. **POSTMASTER:** Send address changes to The Pediatric Clinics of North America, Elsevier Health Sciences Division, Subscription Customer Service, 3251 Riverport Lane, Maryland Heights, MO 63043. **Customer Service: 1-800-654-2452 (US and Canada). From outside of the US and Canada: 1-314-447-8871. Fax: 1-314-447-8029. For print support, E-mail: JournalsCustomerService-usa@elsevier.com. For online support, E-mail: JournalsOnlineSupport-usa@elsevier.com.**

Reprints. For copies of 100 or more, of articles in this publication, please contact the Commercial Reprints Department, Elsevier Inc., 360 Park Avenue South, New York, NY 10010-1710. Tel.: 212-633-3874; Fax: 212-633-3820; E-mail: reprints@elsevier.com.

The Pediatric Clinics of North America is also published in Spanish by McGraw-Hill Inter-americana Editores S.A., Mexico City, Mexico; in Portuguese by Riechmann and Affonso Editores, Rua Comandante Coelho 1085, CEP 21250, Rio de Janeiro, Brazil; and in Greek by Althayia SA, Athens, Greece.

The Pediatric Clinics of North America is covered in MEDLINE/PubMed (Index Medicus), Excerpta Medica, Current Contents, Current Contents/Clinical Medicine, Science Citation Index, ASCA, ISI/BIOMED, and BIOSIS.

PROGRAM OBJECTIVE

The goal of the *Pediatric Clinics of North America* is to keep practicing physicians and residents up to date with current clinical practice in pediatrics by providing timely articles reviewing the state-of-the-art in patient care.

TARGET AUDIENCE

All practicing pediatricians, physicians and healthcare professionals who provide patient care to pediatric patients.

LEARNING OBJECTIVES

Upon completion of this activity, participants will be able to:
1. Discuss the transition from fetus to newborn.
2. Review care considerations for healthy newborns and considerations for the newborn that is sick.
3. Describe the initial assessment and management of the newborn and discharge planning.

ACCREDITATION

The Elsevier Office of Continuing Medical Education (EOCME) is accredited by the Accreditation Council for Continuing Medical Education (ACCME) to provide continuing medical education for physicians.

The EOCME designates this enduring material for a maximum of 15 *AMA PRA Category 1 Credit*(s)™. Physicians should claim only the credit commensurate with the extent of their participation in the activity.

All other health care professionals requesting continuing education credit for this enduring material will be issued a certificate of participation.

DISCLOSURE OF CONFLICTS OF INTEREST

The EOCME assesses conflict of interest with its instructors, faculty, planners, and other individuals who are in a position to control the content of CME activities. All relevant conflicts of interest that are identified are thoroughly vetted by EOCME for fair balance, scientific objectivity, and patient care recommendations. EOCME is committed to providing its learners with CME activities that promote improvements or quality in healthcare and not a specific proprietary business or a commercial interest.

The planning committee, staff, authors and editors listed below have identified no financial relationships or relationships to products or devices they or their spouse/life partner have with commercial interest related to the content of this CME activity:

David H. Adamkin, MD; Brian M. Barkemeyer, MD; Richard L. Bucciarelli, MD; Karen Buchi, MD, FAAP; David A. Clark, MD, FAAP; Melinda B. Clark-Gambelunghe, MD, FAAP; Scott C. Denne, MD; Donald J. Fillipps, MD FAAP; Anjali Fortna; Thomas Gates, MD; Julie Gooding, MD; Kerry Holland; Michael J. Horgan, MD; Brynne Hunter; Indu Kumari; Richard E McClead Jr, MD MHA; Arun K. Pramanik, MD; Nandeesh Rangaswamy; Roberto Parulan Santos, MD, MSCS; Robert A. Sinkin, MD, MPH; Bonita F. Stanton, MD; Justin Stiers, MD; Megan Suermann; Jonathan Swanson, MD, MSc; Debra Tristram BS, MD; Robert M. Ward, MD, FAAP, FCP; Jon F. Watchko, MD.

The planning committee, staff, authors and editors listed below have identified financial relationships or relationships to products or devices they or their spouse/life partner have with commercial interest related to the content of this CME activity:

Darius J. Adams, MD is on Speaker's Bureau for and has a research grant with BioMarin Pharmaceutical Inc.

UNAPPROVED/OFF-LABEL USE DISCLOSURE

The EOCME requires CME faculty to disclose to the participants:
1. When products or procedures being discussed are off-label, unlabelled, experimental, and/or investigational (not US Food and Drug Administration [FDA] approved); and
2. Any limitations on the information presented, such as data that are preliminary or that represent ongoing research, interim analyses, and/or unsupported opinions. Faculty may discuss information about pharmaceutical agents that is outside of FDA-approved labelling. This information is intended solely for CME and is not intended to promote off-label use of these medications. If you have any questions, contact the medical affairs department of the manufacturer for the most recent prescribing information.

TO ENROLL

To enroll in the *Pediatric Clinics of North America* Continuing Medical Education program, call customer service at 1-800-654-2452 or sign up online at http://www.theclinics.com/home/cme. The CME program is available to subscribers for an additional annual fee of USD 290.

METHOD OF PARTICIPATION

In order to claim credit, participants must complete the following:

1. Complete enrolment as indicated above.
2. Read the activity.
3. Complete the CME Test and Evaluation. Participants must achieve a score of 70% on the test. All CME Tests and Evaluations must be completed online.

CME INQUIRIES/SPECIAL NEEDS

For all CME inquiries or special needs, please contact elsevierCME@elsevier.com.

Contributors

CONSULTING EDITOR

BONITA F. STANTON, MD
Vice Dean for Research and Professor of Pediatrics, School of Medicine, Wayne State University, Detroit, Michigan

EDITOR

DAVID A. CLARK, MD, FAAP
Professor and Chairman, Department of Pediatrics, Albany Medical College, Director, Children's Hospital at Albany Medical Center, Albany, New York

AUTHORS

DAVID H. ADAMKIN, MD
Professor of Pediatrics; Director, Division of Neonatal Medicine, Rounsavall Endowed Chair of Neonatology, University of Louisville, Louisville, Kentucky

DARIUS J. ADAMS, MD
Clinical and Biochemical Geneticist, Atlantic Health System, Morristown, New Jersey

BRIAN M. BARKEMEYER, MD
Professor of Pediatrics; Division Head, Neonatology, Louisiana State University Health Sciences Center, New Orleans, Louisiana

RICHARD L. BUCCIARELLI, MD
Professor of Pediatrics, Divisions of Neonatology and Pediatric Cardiology, College of Medicine, University of Florida, Gainesville, Florida

KAREN BUCHI, MD, FAAP
Professor, Pediatrics; Chief, Division of General Pediatrics, Department of General Pediatrics, Salt Lake City, Utah

DAVID A. CLARK, MD, FAAP
Atlantic Health System, Morristown, New Jersey; Professor and Chairman, Department of Pediatrics, Albany Medical College, Director, Children's Hospital at Albany Medical Center, Albany, New York

MELINDA B. CLARK-GAMBELUNGHE, MD, FAAP
Associate Professor, Department of Pediatrics, Albany Medical Center, Albany, New York

SCOTT C. DENNE, MD
Associate Chair of Clinical and Translational Research; Professor of Pediatrics, Indiana University School of Medicine, Indianapolis, Indiana

DONALD J. FILLIPPS, MD, FAAP
Clinical Associate Professor, Division of General Pediatrics, College of Medicine, University of Florida, Gainesville, Florida

THOMAS GATES, MD
Associate Professor of Radiology, LSU Health, Shreveport, Louisiana

JULIE R. GOODING, MD
Assistant Professor of Pediatrics, Department of Pediatrics; Staff Neonatologist, Nationwide Children's Hospital, The Ohio State University, Columbus, Ohio

MICHAEL J. HORGAN, MD
Professor, Division of Neonatology, Department of Pediatrics, Children's Hospital at Albany Medical Center, Albany Medical College, Albany, New York

RICHARD E. McCLEAD Jr, MD, MHA
Professor of Pediatrics, Department of Pediatrics; Associate Chief Medical Officer, Nationwide Children's Hospital, The Ohio State University, Columbus, Ohio

ARUN K. PRAMANIK, MD
Professor of Pediatrics, LSU Health, Shreveport, Louisiana

NANDEESH RANGASWAMY, MD
Assistant Professor of Pediatrics, University of Texas Southwestern, Dallas, Texas

ROBERTO PARULAN SANTOS, MD, MSCS
Associate Professor, Pediatric Infectious Diseases, Bernard & Millie Duker Children's Hospital, Albany Medical Center, Albany, New York

ROBERT A. SINKIN, MD, MPH
Medical Director for Newborn Services, Charles Fuller Professor of Neonatology, Head, Division of Neonatology, Department of Pediatrics, University of Virginia Children's Hospital, Charlottesville, Virginia

JUSTIN STIERS, MD
Fellow, Neonatology, Salt Lake City, Utah

JONATHAN R. SWANSON, MD, MSc
Assistant Professor of Pediatrics; Chief Quality Officer for Children's Services; Medical Director, Neonatal Intensive Care Unit, Division of Neonatology, University of Virginia Children's Hospital, Charlottesville, Virginia

DEBRA TRISTRAM, MD
Professor and Division Chief, Pediatric Infectious Disease, Department of Pediatrics, Albany Medical Center, Albany NY, USA

ROBERT M. WARD, MD, FAAP, FCP
Professor, Pediatrics; Adjunct Professor, Pharmacology/Toxicology; Department of Neonatology, Salt Lake City, Utah

JON F. WATCHKO, MD
Professor of Pediatrics, Obstetrics, Gynecology and Reproductive Sciences; Senior Scientist, Magee-Womens Research Institute, Division of Newborn Medicine, Department of Pediatrics, University of Pittsburgh School of Medicine, Pittsburgh, Pennsylvania

Contents

The fetus to newborn transition is a complex physiologic process that requires close monitoring. Approximately 10% of all newborns require some support in facilitating a successful transition after delivery. Clinicians should be aware of the physiologic processes and pay close regard to the newborn's cardiopulmonary transition at birth to provide appropriate treatment and therapies as required. Trained Personnel in the Neonatal Resuscitation program should be available at the delivery for all newborns to ensure that immediate and appropriate care is provided to achieve the best possible outcomes for those babies not smoothly transitioning to extrauterine life.

This article summarizes the initial assessment of normal newborns and describes a few of the common variations that may occur. These variations require a pediatric provider to reassure anxious new parents and provide follow-up communication with the subsequent primary care provider.

Sensory development is complex, with both morphologic and neural components. Development of the senses begins in early fetal life, initially with structures and then in-utero stimulation initiates perception. After birth, environmental stimulants accelerate each sensory organ to nearly complete maturity several months after birth. Vision and hearing are the best studied senses and the most crucial for learning. This article focuses on the cranial senses of vision, hearing, smell, and taste. Sensory function, embryogenesis, external and genetic effects, and common malformations that may affect development are discussed, and the corresponding sensory organs are examined and evaluated.

Although individual metabolic diseases are relatively uncommon, inherited metabolic diseases collectively represent a more common cause of disease in the neonatal period than is generally appreciated. Newborn screening is among the most successful public health programs today. Every day, newborns considered to be at risk for hypoglycemia are screened. The definition of clinically significant hypoglycemia remains among the most confused and contentious issues in neonatology. There are 2 "competing" methods of defining hypoglycemia that suggest very different levels for management: one based on metabolic–endocrinologic hormones and another that uses outcome data to determine threshold levels of risk.

Cytogenetic anomalies should be considered in individuals with multiple congenital anomalies. DNA methylation analysis is the most sensitive initial test in evaluating for Prader-Willi and Angelman syndromes. The timely identification of cytogenetic anomalies allows for prompt initiation of early intervention services to maximize the potential of every individual as they grow older. Although many of these conditions are rare, keeping them in mind can have a profound impact on the clinical course of affected individuals. This article reviews some of the more common genetic syndromes.

Optimal nutrition in infancy is the foundation of health in later life. Based on the demonstrated health benefits of human milk, breastfeeding should be the primary means of nutrition for most infants. Although many mothers experience some problems with breastfeeding, health professionals can use simple strategies to overcome most of these problems. For infants who cannot breastfeed, standard infant formulas support adequate nutrition and growth. Gastroesophageal reflux is a common feeding-related event and occurs in most infants; it is part of normal physiology and requires no intervention. Gastroesophageal reflux disease occurs in a small number of infants necessitating the use of an algorithm-based evaluation and management strategy.

Preterm births account for 12.5% of all births in the United States. The preterm birth rate has increased by 33% over the last 2 decades. Late and premature infants do not develop the serious and chronic conditions of the extreme premature infant. However, there is growing evidence that these infants are not as healthy as previously thought and do in fact have an increase in morbidity and mortality compared with term infants. This article summarizes the epidemiology of late preterm infants and the associated morbidities associated with their prematurity.

Respiratory disorders are the most frequent cause of admission to the special care nursery both in term and preterm infants. Pediatricians and primary care providers may encounter newborn infants with respiratory distress in their office, emergency room, delivery room, or during physical assessment in the newborn nursery. The authors have proposed a practical approach to diagnose and manage such infants, with suggestions for consulting a neonatologist at a regional center. Their objective is that practicing pediatricians should be able to assess and stabilize such infants, and transfer to or consult a neonatologist, cardiologist, or pulmonologist after reading this article.

applications of pharmacogenomics to the neonatal period are presented, along with pediatric challenges of developmental expression of drug-metabolizing enzymes.

Brian M. Barkemeyer

Hospital discharge is a time of transition for infants and families that requires oversight of common postnatal adaptations, screening tests, and establishment of necessary follow-up care. Preterm infants face additional medical problems that vary in complexity by the degree of prematurity. Infants born at lowest gestational ages are at highest risks for complicated neonatal course and adverse long-term outcomes. Successful transition from hospital to home care is essential to improved outcomes for high-risk infants.

PEDIATRIC CLINICS OF NORTH AMERICA

ISSUE OF RELATED INTEREST

Clinics in Perinatology, December 2013 (Vol. 40, Issue 4)
Moderate Preterm, Late Preterm and Early Term Births
Lucky Jain and Tonse N.K. Raju, *Editors*

NOW AVAILABLE FOR YOUR iPhone and iPad

Foreword

The Healthy and Sick Newborn

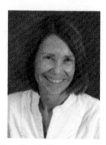

Bonita F. Stanton, MD
Consulting Editor

Few times in the life of parents are associated with as much anticipation, excitement, and anxiety as pregnancy and the newborn period. Likewise, a stunning number of advances have been made over the last several decades in our understanding of and ability to treat and prevent disorders identified during these two critical periods. Practicing pediatricians must be knowledgeable about this new information as they will often be the first to be questioned by a parent, the first to have the opportunity to identify a potential problem, and/or the first to reassure a parent that a condition is a normal variant. For the parents of a neonate who needs additional care, the articles on current approaches to common illnesses, medications, and diagnostic procedures will enable the pediatrician to offer comfort through knowledge-based explanation.

This thoughtful and carefully compiled issue thoroughly reviews normal fetal and neonatal growth and development, screening procedures, and the identification of abnormalities. This is a "must read" issue for pediatricians who have contact with families during the prenatal period and/or with neonates and their families. Written in a practical manner, the issue carefully reviews established procedures and approaches as well as describes new diagnostic approaches and criteria.

A careful reading of these articles will well equip you to make a substantial difference in the life of young parents as they welcome their newborn into the world!

Bonita F. Stanton, MD
School of Medicine
Wayne State University
1261 Scott Hall
540 East Canfield, Suite 1261
Detroit, MI 48201, USA

E-mail address:
bstanton@med.wayne.edu

Pediatr Clin N Am 62 (2015) xiii
http://dx.doi.org/10.1016/j.pcl.2015.01.002
0031-3955/15/$ – see front matter © 2015 Published by Elsevier Inc.

pediatric.theclinics.com

Preface

The Problem Baby: Too Much Information

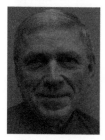

David A. Clark, MD
Editor

The medical care of acutely ill neonates has become increasingly complex. Advances in virtually every basic science discipline have refined our understanding of the basic physiology underpinning the ever more complex therapy. This is especially true of breakthroughs in the subtleties of brain development, genetic and metabolic disease, epigenetic influences on fetal and early childhood organ maturation, pulmonary physiology, and the gastrointestinal tract, including nutrition, to name a few.

The medical literature has mushroomed beyond the capability of even the most avid reader to fully master. A search for the term newborn or neonate in PubMed yielded 378,177 citations, and a similar search in Google Scholar (the academic subset of the massive search engine) resulted in 411,000+ citations for neonate and 1,580,000+ hits for newborn. Even a limited topic such as neonatal necrotizing enterocolitis produced over 2800 PubMed responses. The most useful reference textbooks on Neonatology exceed 1500 pages written in the ever more technical language of neonatologese.

The authors of the articles in this issue were challenged to distill the vast amount of information to a subset of practical and useful concepts to assist the primary care provider. They bring over 300 years of combined experience in caring for critically ill newborns. In addition, they have authored over 1000 peer-reviewed publications, trained more than 3000 pediatricians, and have been mentors to at least 400 neonatal-perinatal fellows.

Pediatr Clin N Am 62 (2015) xv–xvi
http://dx.doi.org/10.1016/j.pcl.2015.01.001
0031-3955/15/$ – see front matter © 2015 Published by Elsevier Inc.

pediatric.theclinics.com

I thank the authors and their colleagues for their willingness to devote time from their hectic schedules to share their insights and experience in order to provide a handy, quick reference to the many "front-line" physicians evaluating neonates.

David A. Clark, MD
Albany Medical College
Children's Hospital at Albany Medical Center
MC88, 43 New Scotland Avenue
Albany, NY 12208, USA

E-mail address:
clarkd@mail.amc.edu

Erratum

An error was made in the December 2014 (Volume 61, Number 6) and February 2015 (Volume 62, Number 1) issues of *Pediatric Clinics of North America* on the Forthcoming Issues page. Dr Gyula Acsadi's name is spelled incorrectly as Guyla Acsadi.

Pediatr Clin N Am 62 (2015) xvii
http://dx.doi.org/10.1016/j.pcl.2015.02.001
0031-3955/15/$ – see front matter © 2015 Published by Elsevier Inc.

Transition from Fetus to Newborn

Jonathan R. Swanson, MD, MSc, Robert A. Sinkin, MD, MPH*

KEYWORDS

- Neonate • Transition • Resuscitation • Physiology • Neonatal resuscitation program
- Fetal circulation

KEY POINTS

- The fetus to newborn transition is complex and depends on several factors, including maternal health and chronic medical conditions, the status of the placenta, gestational duration, presence of fetal anomalies, and delivery room care.
- Although the vast majority of infants do well, approximately 10% require intervention to facilitate the transition from fetus to newborn.
- Clinicians caring for newborns should be well-versed in the recommendations of the Neonatal Resuscitation Program.

INTRODUCTION

The adaptation from the intrauterine to extrauterine environment is complex and likely among the most remarkable and difficult physiologic transitions known, all the more noteworthy because it is also a normal and required process for our species. Although all systems of the human body undergo extensive changes, the initial and most crucial adaptations occur in the pulmonary and cardiovascular systems (**Box 1**). Clinicians who take care of newborns during this transition must be prepared to help neonates having difficulty during this changeover. Maternal medical and fetal conditions can have a profound effect on a successful transition. Understanding how these issues affect a neonate's ability to adapt ex utero are essential for informing a clinician's ability to shepherd a newborn through this process. Up to 10% of newborns require some clinical intervention during birth, and approximately 1% require more extensive resuscitation.[1] It is imperative that clinicians be prepared to provide needed interventions and understand why some neonates have difficulty transitioning.

Disclosures: None.
Division of Neonatology, Department of Pediatrics, University of Virginia Children's Hospital, Box 800386, Charlottesville, VA 22908, USA
* Corresponding author.
E-mail address: rsinkin@virginia.edu

Box 1
Requirements for a normal fetal to newborn transition

- Fetal lung fluid resorption
- Expansion of lungs and establishment of functional residual capacity
- Increased systemic vascular resistance
- Decreased pulmonary vascular resistance and increased pulmonary blood flow
- Closure of right to left shunts

FETUS TO NEWBORN TRANSITION PHYSIOLOGY

The fetus to newborn physiologic transition begins in utero. This transition depends on several factors, including maternal health and chronic medical conditions, the status of the placenta, gestational duration, and the presence of fetal anomalies. The physiology of this transition is complex and requires an understanding of the cardiovascular and pulmonary systems in utero and ex utero.

Fetal Cardiopulmonary Physiology

In utero, the fetus depends on the placenta for all gas exchange and nutrient delivery from the maternal circulation. The placenta has low vascular resistance and receives approximately 40% of fetal cardiac output.[2] Because the fetal lungs are not required for gas exchange, only approximately 10% of cardiac output passes through the pulmonary circulation.[3] Blood flows through the umbilical artery to the placenta, where it is oxygenated and then delivered back to the fetus through the umbilical vein with an oxygen saturation of approximately 80% (PaO_2 30–35 mmHg).[4] Blood in the umbilical vein is mixed with portal venous blood from the fetus, and reaches the right atrium via the inferior vena cava with an oxygen saturation of about 67%.[4] Owing to the dynamics of blood flow and the anatomic location of the foramen ovale, this relatively well-oxygenated blood is preferentially shunted across the foramen into the left atrium and subsequently pumped from the left ventricle into the aorta. This fetal shunt allows for the favored delivery of more highly oxygenated blood to the brain (carotid arteries) and heart (coronary arteries). Similarly, blood returning to the heart via the superior vena cava is directed to the right ventricle, where it is pumped into the pulmonary artery. Owing to relative fetal hypoxia, the pulmonary arteries are vasoconstricted, resulting in high pulmonary vascular resistance. Secondary to this high resistance and the low systemic resistance (secondary to the placenta), the majority of red blood cells traverse the ductus arteriosus to the descending aorta where they are delivered to the placenta for reoxygenation.

Fetal lung growth and maturation revolve around fetal lung fluid. This fluid is detected as early as the first trimester, although secretion depends on gestational age until its significantly reduced production before labor.[5,6] The active transport of chloride has been elucidated as the mechanism of fetal lung fluid secretion.[7] Owing in part to closed vocal cords, the secretion of fetal lung fluid results in increased bronchoalveolar intraluminal pressure, allowing developing lung airway structures to stay open while also contributing to elevated pulmonary vascular resistance.

Fetus to Newborn Cardiovascular and Pulmonary Changes

Many textbooks promote the incorrect belief that the fetus to newborn transition begins when the umbilical cord is clamped or cut; however, transition is initiated before the onset of labor. The successful transition begins with fetal lung fluid clearance. Cortisol production, which plays a role in multiple organ systems preparing the fetus for transition to ex utero, increases dramatically at the end of the third trimester as the fetal adrenal gland matures. One mechanism by which cortisol prepares the fetus is via its effect on pulmonary maturation. Surfactant production increases, which allows for a reduction in alveolar surface tension while maintaining alveolar expansion.[8] Cortisol likewise increases β-adrenergic receptors within the lung and increases the transcription of genes that produce epithelial sodium channels.[6,9] Epithelial sodium channels transform the lung from a chloride-secreting organ into one that reabsorbs sodium, thereby pulling fetal lung fluid out of the alveolar air spaces and into the interstitium and intravascular spaces. Studies in sheep have demonstrated that this transition begins before the onset of labor, but then significantly increases during labor. Bland and colleagues[10] found that sheep delivered after labor had 45% less lung fluid than those delivered without going through labor.

After delivery, the remainder of the fetal lung fluid is resorbed via several mechanisms. Increased blood oxygen concentration increases epithelial sodium channels gene expression, which improves the ability of the epithelium to transport sodium and water into the interstitium.[11,12] The initial breaths of the infant also generate elevated intrapulmonary pressure, which drives alveolar fluid into the interstitium. Pressures between −50 and 70 cm H_2O have been measured in term infants in the delivery room.[13] Finally, although it was previously believed that the thoracic squeeze while the fetus travels through the birth canal cleared fetal lung fluid, it is now thought that this mechanism plays a very minor role.[14]

In the near-term fetus, cardiac output is approximately 450 mL/kg per minute with two-thirds of the output performed by the right ventricle.[15] Soon after birth, however, there is a marked increase in cardiac output by both the right and left ventricles, increasing blood flow to the lungs, heart, kidney, and intestines.[9,16] Although this marked increase is secondary to multiple factors, the increased levels of cortisol, as described, likely plays a major role.

Another cardiovascular change after delivery includes the closure of several vascular shunts (**Table 1**). Once an infant starts to breathe, oxygen content within the blood is higher than it is in utero. This reduction in hypoxia leads to vasoconstriction of the umbilical artery and, because oxygen is a potent pulmonary dilator,

Table 1
Fetal vessels and cardiovascular shunts

Vessels	In Utero Function	Response to Delivery
Umbilical artery	Blood from descending aorta to placenta	Vasoconstrict with increased oxygenation
Umbilical vein	Blood from placenta to inferior vena cava	Collapse with absent blood flow
Ductus arteriosus	Shunt from pulmonary artery to descending aorta	Functionally closes with increased oxygenation and loss of prostaglandin E2 from placenta
Ductus venosus	Shunt from umbilical vein to inferior vena cava	Collapse with absent blood flow
Foramen ovale	Allows blood flow between right and left atria	Closes when systemic pressure is greater than pulmonary pressure
Pulmonary arteries	Minimal—vasoconstricted in hypoxic environment	Vasodilate with elevated oxygen levels

pulmonary vascular resistance falls. This allows for an increase in pulmonary blood flow, further increasing oxygen delivery throughout the body. In a duration of approximately 10 minutes, a newborn's oxygen saturation increases from a fetal level of approximately 60% to well over 90% (**Box 2**).[1,17] Additionally, as oxygenation improves, calcium channels are activated in the smooth muscle of the ductus arteriosus leading to ductal constriction, limiting blood flow and functionally closing the ductus arteriosus. As systemic vascular resistance increases and pulmonary vascular resistance decreases, the pressure gradient at the atrial level changes and the foramen ovale physiologically closes, stopping the right-to-left atrial shunt.

The timing of umbilical cord clamping also plays a role in the success of this transition and recent data suggest that transition may be adversely effected by premature cord cutting or clamping. Charles Darwin's grandfather, Erasmus Darwin, a British physician, noted in 1801:

Another thing very injurious to the child, is the tying and cutting of the navel string too soon; which should always be left till the child has not only repeatedly breathed but till all pulsation in the cord ceases. As otherwise the child is much weaker than it ought to be, a portion of the blood being left in the placenta, which ought to have been in the child.[18]

Although the umbilical artery constricts with increasing oxygenation, preventing further blood flow to the placenta from the newborn, the umbilical vein remains dilated, allowing blood to continue to flow from the placenta in the direction of gravity. There is increasing evidence that delaying cord clamping until the onset of respirations is important and beneficial in newborn transition. In preterm lambs, Bhatt and colleagues[19] demonstrated that delaying cord clamping for 3 to 4 minutes until ventilation was established resulted in improved cardiac function. Lambs whose cords were immediately clamped had a significant, although transient, increase in pulmonary and carotid artery pressures and blood flow, and a significant decrease in right ventricular output and heart rate. Lambs whose cords were clamped after establishing ventilation had no change in heart rate and ultimately a much more stable cardiovascular transition at birth. In a cohort study of more than 15,000 infants in Tanzania, neonates were more likely to die or require hospital admission when cord clamping occurred before or immediately after onset of spontaneous respirations compared with infants who were breathing before cord clamping.[20] For every 10 seconds cord clamping was delayed after initiation of spontaneous respiration, the risk of death or admission

---

Box 2
Targeted preductal oxygen saturation after birth

- 1 minute: 60%–65%
- 2 minutes: 65%–70%
- 3 minutes: 70%–75%
- 4 minutes: 75%–80%
- 5 minutes: 85%–90%
- 10 minutes: 85%–95%

From Kattwinkel J, Perlman JM, Aziz K, et al. Part 15: neonatal resuscitation: 2010 American Heart Association guidelines for cardiopulmonary resuscitation and emergency cardiovascular care. Circulation 2010;122:S909–19; with permission.

decreased by 20% across birth weight groups. This evidence suggests that the cardiopulmonary transition of a neonate is much smoother and more stable when cord clamping occurs after the establishment of ventilation. Several trials evaluating this process are currently registered at Clinicaltrials.gov.

NEONATAL PROBLEMS OF TRANSITION

As previously cited, although the majority of infants successfully transition from intra-uterine to extrauterine life, approximately 10% require some resuscitation at birth owing to difficulty in adaptation.[1] The issues surrounding these difficulties can be divided into several categories, of which the clinician should be aware to anticipate the potential need for resuscitative support both in the delivery room and in the early hours and days after birth.

Maternal Conditions Affecting the Newborn Transition

Maternal conditions can significantly affect a newborn's ability to transition effectively; clinicians should be aware of them whether they are chronic medical conditions, or issues that arise during prenatal screening or over the course of the pregnancy (**Box 3**). Although it is beyond the scope of this article, clinicians should be well aware of chronic medical conditions that require early initiation of therapy to the newborn. This includes several chronic infections, such as maternal human immunodeficiency virus and hepatitis B virus infection. Other conditions include Rh incompatibility, which can lead to hemolytic disease of the newborn, and immune thrombocytopenic purpura, which may lead to cerebral and other organ bleeding, secondary to thrombocytopenia. Additionally, prenatal screening results may require the clinician to manage the newborn differently. The prenatal findings of fetal hydronephrosis or echogenic cardiac foci may suggest further imaging is needed. Therefore, clinicians caring for the newborn should be knowledgeable of the entire maternal medical history, both prepregnancy and prenatal.

Certain, more acute maternal medical conditions may also cause difficulties in transition for the newborn for which the newborn clinician should be aware and anticipate the need for resuscitative measures. Hypertensive disorders in pregnancy including gestational hypertension, preeclampsia, eclampsia, hemolysis, elevated liver enzymes, low platelets (HELLP syndrome), or previously diagnosed chronic hypertension, are not uncommon worldwide.[21] Preeclampsia complicates up to 10% of pregnancies in the United States alone and is thought to be even greater in underdeveloped countries.[22] This spectrum of hypertensive disorders can all contribute to intrauterine growth restriction (decreased birth weight/small for gestational age status)

Box 3
Fetal to newborn transition difficulties—maternal conditions

- Hypertensive disorders (primary [essential] and secondary hypertension, preeclampsia, hemolysis, elevated liver enzymes, low platelets [HELLP])
- Diabetes mellitus
- Perinatal substance abuse
- Lupus
- Myasthenia gravis
- Advanced maternal age

likely secondary to decreased uteroplacental blood flow and ischemia. Fetal intrauterine growth restriction is a significant risk factor for fetal demise and neonatal death.[22–25] Associated with these hypertensive disorders are 2 common hematologic manifestations in the neonate: neutropenia (absolute neutrophil count <500/μL) and thrombocytopenia (platelet count <150,000/μL). Newborns of mothers with preeclampsia have up to a 50% incidence of neutropenia, but it is generally thought to be self-limited.[26,27] Although the pathogenesis of neonatal thrombocytopenia in preeclampsia is unknown, it may be clinically significant, necessitating 1 or more platelet transfusions.[28] Therefore, newborns of preeclamptic women should be monitored closely with examination of a complete blood count with differential even if asymptomatic. Finally, if low birth weight, clinicians should monitor the neonate's ability to tolerate feedings and maintain thermoregulatory homeostasis while transitioning; such difficulties are not infrequent and often require admission to special care nurseries.[29,30]

Maternal diabetes mellitus can also have a profound influence on the fetus to newborn transition. Glucose levels in the fetus are entirely dependent upon facilitated diffusion across the placenta from the maternal serum. When the fetus lives in a chronic state of abnormally elevated glucose levels (poorly controlled diabetes), fetal insulin levels increase and glucagon levels decrease. This can result in hyperinsulinsim in the fetus. At birth, after the maternal glucose supply is acutely interrupted, newborn insulin levels decrease and glucagon levels increase. However, insulin levels may not decrease quickly enough in the setting of the acute glucose shortage, resulting in hypoglycemia. Frequent checking of blood glucose levels in the newborn is warranted to detect hypoglycemia and to ensure appropriate response to treatment.[31] Early breastfeeding (within 1 hour of delivery) to prevent hypoglycemia has been studied and should be encouraged.[32] Additionally, when hypoglycemic events do occur, dextrose gel therapy may be considered to prevent recurrent events.[33]

Other conditions associated with maternal diabetes are not insignificant. Uncontrolled diabetes results in increased risk of newborn hyperbilirubinemia, polycythemia, asymmetric septal hypertrophy, and hypocalcemia, all of which must be anticipated by the clinician responsible for the newborn to treat or prevent long-term morbidity.[34] Macrosomic neonates of diabetic mothers are also at greater risk of birth injuries and hypoxic–ischemic encephalopathy.[35] Focusing on ensuring adequate cardiorespiratory transition at birth, infants of diabetic mothers are at higher risk of developing respiratory distress syndrome (RDS) compared with similarly aged infants of nondiabetic mothers.[36–38] The pathogenesis of RDS in infants of diabetic mothers stems from a relative surfactant deficiency. In a study examining more than 3000 deliveries after 34 weeks' gestation, gestational diabetes was identified as an independent risk factor for admission to a neonatal intensive care unit or the need for ventilator support at 24 hours of age with an adjusted odds ratio of 11.55.[38] Although the authors did not evaluate the immediate need for aggressive resuscitation, it is likely that many of the neonates receiving ventilator support required significant respiratory support in the delivery room.

Clinicians should also be aware of other maternal conditions that can affect a neonate's ability to transition effectively from the in utero environment. Mothers of advanced maternal age (>35 years) are at greater risk not only for maternal morbidities, but their newborns face greater risks for neonatal morbidities and mortality. The risks of preterm birth, small for gestational age stature, low Apgar score, fetal death, and neonatal death increase as maternal age advances over the age of 30.[39] There is also increased risk of gestational diabetes and hypertensive disorders in mothers over the age of 45 years.[40]

Maternal substance abuse is another significant contributor to increased perinatal morbidities. In a single-center study of 85 pregnancies complicated by illicit drug abuse, premature delivery, congenital anomalies, low birth weight, and Apgar scores of less than 7 were all increased in neonates of mothers abusing drugs.[41] In addition, there was an increased risk of maternal hepatitis infections and neonatal abstinence syndrome. Clinicians should be well aware of the potential need for closer observation in these infants.

Another chronic medical condition that can affect neonatal management is myasthenia gravis. Antibodies to acetylcholine receptors (typically immunoglobulin G, which crosses the placenta) are found in up to 90% of mothers with myasthenia gravis. Approximately 10% to 20% of newborns born to these mothers can present with sequelae, including arthrogryposis, respiratory distress, and poor feeding.[42,43] Symptoms typically occur 12 to 48 hours after birth and can last for several weeks, although earlier symptomatology can occur. Finally, maternal lupus is the most likely cause of fetal heart block that can cause significant cardiopulmonary disease at birth owing to poor cardiac output. It is paramount that clinicians understand and are knowledgeable about the maternal medical history of the newborns that are under their care.

Fetal/Newborn Conditions Affecting Transition

Several conditions in the fetus and newborn can adversely affect the transition from intrauterine to extrauterine life (**Box 4**). The most problematic transitional medical condition for the clinician is persistent pulmonary hypertension of the newborn (PPHN, formerly called persistent fetal circulation). PPHN is characterized by elevated pulmonary vascular resistance that results in extrapulmonary shunting across the ductus arteriosus and continued right-to-left shunting through the foramen ovale, leading to significant hypoxemia. Risk factors that are independently associated with PPHN include late preterm or postterm birth, large for gestational age, and cesarean delivery.[44] Maternal risk factors include black or Asian race, diabetes, and asthma.[44] Although direct causation has not been shown with these risk factors, clinicians need to be alert to the increased susceptibility to developing PPHN and the need for close monitoring and interventions required in the immediate neonatal period for these newborns to minimize its potential morbidity.

Box 4
Fetal to newborn transition difficulties—fetal/infant conditions

- Congenital anomalies
  - Heart defects
  - Diaphragmatic hernia
  - Airway anomalies
- Pulmonary hypoplasia
- Sepsis/pneumonia
- Persistent pulmonary hypertension
- Prematurity
- Intrauterine growth restriction/small for gestational age
- Large for gestational age

Respiratory distress in the newborn period can also present as a result of poor respiratory effort, airway malformations, and impaired lung function. Poor respiratory effort in the newborn can result in delayed clearance of fetal lung fluid, as described previously. This respiratory depression can be secondary to a variety of factors, including maternal analgesia, congenital neuromuscular disorders, and neonatal encephalopathy. Congenital anomalies of the airway, although rare, may mechanically block the bronchi or trachea, preventing adequate lung inflation and resulting in continued elevations in pulmonary vascular resistance. Some causes include choanal atresia, laryngeal webs, and, more commonly, the presence of meconium or mucus in the airway. Routine oral or nasopharyngeal suctioning of infants is no longer recommended because it can be associated with cardiorespiratory complications.[45] Current practice and recommendations in the Neonatal Resuscitation Program (NRP) for infants born through meconium-stained fluid includes tracheal suctioning in nonvigorous infants.[1] However, the evidence available for even this scaled-down intervention does not support or refute this activity; it is likely that this recommendation may change in subsequent editions of the NRP.[45]

Impaired lung function in the neonate results from several mechanisms, including the presence of air leaks, pulmonary hypoplasia (secondary to prolonged oligohydramnios or congenital diaphragmatic hernia), and intrinsic lung disease. Congenital pneumonia is rare but typically presents immediately after delivery. It is acquired either through aspiration of infected amniotic fluid or via vertical transmission from maternal vaginal or blood infections. More commonly affecting the neonatal transition are RDS and transient tachypnea of the newborn. RDS is associated with decreased lung volumes, air bronchograms, and ground glass appearance on radiographic studies. Clinically, infants present with grunting, retractions, and tachypnea. If left untreated, the reduced lung volumes and hypoxemia may lead to continued elevation of pulmonary artery pressures. Transient tachypnea of the newborn is more commonly associated with inadequate or delayed clearance of fetal lung fluid. As described, transient tachypnea of the newborn can be seen in neonates delivered without labor (scheduled cesarean section) or born precipitously. Tachypnea typically resolves within the first 48 hours but may persist beyond 72 hours of age. Radiographic findings include perihilar streaking and intralobar fluid.

Fetal conditions may also affect where and when delivery should take place. Newborns with conditions discovered prenatally that require early surgical correction should be delivered at a tertiary facility equipped to handle emergencies and complications. Such conditions may include congenital diaphragmatic hernia, congenital heart defects, airway anomalies, gastroschisis, omphalocele, and renal agenesis. The most advanced neonatal intensive care units typically have the capability to provide cardiopulmonary bypass and extracorporeal membrane oxygenation for these neonates should they be necessary.

Delivery Issues Affecting the Newborn Transition

Clinicians taking care of newborns should work with their obstetric colleagues to eliminate elective deliveries before 39 weeks' gestation (**Box 5**). Respiratory morbidity, including RDS and transient tachypnea, are increased if delivery is electively done before this gestational age.[46,47] The American College of Obstetricians and Gynecologists has endorsed the elimination of nonmedically indicated deliveries before 39 weeks owing to these morbidities and this proactive recommendation has also become a National Quality Forum project.[48,49]

Additionally, elective cesarean deliveries are accompanied by an increased risk of newborn respiratory distress. Term infants delivered electively in this manner have

---

Box 5
Fetal to newborn transition difficulties—delivery issues

- Maternal analgesia
- Meconium-stained amniotic fluid
- Instrumentation (forceps, vacuum)
- Cesarean delivery
- Complex and breech fetal presentations

---

almost twice the incidence of RDS (2.1% vs 1.4%; $P<.01$) and transient tachypnea (4.1% vs 1.9%; $P<.01$) compared with infants born vaginally after a prior cesarean birth.[50] Other studies have corroborated these findings in other populations.[51,52] Due to the risks of retained lung fluid, surfactant deficiency, and subsequent pulmonary hypertension, some authors have argued for administration of antenatal corticosteroids to women undergoing elective cesarean delivery even at term gestation.[53,54]

Maternal administration of magnesium as a therapy for preeclampsia, as a tocolytic, and/or to prevent neurodevelopmental impairment in premature infants can also affect the transitioning neonate. Side effects of maternal magnesium administration in the neonate include poor respiratory effort, and delayed peristalsis and gastric emptying. Similar to the effects of maternal general anesthesia at cesarean deliveries, comparable side effects in the neonate may be manifested including respiratory depression and hypotonia. In 1 study, although the 5-minute Apgar scores were similar, the need for resuscitation was more common in neonates exposed to general anesthesia.[55]

NEWBORN RESUSCITATION

Although the vast majority of newborns do not require resuscitation at birth, with an annual US birth number of approximately 4 million, up to 400,000 babies will need help in the transition to extrauterine life each year. Three risk assessment questions by the clinician can generally affirm whether or not newborn resuscitation will be needed: (1) Is the baby term? (2) is the baby crying or breathing? and (3) does the baby have good muscle tone?[1] If the clinician can answer "yes" to all 3 of these questions, the baby should be placed skin to skin on the mother as soon as possible with continued observation recommended. If the answer to any of these questions is "no," then the clinician should closely monitor the baby or begin the initial steps in stabilizing and/or resuscitating the baby with the appropriate equipment (**Box 6**) as indicated.[1]

Thermoregulation

The goal for any infant should be normothermia. Several therapies have been recommended by the NRP, American College of Obstetricians and Gynecologists, and the American Academy of Pediatrics including prewarming the delivery room to 26°C, using plastic wrap around the infant, placing the infant on an exothermic mattress, and placing the baby under a radiant warmer.[1,56] It should be noted that for newborns requiring resuscitation secondary to hypoxic–ischemic encephalopathy, the goal should be to avoid iatrogenic hyperthermia, which has been shown in animal studies to increase the progression of neuronal damage.[57] Clinicians should work with their tertiary referral centers to determine the optimal ways to reduce hyperthermia and potentially induce mild hypothermia.[58]

Box 6
Recommended newborn resuscitation equipment

Respiratory equipment
- Oxygen supply
- Masks (assorted sizes)
- Neonatal bag and tubing or other oxygen delivery device
- Endotracheal tubes (size 2.5–4 mm)
- Laryngoscope (blade sizes 0 and 1)
- Carbon dioxide detector
- Tape and scissors

Suction equipment
- Bulb syringe
- Suction device
- Suction catheters (size 6–10 French)
- Meconium aspirator

Fluids/medications
- Epinephrine (1:10,000 concentration)
- Intravenous catheters
- Normal saline solution
- 10% Dextrose in water solution
- T-connectors
- Syringes (1–20 mL sizes)

Other equipment
- Umbilical catheters (2.5 and 5 French)
- Sterile procedure trays (forceps, scalpel, hemostat, etc)

Airway Clearance

Routine suctioning of term infants without evidence of obstruction or meconium is not recommended.[1] Suctioning of the nasal passage or oropharynx can cause bradycardia and infants may take longer to reach targeted oxygen saturation; there is also limited evidence that suctioning provides any respiratory benefit.[59,60] In nonvigorous infants who are born through meconium-stained fluid, endotracheal suction is still recommended, as noted previously. Gastric suctioning is of limited value. In a study of more than 300 infants randomized to either suctioning or no suctioning, no benefit and possible adverse effects with suctioning were demonstrated.[61]

Supplemental Oxygen

Insufficient or excessive oxygen can be harmful to neonates during resuscitation. Several randomized, controlled studies have been performed comparing 100% oxygen with room air during resuscitation. Two meta-analyses of these studies have demonstrated that neonates resuscitated with room air have increased survival; there is also growing evidence that even brief periods of too much oxygen have adverse effects well beyond the neonatal period.[62,63] No studies have been published to date examining resuscitations started with different oxygen concentrations. The NRP recommends that preductal oxygen saturations be targeted in all neonates based on how many minutes old they are (see **Box 2**).[1] In centers where blended oxygen is not available, the recommendation is to start resuscitations with room air. In centers where blended oxygen is available, titrating the oxygen concentration to the targeted saturation levels using pulse oximetry is recommended.

Assisted Ventilation

If, after 30 seconds of warming, drying, and stimulating, a neonate needing resuscitation has a heart rate below 100 beats per minute or has apnea/gasping, positive pressure ventilation is indicated.[1] Other newborns who may benefit from positive end-expiratory pressure include those with tachypnea, grunting, retracting, or persistent cyanosis. To deliver adequate distending pressure to create a functional residual capacity, initial pressures should be high enough to provide chest expansion; 20 cm H_2O may be effective, although some neonates may require up to 40 cm H_2O.[1] The best measure of adequate ventilation is a rapid improvement in heart rate. Clinicians should be aware of the amount of pressure used and should be ready to adjust pressures based on the newborn's response. There is no current recommendation on what type of oxygen delivery device should be used, but no matter which device a clinician chooses, knowledge of its proper use and ability to troubleshoot is mandatory. Finally, there are limited data on the use of laryngeal mask airways, but they may be considered if facemask ventilation is unsuccessful and endotracheal intubation is either not feasible or unsuccessful.

Chest Compressions

Once an airway is established or secured and the heart rate remains below 60 beats per minute despite effective ventilation for at least 30 seconds, chest compressions should be initiated. The NRP recommends the 2 thumb-encircling technique (vs the 2-finger technique) on the lower one-third of the sternum providing compressions to a depth of one-third of the anterior–posterior diameter of the chest.[1] Proper technique also involves coordination between ventilation and compressions, avoiding their simultaneous delivery at a ratio of 3 compressions to every ventilation, yielding approximately 120 events per minute.

Medications and Volume Expansion

The only medication currently recommended in neonatal resuscitation is epinephrine. If the heart rate remains at less than 60 with adequate ventilation and 100% oxygen, chest compressions, epinephrine, and volume expansion with isotonic saline should be considered.[1] Intravenous administration of epinephrine should be used as soon as venous access is obtained at a dose of 0.01 to 0.03 mg/kg per dose. If venous access cannot be established or while access is being obtained, doses of 0.05 to 0.1 mg/kg via the endotracheal tube can be attempted, although there is limited evidence of its effectiveness by this route.[1] Placement of an emergency umbilical venous catheter should be used for intravenous administration of epinephrine or volume expansion. The catheter should be placed only to the point where blood flow is returned. Volume expansion with 10 mL/kg of normal saline can be given when the baby's heart rate has not responded adequately to resuscitation or when blood loss is known or suspected.

Special Considerations

It is always difficult to know when resuscitative efforts should be withheld or discontinued. Practice and attitudes vary based on available resources and location. In a neonate who has been provided adequate resuscitation but whose heart rate remains undetectable for 10 minutes, it is appropriate and acceptable to consider stopping resuscitation efforts.[1] When withholding resuscitation, decisions should be made with regard to regional outcomes. There remains controversy on initiating and/or withholding resuscitation at extremely young gestational ages. Recently, a joint workshop between the American Academy of Pediatrics, American College of Obstetricians and Gynecologists, the Society for Maternal-Fetal Medicine, and the National Institute for Child Health and Development on periviable birth recommended aggressive resuscitation for infants greater than 23 weeks' gestation unless the neonate is considered to be nonviable based on individual circumstances, such as having a lethal genetic disorder.[64] Infants born between 22 0/7 and 22 6/7 weeks could be resuscitated after antenatal counseling between clinicians and the family and if there is a potential for error in gestational age assessment. Clinicians should remember that obstetric dating may be quite variable, depending on the technique and timing of the dating calculation used. Parental desires regarding initiation of resuscitation should always be taken into consideration in neonates born before 25 weeks' gestation.[1]

SUMMARY

The fetus to newborn transition is a complex physiologic process that requires close monitoring. Approximately 10% of all newborns require some support in facilitating a successful transition after delivery. Clinicians should be aware of the physiologic processes and pay close regard to the newborn's cardiopulmonary transition at birth to provide appropriate treatment and therapies as required. Personnel trained in the NRP should be available at the delivery for all newborns to ensure that immediate and appropriate care can be provided to achieve the best possible outcomes for those babies during this period of vulnerability.

REFERENCES

1. Kattwinkel J, Perlman JM, Aziz K, et al. Part 15: neonatal resuscitation: 2010 American Heart Association guidelines for cardiopulmonary resuscitation and emergency cardiovascular care. Circulation 2010;122:S909–19.
2. Wladimiroff JW, McGhie J. Ultrasonic assessment of cardiovascular geometry and function in the human fetus. Br J Obstet Gynaecol 1981;88:870–5.
3. Mielke G, Benda N. Cardiac output and central distribution of blood flow in the human fetus. Circulation 2001;103:1662–8.
4. Blackburn S. Maternal, fetal and neonatal physiology: a clinical perspective. 3rd edition. St Louis (MO): Elsevier Saunders; 2007.
5. McCray PB Jr, Bettencourt JD, Bastacky J. Developing bronchopulmonary epithelium of the human fetus secretes fluid. Am J Physiol 1992;262:L270–9.
6. Andersson S, Pitkanen O, Janer C, et al. Lung fluid during postnatal transition. Chin Med J 2010;123:2919–23.
7. Krochal EM, Ballard ST, Yankaskas JR, et al. Volume and ion transport by fetal rat alveolar and tracheal epithelia in submersion culture. Am J Physiol 1989;256:F397–407.
8. Garbrecht MR, Klein JM, Schmidt TJ, et al. Glucocorticoid metabolism in the human fetal lung: implications for lung development and the pulmonary surfactant system. Biol Neonate 2006;89:109–19.

9. Hillman N, Kallapur SG, Jobe A. Physiology of transition from intrauterine to extra-uterine life. Clin Perinatol 2012;39:769–83.
10. Bland RD, Hansen TN, Haberkern CM, et al. Lung fluid balance in lambs before and after birth. J Appl Physiol Respir Environ Exerc Physiol 1982;53:992–1004.
11. Bland RD, Nielson DW. Developmental changes in lung epithelial ion transport and liquid movement. Annu Rev Physiol 1992;54:373–94.
12. O'Brodovich HM. Immature epithelial Na+ channel expression is one of the path-ogenetic mechanisms leading to human neonatal respiratory distress syndrome. Proc Assoc Am Physicians 1996;108:345–55.
13. Vyas H, Field D, Milner AD, et al. Determinants of the first inspiratory volume and functional residual capacity at birth. Pediatr Pulmonol 1986;2:189–93.
14. Goldsmith JP. Delivery room resuscitation of the newborn. In: Martin RJ, Fanaroff AA, Walsh MC, editors. Neonatal-perinatal medicine: diseases of the fetus and infant. 9th edition. St Louis (MO): Elsevier Mosby; 2011. p. 449–54.
15. Heymann MA, Iwamoto HS, Rudolph AM. Factors affecting changes in the neonatal systemic circulation. Annu Rev Physiol 1981;43:371–83.
16. Behrman RE, Lees MH. Organ blood flows of the fetal, newborn and adult rhesus monkey: a comparative study. Biol Neonate 1971;18:330–40.
17. Dawson JA, Kamlin CO, Vento M, et al. Defining the reference range for oxygen saturation for infants after birth. Pediatrics 2010;125:e1340–7.
18. Darwin E. Zoonomia, vol. III. 3rd edition. London: Johnson; 1801.
19. Bhatt S, Alison BJ, Wallace EM, et al. Delaying cord clamping until ventilation onset improves cardiovascular function at birth in preterm lambs. J Physiol 2013;591:2113–26.
20. Ersdal HL, Linde J, Mduma E, et al. Neonatal outcome following cord clamping after onset of spontaneous respiration. Pediatrics 2014;134:265–72.
21. Abalos E, Cuesta C, Carroli G, et al. Pre-eclampsia, eclampsia and adverse maternal and perinatal outcomes: a secondary analysis of the World Health Orga-nization Multicountry Survey on Maternal and Newborn Health. BJOG 2014;121(Suppl 1):14–24.
22. Backes CH, Markham K, Moorehead P, et al. Maternal preeclampsia and neonatal outcomes. J Pregnancy 2011;2011:214365. http://dx.doi.org/10.1155/2011/214365.
23. Simpson LL. Maternal medical disease: risk of antepartum fetal death. Semin Perinatol 2002;26:42–50.
24. Resnik LO, Hansman C, Dressler M, et al. Intrauterine growth as estimated from liveborn birth-weight data at 24 to 42 weeks of gestation. Pediatrics 1963;32:793–800.
25. Aucott SW, Donohue PK, Northington FJ. Increased morbidity in severe early intrauterine growth restriction. J Perinatol 2004;24:435–40.
26. Koenig JM, Christensen RD. Incidence, neutrophil kinetics, and natural history of neonatal neutropenia associated with maternal hypertension. N Engl J Med 1989;321:557–62.
27. Mouzinho A, Rosenfeld CR, Sanchez PJ, et al. Effect of maternal hypertension on neonatal neutropenia and risk of nosocomial infection. Pediatrics 1992;90:430–5.
28. Castle V, Andrew M, Kelton J. Frequency and mechanism of neonatal thrombocy-topenia. J Pediatr 1986;108:749–55.
29. Jadcherla SR, Kliegman RM. Studies of feeding intolerance in very low birth weight infants: definition and significance. Pediatrics 2002;109:516–7.

30. Parry M, Davies MW. The low birthweight, term infant and the need for admission to special care nurseries. J Paediatr Child Health 2013;49:1019–24.
31. Rozance PJ. Update on neonatal hypoglycemia. Curr Opin Endocrinol Diabetes Obes 2014;21:45–50.
32. Maayan-Metzger A, Schushan-Eisen I, Lubin D, et al. Delivery room breastfeeding for prevention of hypoglycemia in infants of diabetic mothers. Fetal Pediatr Pathol 2014;33:23–8.
33. Harris DL, Weston PJ, Signal M, et al. Dextrose gel for neonatal hypoglycemia (the Sugar Babies Study): a randomized, double-blind, placebo-controlled trial. Lancet 2013;382:2077–83.
34. Barnes-Powell LL. Infants of diabetic mothers: the effects of hyperglycemia on the fetus and neonate. Neonatal Netw 2007;26:283–90.
35. Das S, Irigoyen M, Patterson MB, et al. Neonatal outcomes of macrosomic births in diabetic and non-diabetic women. Arch Dis Child Fetal Neonatal Ed 2009;94: F419–22.
36. Hay WW Jr. Care of the infant of the diabetic mother. Curr Diab Rep 2012;12: 4–15.
37. Badran EF, Abdalgani MM, Al-Lawama MA, et al. Effects of perinatal risk factors on common neonatal respiratory morbidities beyond 36 weeks of gestation. Saudi Med J 2012;33:1317–23.
38. Vignoles P, Gire C, Mancini J, et al. Gestational diabetes: a strong independent risk factor for severe neonatal respiratory failure after 34 weeks. Arch Gynecol Obstet 2011;284:1099–104.
39. Waldenstrom U, Aasheim V, Nilsen AB, et al. Adverse pregnancy outcomes related to advanced maternal age compared with smoking and being overweight. Obstet Gynecol 2014;123:104–12.
40. Carolan M. Maternal age >45 years and maternal and perinatal outcomes: a review of the evidence. Midwifery 2013;29:479–89.
41. Vucinovic M, Roje D, Vucinovic Z, et al. Maternal and neonatal effects of substance abuse during pregnancy: our ten-year experience. Yonsei Med J 2008; 49:705–13.
42. Barlow CF. Neonatal myasthenia gravis. Am J Dis Child 1981;135:209.
43. Varner M. Myasthenia gravis and pregnancy. Clin Obstet Gynecol 2013;56: 372–81.
44. Hernandez-Diaz S, Van Marter LJ, Werler MM, et al. Risk factors for persistent pulmonary hypertension of the newborn. Pediatrics 2007;120:e272–82.
45. Perlman JM, Wyllie J, Kattwinkel J, et al. Part 11: neonatal resuscitation: 2010 international consensus on cardiopulmonary resuscitation and emergency cardiovascular care science with treatment recommendations. Circulation 2010; 122(Suppl 2):S516–38.
46. Ertugrul S, Gun I, Mungen E, et al. Evaluation of neonatal outcomes in elective repeat cesarean delivery at term according to weeks of gestation. J Obstet Gynaecol Res 2013;39:105–12.
47. Clark S, Miller D, Belfort M, et al. Neonatal and maternal outcomes associated with elective delivery. Am J Obstet Gynecol 2009;200:156.e1–4.
48. ACOG Committee on Practice Bulletins – Obstetrics. American College of Obstetricians and Gynecologists. ACOG Practice bulletin No 107: Induction of labor. Obstet Gynecol 2009;114:386–97.
49. National Quality Forum. NQF #0469 PC-01 elective delivery. Perinatal and Reproductive Health Project Bulletin. October 24, 2008.

50. Jain L, Eaton DC. Physiology of fetal lung fluid clearance and the effect of labor. Semin Perinatol 2006;30:34–43.
51. Werner EF, Savitz DA, Janevic TM, et al. Mode of delivery and neonatal outcomes in preterm, small-for-gestational age newborns. Obstet Gynecol 2012;120:560–4.
52. Werner EF, Han CS, Savitz DA, et al. Health outcomes for vaginal compared with cesarean delivery of appropriately grown preterm neonates. Obstet Gynecol 2013;121:1195–200.
53. Ramachandrappa A, Jain L. Elective cesarean section: its impact on neonatal respiratory outcome. Clin Perinatol 2008;35:373–93.
54. Riley CA, Boozer K, King TL. Antenatal corticosteroids at the beginning of the 21st century. J Midwifery Womens Health 2011;56:591–7.
55. Dasgupta S, Chakraborty B, Saha D, et al. Comparison of neonatal outcome in women with severe pre-eclampsia undergoing cesarean section under spinal or general anesthesia. J Indian Med Assoc 2011;109:166–70.
56. Lockwood CJ, Lemons JA, editors. Guidelines for perinatal care. 6th edition. Elk Grove Village (IL): American Academy of Pediatrics and the American College of Obstetricians and Gynecologists; 2007.
57. Zhu C, Wang X, Xu F, et al. Intraischemic mild hypothermia prevents neuronal cell death and tissue loss after neonatal cerebral hypoxia-ischemia. Eur J Neurosci 2006;23:387–93.
58. Fairchild K, Sokora D, Scott J, et al. Therapeutic hypothermia on neonatal transport: 4-year experience in a single NICU. J Perinatol 2010;30:324–9.
59. Gungor S, Kurt E, Teksoz E, et al. Oronasopharyngeal suction versus no suction in normal and term infants delivered by elective cesarean section: a prospective randomized controlled trial. Gynecol Obstet Invest 2006;61:9–14.
60. Graves BW, Haley MM. Newborn transition. J Midwifery Womens Health 2013;58: 662–70.
61. Kiremitci S, Tuzun F, Yesilirmak DC, et al. Is gastric aspiration needed for newborn management in delivery room? Resuscitation 2011;82:40–4.
62. Davis PG, Tan A, O'Donnell CP, et al. Resuscitation of newborn infants with 100% oxygen or air: a systematic review and meta-analysis. Lancet 2004;364:1329–33.
63. Rabi Y, Rabi D, Yee W. Room air resuscitation of the depressed newborn: a systematic review and meta-analysis. Resuscitation 2007;72:353–63.
64. Raju TN, Mercer BM, Burchfield DJ, et al. Periviable birth: executive summary of a joint workshop by the Eunice Kennedy Shriver National Institute for Child Health and Development, Society for Maternal-Fetal Medicine, American Academy of Pediatrics, and American College of Obstetricians and Gynecologists. J Perinatol 2014;34:333–42.

Initial Assessment and Management of the Newborn

 CrossMark

Julie R. Gooding, MD, Richard E. McClead Jr, MD, MHA*

KEYWORDS

- Newborn assessment • Physical examination • Normal variation • Gestational age
- Birth trauma • Congenital anomalies

KEY POINTS

- It is important for primary providers to recognize normal variations and reassure anxious parents when these common variants are present.
- When a newborn practitioner is not providing the subsequent follow-up care, communication with the infant's primary care provider regarding these findings as well as the pertinent perinatal history is critical.
- The after-visit or discharge summary provided to a parent may not be adequate to conveying findings. A phone call, especially when an infant remains at risk for hyperbilirubinemia or group B streptococcal disease, is the most efficient means of communication.

It is evident that the physical findings obtained at single examinations during the first six hours of life in health neonates may vary considerably.
—*Murdina M. Desmond and colleagues[1]*

INTRODUCTION

Birth is an exciting time for new parents. It is also a time of great anxiety and concern: "Is my baby healthy?" "How much does my baby weigh?" "Can my baby stay with me?" "Will our baby go home with us?" For many new parents, this is their first encounter with the health care system as a family. Many parents may not have thought about the need to choose a pediatrician. Some parents think their obstetrician will care for the baby. Some parents may have a pediatrician, but their pediatrician is not on staff at the hospital where they delivered. Instead, an unfamiliar pediatrician or

---

Disclosure: Neither author has any conflicts or financial relationships to disclose.
Department of Pediatrics, Nationwide Children's Hospital, The Ohio State University, 700 Children's Drive, Columbus, OH 43205, USA
* Corresponding author.
E-mail address: Richard.McClead@nationwidechildrens.org

http://dx.doi.org/10.1016/j.pcl.2014.12.001
0031-3955/15/$ – see front matter
pediatric.theclinics.com

neonatologist provides care for the infant when in the well-baby nursery. Physicians providing care for well newborns need to be aware and sensitive to these parental concerns.

As noted by Warren and Phillipi,[2] "care of the family should be accessible, continuous, comprehensive, family-centered, coordinated, compassionate, and culturally effective." The ability of pediatricians to meet these ideals might be limited, however, by demands and expectation for families and by the health care system. For instance, families may want to be discharged before the newborn has had a sufficient period of observation. Although most major problems present in the first 12 hours of life, problems, such as significant hyperbilirubinemia, certain ductal-dependent cardiac lesions, and gastrointestinal disorders, may take longer to present. "The hospital stay of the mother and her healthy term newborn infant should be long enough to allow identification of early problems and to ensure that the family is able and prepared to care for the infant at home."[3] Although regulations permit healthy term infants to remain hospitalized 48 hours after a vaginal birth and 96 hours after a cesarean delivery, it is uncommon for families with healthy newborns to want to stay the allotted time for observation. This might be a problem when an infant must be observed for 48 hours per group B streptococcal disease prevention guidelines.[4]

The normal variations that newborns exhibit can also create anxiety for new parents. These variations result from a variety of factors, including mode of delivery, medications administered during labor and delivery, and changes related to transition from an intrauterine to extrauterine environment. It is the pediatrician's role to identify abnormal clinical findings that may have implications in a newborn's course as well as to reassure parents of normal newborn variations.

This article discusses some of these variations related to gestational age assessment, sizing, and physical examination not discussed elsewhere in this issue. Some of the common physical findings that may require additional evaluation and treatment are also discussed.

INITIAL ASSESSMENT OF THE NEWBORN

The initial assessment of a normal, healthy newborn by a pediatrician should take place in the first 24 hours after birth. Attention should be paid to the maternal record, including antenatal history, labor and delivery course, postpartum record, and parental interview, to evaluate for risk factors or pregnancy complications that can affect an infant's well-being and subsequent development. A thorough examination of each organ system should be performed and any variation of normal identified and discussed with the parents.

Assessing Gestational Age and Growth

Assessing newborn infants includes determining the gestational age of infants and obtaining measurements that include weight, length, and head circumference. Using a systematic method to assess the gestational age of infants is important when the dates are uncertain or if prenatal care was not obtained in the first trimester. The Ballard scoring system is a gestational age assessment tool that uses standardized physical examination findings to score infants in the areas of physical and neurologic maturity (**Fig. 1**). Scores in each area are combined and a maturity rating score is assigned that approximates infant gestational age in weeks. In general, this gestational assessment is accurate to within approximately 2 weeks. These results can be compared with results determined from last menstrual period dating or by prenatal ultrasound if available.

Physical maturity

	0	1	2	3	4	5
Skin	Gelatinous, red, transparent	Smooth, pink, visible veins	Superficial peeling and/or rash, few veins	Cracking, pale area, rare veins	Parchment, deep cracking no vessels	Leathery, cracked, wrinkled
Lanugo	None	Abundant	Thinning	Bald areas	Mostly bald	
Plantar creases	No crease	Faint red marks	Anterior transverse crease only	Creases anterior two thirds	Creases cover entire sole	
Breast	Barely perceptible	Flat areola, no bud	Stippled areola, 1–2 mm bud	Raised areola, 3–4 mm bud	Full areola, 5–10 mm bud	
Ear	Pinna flat, stays folded	Slightly curved pinna, soft, slow recoil	Well-curved pinna, soft but ready recoil	Formed and firm with instant recoil	Thick cartilage, ear stiff	
Genitals: male	Scrotum empty, no rugae		Testes descending, few rugae	Testes down, good rugae	Testes pendulous, deep rugae	
Genitals: female	Prominent clitoris and labia minora		Majora and minora equally prominent	Majora large, minora small	Clitoris and minora completely covered	

Maturity rating

Score	Weeks
5	26
10	28
15	30
20	32
25	34
30	36
35	38
40	40
45	42
50	44

Neuromuscular maturity

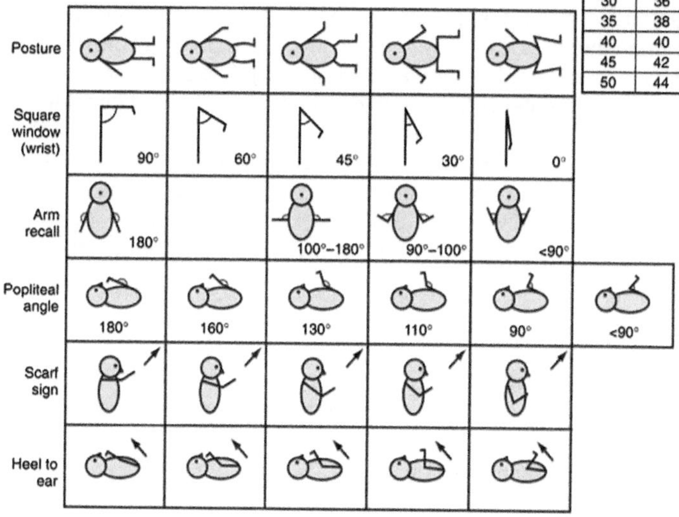

Posture						
Square window (wrist)	90°	60°	45°	30°	0°	
Arm recall	180°		100°–180°	90°–100°	<90°	
Popliteal angle	180°	160°	130°	110°	90°	<90°
Scarf sign						
Heel to ear						

Fig. 1. New Ballard scoring tool to assess gestational age. Scores from neuromuscular and physical domains are added to obtain total score and estimate gestational age. (*From* Ballard JL, Khoury JC, Wedig K, et al. New Ballard core, expanded to include extremely premature infants. J Pediatr 1991;119(3):417–23; with permission.)

The American College of Obstetricians and Gynecologists (ACOG) and the Society for Maternal-Fetal Medicine have proposed new terminology to describe infants previously considered "term." New designations have been established because research shows that infants between 39 0/7 and 40 6/7 weeks of gestation have lower morbidities than infants delivered before or after this gestational age[5]:

- Early term (37 0/7 weeks of gestation through 38 6/7 weeks of gestation)
- Full term (39 0/7 weeks of gestation through 40 6/7 weeks of gestation)
- Late term (41 0/7 weeks of gestation through 41 6/7 weeks of gestation)
- Post term (42 0/7 weeks of gestation and beyond)

Once gestational age has been determined, an infant's weight, length, and head circumference measurements are plotted on a growth chart to determine the percentile compared with other infants of the same gestational age. Recommendations from the Centers for Disease Control and Prevention (CDC) in 2010 are to use the World Health Organization (WHO) growth chart for infants 0 to 24 months of age.[6] The WHO growth charts are recommended because they are based on infants who were predominantly breastfed for the first 4 months of life and were still receiving breast milk at 12 months. Thus, these growth charts represent infant growth under optimal conditions. Charts based on weight for age, length for age, weight for length, and head circumference for age are available for boys and girls from birth until 24 months of age (**Figs. 2** and **3**).

Infants who fall outside the normal weight range (or 2 SDs above or below the mean) for gestational age are considered large for gestational age (LGA) (>90th percentile) or small for gestational age (SGA) (<10th percentile) (**Fig. 4**). Intrauterine growth restriction occurs when the fetus is unable to reach its growth potential due to maternal, uteroplacental, or fetal factors that prevent adequate gas exchange or nutrient delivery. These infants are at greater risk of morbidity and mortality than constitutionally SGA infants.[7] Causes of IUGR are shown in **Box 1**.

Identification of IUGR in pregnancy by an obstetrician should alert pediatricians that an infant is at higher risk of complications than other infants of the same gestational age. Infants who are constitutionally SGA may be admitted to the well-baby nursery. These small infants are at risk, however, for a variety of problems, including

- Abnormal temperature regulation due to decreased fat stores
- Poor feeding due to decreased muscle tone and stamina
- Hypoglycemia due to decreased glycogen stores
- Polycythemia from chronic in utero hypoxia
- Hypoxic-ischemic encephalopathy due to uteroplacental insufficiency and intolerance to labor
- Meconium aspiration syndrome due to perinatal stress

Complications of SGA extend past the immediate neonatal period with recent evidence suggesting that SGA infants may be at higher risk of lower IQ, obesity, diabetes, and cardiovascular disease in early adulthood and should be closely monitored for these conditions by a primary care physician.[8-10]

LGA infants most commonly result from maternal diabetes or are caused by genetic predisposition to large size or large maternal weight gain during pregnancy (**Fig. 5**). Infants who are LGA are at risk for birth trauma, increased rate of cesarean delivery, hypoglycemia, and respiratory distress.

Over the last quarter of the twentieth century there was an increase in the mean birth weight of infants born in the United States and other Western countries.[11-13] A study of Canadian infants indicates that this finding is associated with an increase in maternal

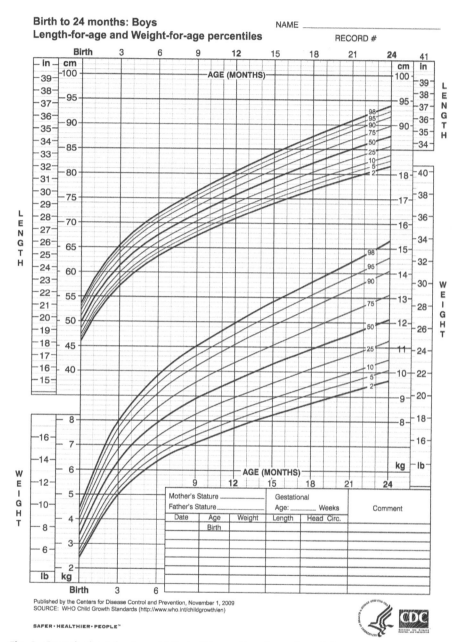

Birth to 24 months: Boys
Length-for-age and Weight-for-age percentiles

NAME _____

RECORD # _____

Published by the Centers for Disease Control and Prevention, November 1, 2009
SOURCE: WHO Child Growth Standards (http://www.who.int/childgrowth/en)

SAFER · HEALTHIER · PEOPLE™

Fig. 2. Growth chart for boys birth to 24 months of age: length-for-age and weight-for-age percentiles (Figure is in the public domain and includes appropriate attributions). (*From* Centers for Disease Control and Prevention. Available at: http://www.cdc.gov/growthcharts/data/who/grchrt_boys_24lw_100611.pdf. Accessed January 8, 2015.)

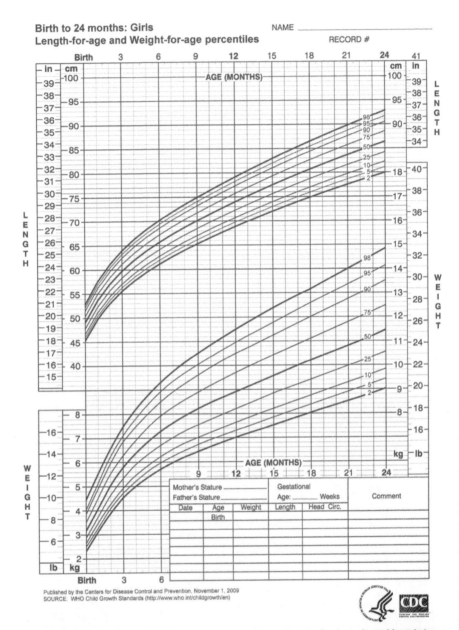

Fig. 3. Growth chart for girls birth to 24 months of age. Weight for length and head circumference for age. (Figure is in the public domain and includes appropriate attribution). (*From* Centers for Disease Control and Prevention. Available at: http://www.cdc.gov/growthcharts/data/who/grchrt_girls_24lw_9210.pdf. Accessed January 8, 2015.)

prepregnancy body mass index, gestational weight gain, and gestational diabetes and a decrease in maternal smoking and post-term deliveries.[14] As a consequence, the proportion of LGA infants has increased whereas that of SGA infants has decreased. Infants whose birth weights exceed 4500 g have significant increased risk of morbidity

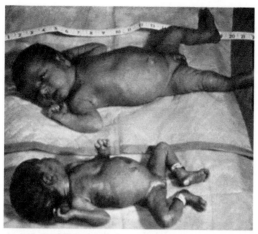

Fig. 4. SGA and appropriate–for–gestational age discordant twin infants. SGA twin due to abnormal placentation compared with appropriately grown twin. (*From* Brozansky BS, Riley MM, Bogen DL. Neonatology. In: Zitelli BJ, McIntire SC, Nowalk AJ, editors. Atlas of Pediatric Diagnosis, 6th edition. Philadelphia: Elsevier Saunders, 2012; with permission.)

Box 1
Causes of intrauterine growth restriction

Maternal factors

    High blood pressure (chronic or pregnancy induced)

    Chronic kidney disease

    Advanced diabetes (class F or higher)

    Cardiac or respiratory disease

    Malnutrition

    Infection (toxoplasmosis, other viruses, rubella, cytomegalovirus, herpes viruses)

    Substance abuse (alcohol, illicit drugs, tobacco)

    Clotting disorders

    Autoimmune disease

    Chronic exposure to high altitudes

Uterine or placental factors

    Abnormal placentation

    Chronic placental abruption

    Abnormal cord insertion or cord anomalies

Fetal factors

    Multiple gestations

    Infection (cytomegalovirus, rubella)

    Birth defects

    Chromosomal anomalies

Data from Gabbe S. Intrauterine growth restriction. In: Gabbe S, editor. Obstetrics: normal and problem pregnancies. 6th edition. Philadelphia: Saunders; 2012. p. 706–41.

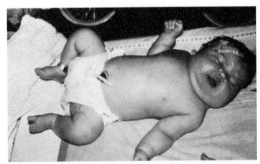

Fig. 5. LGA infant of a diabetic mother. (*From* Brozansky BS, Riley MM, Bogen DL. Neonatology. In: Zitelli BJ, McIntire SC, Nowalk AJ, editors. Atlas of Pediatric Diagnosis, 6th edition. Philadelphia: Elsevier Saunders, 2012; with permission.)

and mortality. Birth trauma is more likely and their mothers are at increased risk for genitourinary injury and other intrapartum and postpartum complications.[12] LGA infants may also be at risk for long-term health effects.[15]

PHYSICAL EXAMINATION OF THE NEWBORN

The first physical examination performed by a pediatrician should be performed in the mother's room to limit separation of mother and infant. The room should be warm and quiet with ample lighting. Initial impressions of the infant in a quiet state should be recorded followed by a systematic examination. Gestational age assessment information is important because premature infants have special considerations.

BIRTH TRAUMA

Most newborn infants tolerate delivery with little to no physical trauma. Occasionally, temporary or permanent trauma to a newborn occurs. Recognition of trauma necessitates a careful physical and neurologic evaluation of the infant to establish whether additional injuries are present. Symmetry of structure and function should be assessed; the cranial nerves should be examined; and specifics, such as individual joint range of motion and scalp/skull integrity, should be evaluated.

Risk factors for birth trauma include the following:

- LGA infants, especially infants who weigh more than 4500 g
- Instrumental deliveries, especially forceps or vacuum
- Vaginal breech delivery
- Abnormal or excessive traction during delivery

EXTRACRANIAL INJURIES
Caput Succedaneum

Scalp edema that results from the normal process of a vertex vaginal delivery is called caput succedaneum (**Fig. 6**). This edema is seen most commonly over the presenting part of a newborn's head, crosses suture lines, and resolves without intervention within several days. Bruising may accompany scalp edema especially in cases of vacuum extraction (**Fig. 7**).

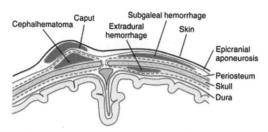

Fig. 6. Layers of scalp/skull. Sites of extracranial hemorrhages in the newborn. (*From* Brozansky BS, Riley MM, Bogen DL. Neonatology. In: Zitelli BJ, McIntire SC, Nowalk AJ, editors. Atlas of Pediatric Diagnosis, 6th edition. Philadelphia: Elsevier Saunders, 2012; with permission.)

Cephalohematoma

Cephalohematomas are caused by rupture of vessels and collection of blood under the periosteum of the calvarial bones. In contrast to caput succedaneum, most cephalohematomas are unilateral, involve the parietal or occipital bones, and do not cross suture lines. The incidence of cephalohematomas is 1% to 2% of all deliveries but are more common in vacuum- or forceps-assisted deliveries.[16] Cephalohematomas are fluctuant on palpation and the lesions resolve over months as the hematoma is broken down (**Fig. 8**). Complications of cephalohematomas include elevated bilirubin levels and should be considered risk factors when evaluating infants for jaundice per American Academy of Pediatrics (AAP) Clinical Practice Guideline and Bhutani nomogram.[17,18]

Subgaleal Hemorrhage

Subgaleal hemorrhage (SGH) is a rare but often lethal complication of the birth process and results from tearing or shearing of the emissary vessels between the dural sinuses and the scalp veins as a result of traction to the scalp during delivery. Blood accumulates in the loose areolar tissue in the space between the periosteum of the skull and the epicranial aponeurosis. The injury occurs when the emissary veins between the scalp and dural sinuses are sheared or severed as a result of traction on the scalp during delivery.

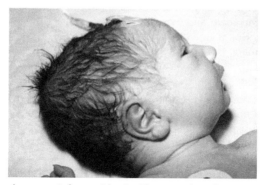

Fig. 7. Caput succedaneum. Infant with significant scalp edema secondary to passage through the birth canal. (*From* Brozansky BS, Riley MM, Bogen DL. Neonatology. In: Zitelli BJ, McIntire SC, Nowalk AJ, editors. Atlas of Pediatric Diagnosis, 6th edition. Philadelphia: Elsevier Saunders, 2012; with permission.)

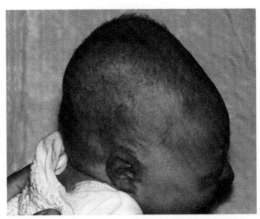

Fig. 8. Cephalohematoma. Infant with bilateral cephalohematomas. Note that the palpable sagittal suture confirms the periosteal location of the hematomas. (*From* Brozansky BS, Riley MM, Bogen DL. Neonatology. In: Zitelli BJ, McIntire SC, Nowalk AJ, editors. Atlas of Pediatric Diagnosis, 6th edition. Philadelphia: Elsevier Saunders, 2012; with permission.)

SGH presents as a boggy, fluctuant swelling of the head often with accompanying fluid wave that extends forward to the orbital margins, backward to the nuchal ridge, and to the level of the ears laterally. In term babies, this subaponeurotic space may hold as much as 260 mL of blood.[19] An infant's head circumference can increase rapidly. Affected infants may appear normal at birth but then develop tachycardia and pallor in the well-baby nursery where they can decompensate quickly due to hypovolemic shock. Early recognition and volume expansion are essential for survival.

The incidence of moderate to severe SGH has been estimated to occur in 1.5 per 10,000 births and although it can occur spontaneously, it is more commonly caused by vacuum extraction and forceps delivery.[20,21]

SOFT TISSUE INJURIES
Lacerations

Fetal laceration has been reported as the most common birth injury associated with cesarean delivery (**Fig. 9**). Lacerations occur most often on the presenting part of the fetus, typically the scalp and face. Most lacerations are minor and repaired with thin adhesive strips. Some lacerations, however, especially those involving the face, may require consultation from plastic surgery.

Bruising and Petechiae

Superficial bruising and petechiae found on the presenting part are common and self-limited and occur after difficult deliveries. Extensive bruising places newborns at risk for severe hyperbilirubinemia and should be followed closely for progressive jaundice. Infants who are delivered in the breech position can present with severe vaginal or scrotal edema and bruising (**Fig. 10**). A urology consultation in cases of severe scrotal swelling for the drainage of a hematoma surrounding the testes may be needed in rare cases.

No additional work-up is needed in cases of petechiae present at birth that do not progress and are not associated with other bleeding. Appearance of new petechiae should alert the pediatrician for the need to evaluate for a possible bleeding disorder.

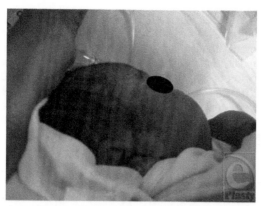

Fig. 9. Facial laceration. The female newborn, weighing 3.25 kg, accidentally sustained a laceration over the right side of the face and temporal region. (*From* Saraf S. Facial laceration at caesarean section: experience with tissue adhesive. ePlasty 2009;9:e3. Epub 2009 Jan 9; with permission.)

Torticollis can result from manual stretching of the neck that causes bleeding into the sternocleidomastoid muscle after delivery. A hematoma of the muscle may be noticeable at birth. Infants with torticollis present in the 4th week of life with tilting of the head toward the side of the affected muscle and rotation toward the opposite side. Treatment with stretching exercises results in a 90% rate of recovery.[22]

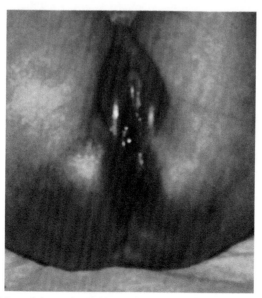

Fig. 10. Severe bruising of the perineum secondary to breech presentation. (*From* Brozansky BS, Riley MM, Bogen DL. Neonatology. In: Zitelli BJ, McIntire SC, Nowalk AJ, editors. Atlas of Pediatric Diagnosis, 6th edition. Philadelphia: Elsevier Saunders, 2012; with permission.)

Subcutaneous Fat Necrosis

It is common for infants delivered with the aid of forceps to have forceps marks after delivery. Most commonly, these marks fade within 1 to 2 days without additional complications. Occasionally, subcutaneous fat necrosis results at the site as a well-circumscribed, discolored, firm nodule (**Fig. 11**), which is the result of ischemia to the adipose tissue. Typically, these nodules resolve by 6 to 8 weeks of age. Infants diagnosed with severe subcutaneous fat necrosis require long-term follow-up for the development of hypercalcemia, which can occur up to 6 months after the initial presentation of the skin lesions.

Nasal Deformities

Abnormalities of the nose are common after delivery, particularly if infants are delivered vaginally. Most deformations of the nose are transient and resolve within 48 hours after birth. In cases of true dislocation of the triangular cartilage of the nasal septum, closed reduction by an otolaryngologist in the newborn nursery can be accomplished and prevents permanent deformity as well as nasal and systemic complications from an impaired airway.[23]

NEUROLOGIC INJURY
Brachial Plexus

Neonatal brachial plexus palsy results from traction to the brachial plexus that results from the forces of labor, fetal position and maternal pushing, or by the provider during delivery. Most cases are unilateral and involve the following nerves:

- C5 to C7 injury (Erb's palsy).

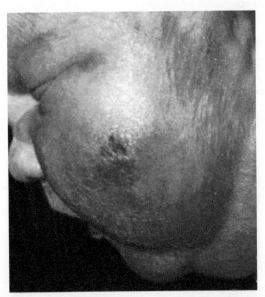

Fig. 11. Subcutaneous fat necrosis. Discolored nodular lesion on the cheek characteristic of subcutaneous fat necrosis secondary to forceps trauma. (*From* Brozansky BS, Riley MM, Bogen DL. Neonatology. In: Zitelli BJ, McIntire SC, Nowalk AJ, editors. Atlas of Pediatric Diagnosis, 6th edition. Philadelphia: Elsevier Saunders, 2012; with permission.)

Clinically, the infants presents with adduction and internal rotation of the upper arm, extension and pronation of the forearm and flexion of the wrists and fingers. This involvement gives the classic waiter's tip posture (**Fig. 12**).

- Severe damage to all C5 to T1 roots is characterized by a flail arm and Horner syndrome.
- C8 to T1 injury (Klumpke palsy) is the most infrequent pattern and manifests as isolated hand paralysis and Horner syndrome.

In most cases of brachial plexus injury, a full recovery occurs over several months; physical therapy may be beneficial to improve function. In a study of 1383 infants with a brachial plexus injury, 94.4% without an ipsilateral clavicular fracture had complete resolution. In addition to the palsy had even better recovery rates than those who did not have a fracture. This retrospective study assumed, however, that infants that never returned to the brachial plexus injury clinic had a full recovery.[24]

Facial Nerve Palsy

Injury to the facial nerve is attributed most commonly to compression of the nerve secondary to a forceps assisted delivery or via a prominent maternal sacral promontory. Infants present with diminished movement on the affected side of the face, inability to fully close the eye, and an inability to contract the lower facial muscles. During crying, the mouth is drawn to the unaffected side. Spontaneous resolution occurs within the first 2 weeks of life.

Diaphragmatic Paralysis

Infants with brachial plexus injury can have associated phrenic nerve involvement and injury. Infants present with respiratory distress on the first day of life and chest radiograph demonstrates decreased diaphragmatic excursion on the side of the injury. Most cases resolve spontaneously with supportive care within the first 6 to 12 months of life, but occasional plication of the diaphragm is necessary for recovery.

Laryngeal Nerve Injury

Laryngeal nerve injury during birth may cause vocal cord paralysis. Symptoms include stridor; respiratory distress; hoarse, faint, or absent cry; dysphagia; and aspiration. Otolaryngology consultation and visualization of the vocal cords by direct

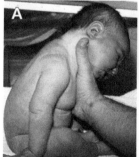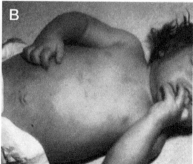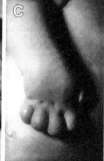

Fig. 12. Brachial plexus injuries. (*A*) Traction injury to C5, C6, and C7 spinal cord segments results in characteristic waiter's tip abnormality of Erb's palsy. (*B, C*) Injuries to segments C7 and T1 result in the claw hand of Klumpke's palsy. (*From* Brozansky BS, Riley MM, Bogen DL. Neonatology. In: Zitelli BJ, McIntire SC, Nowalk AJ, editors. Atlas of Pediatric Diagnosis, 6th edition. Philadelphia: Elsevier Saunders, 2012; with permission.)

laryngoscopy are necessary for diagnosis. Treatment depends on the severity of the injury, with most cases of paralysis resolving over time.

OTHER ASSOCIATED INJURIES
Fractured Clavicle

The evaluation of newborns for suspected clavicular fracture includes

- History of difficult delivery (LGA infant, cephalopelvic disproportion)
- Physical examination with crepitus along clavicle
- Radiograph demonstrating fracture
- Evaluation for other injuries (brachial plexus)

Clavicular fractures heal spontaneously with no long-term sequelae. For comfort, the arm on the affected side can be placed in a long-sleeved garment and pinned to the chest with the elbow at 90° flexion. Clinical assessment is usually satisfactory to assess healing, but repeat radiograph 2 weeks after birth confirms diagnosis.

Fractured Humerus

Humeral fractures are rare in newborn infants but are the most common long bone fracture, with a reported incidence of 0.2 per 1000 deliveries.[25] Most fractures occur at the proximal third of the humerus and are transverse and complete. Infants with humeral fractures present with decreased movement of the affected arm, decreased Moro reflex, localized swelling, and an increased pain response on palpation. Because brachial plexus injuries often accompany humeral fractures, clinicians should perform a thorough neurologic examination. An orthopedic consultation and immobilization of the arm are required for treatment. Radiographs of the affected arm should be followed at 3 to 4 weeks to ensure healing.

Skull Fracture

There are 2 types of skull fractures that result from birth trauma:

- Linear
  - Secondary to pressure on the fetal skull against maternal structures
  - Rarely associated with neurologic sequelae
  - Plain film of the skull for diagnosis
  - No specific therapy indicated
- Depressed (**Fig. 13**)
  - Most commonly due to forceps delivery
  - Increased risk of intracranial bleeding and cephalohematoma
  - CT scan of the head to evaluate for intracranial lesions
  - Neurosurgery consultation for intracranial processes

NEUROLOGIC ASSESSMENT

A comprehensive neurologic assessment of newborns is essential in determining the presence and location of a disturbance, the diagnosis, and long-term outcomes.
Factors influencing the neurologic examination

- Gestational age of infant
  - Various aspects of examination change with maturity
  - Assess gestational age using New Ballard Score[26–28]
- Level of alertness

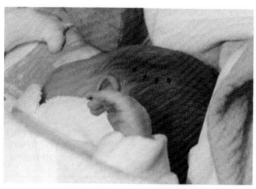

Fig. 13. Depressed (ping pong) skull fracture in the left temporoparietal region due to birth trauma. (*Courtesy of* Prof. Dr. med. Thomas M. Berger, Case of the Month (COTM) series of the Swiss Society of Neonatology [COTM: November 2006 at www.neonet.ch. Accessed January 8, 2015.])

GENERAL ASSESSMENT
Level of alertness
- Level 1: quiet sleep
- Level 2: active sleep
- Level 3: quiet awake (optimal time for assessment)
- Level 4: alert and active
- Level 5: crying

The level of alertness is one of the most sensitive indicators of neurologic injury in newborns. Gestational age, timing of last feeding, and frequency of disturbances all must be taken into consideration when assessing infants.[29]

MOTOR FUNCTION

The evaluation of motor function in term infants should include muscle tone and limb posture, motility, deep tendon reflexes, and the plantar response.

Muscle Tone and Posture

Muscle tone should be assessed with an infant's head in midline position while in an optimal alertness state. Tone should be measured by the resistance of passive movement of the limbs and should be symmetric in all 4 extremities. Flexion of all 4 limbs is the normal posture in a full-term infant and varies with gestational age.

Primitive Reflexes

The list of primitive reflexes is extensive. A sampling of a few with descriptions of the maneuvers to illicit the reflexes and the expected responses are listed in **Table 1** (see video of normal and abnormal components of the neonatal neurologic examination at: http://library.med.utah.edu/pedineurologicexam/html/newborn_n.html).

CONGENITAL ANOMALIES OF THE EXTREMITIES
- Digits
  - Supernumerary digits
    - Typically located lateral to the fifth digit on the hand or foot
    - Attached by a pedicle and contains no bones

Table 1
Primitive reflexes

Reflex	Examination Maneuver	Infant Response
Moro/startle	Elicited by sudden dropping of the head in relation to the trunk. (Examiner should catch head.)	Opening of hands and extension and abduction of the upper extremities followed by anterior flexion of the upper extremities and an audible cry.
Tonic neck/ fencing position	Place infant supine and turn his or her head to one side.	Extension of the upper extremity on the side to which the face is rotated and flexion of the opposite extremity.
Stepping	Hold infant upright and place dorsum of feet to a flat surface.	Infant makes alternating stepping movements.
Sucking	Touch or stroke baby's lips.	Mouth opens and sucking movements begin.
Rooting	Stroke infant's cheek and corner of the mouth.	Infant's head turns toward the stimulus and the mouth opens.
Palmar grasp	Finger placed in infant's open palm.	Infant grasps the finger and holds tighter with attempts to withdraw. Full-term neonate can support full body weight if lifted slightly.
Truncal incurvation or Galant reflex	Hold infant prone, in suspended position, with palm of hand against infant's chest. Apply firm pressure with the thumb or cotton swab parallel to the spine in the thoracic region.	Infant flexes the pelvis toward the side of the stimulus.

Descriptions of the examiner maneuvers and the infant responses were drawn from the PediNeuro-Logic Exam Web site and are used by permission of Paul D. Larsen, MD, University of Nebraska Medical Center, Omaha, NE and Suzanne S. Stensaas, PhD, University of Utah School of Medicine, Salt Lake City, UT. Additional materials were drawn from resources provided by Alejandro Stern, Stern Foundation, Buenos Aires, Argentina; Kathleen Digre, MD, University of Utah, Salt Lake City, UT; and Daniel Jacobson, MD, Marshfield Clinic, Marshfield, WI. The movies are licensed under a Creative Commons Attribution-NonCommerical-ShareAlike 2.5 License. (Available at: http://library.med.utah.edu/pedineurologicexam/html/newborn_n.html; Accessed January 8, 2015.)

- Resolve with suture ligation after approximately 1 week
  - Polydactaly
    - Duplication of digits
    - More common on lower extremities
    - May be familial or associated with other malformations
  - Syndactaly
    - Common
    - Fusion of soft tissues between digits
    - Surgical correction after 3 years of age to allow for function of digits
- Amniotic bands (**Fig. 14**)
  - Structural disruption most commonly involving the limbs but can affect trunk and craniofacial region
  - Constriction rings of amnion can lead to amputation
  - Most cases sporadic with low recurrence risk
- Club feet (talipes equinovarus)
  - Can involve 1 or both feet

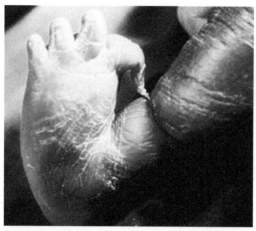

Fig. 14. Amniotic bands. Note amputation of toes and constriction of lower extremity by amniotic bands. (*From* Zitelli BJ, McIntire SC, Nowalk AJ, editors. Zitelli and Davis atlas of pediatric physical diagnosis. 6th edition. Amsterdam: Mosby, Elsevier; 2012. p. 61 [Fig. 2-52]; with permission.)

- ○ Physical examination
  - ■ Foot in plantar flexion
  - ■ Hindfoot in fixed inversion
  - ■ Forefoot adducted and supinated
- ○ Occur in 1 to 3 per 1000 white infants
- ○ 2:1 Male-to-female ratio
- ○ May be idiopathic or genetic
- • Congenital hip dysplasia[30]
  - ○ Displacement of femoral head from acetabulum
  - ○ Incidence 1 in 1000 live births
  - ○ More common in female infants
  - ○ Presents with limited hip abduction, asymmetric gluteal folds, or leg length discrepancy
  - ○ Positive Ortolani sign or Barlow maneuver on physical examination (See video at: https://www.youtube.com/watch?v=imhI6PLtGLc produced by Nabil Ebraheim, MD, University of Toledo Medical Center, Toledo, Ohio.)
  - ○ Diagnosis: physical examination and/or ultrasound of the hip
  - ○ Asymmetric gluteal folds (**Fig. 15**)
  - ○ Treatment: splinting with Pavlik harness (**Fig. 16**)

UMBILICAL CORD

At delivery, the clamped umbilical cord is inspected to detect any alterations of the normal characteristics (thickness, length, and coiling) of the cord, which can be associated with an increased risk of significant pathology in newborn infants.

Abnormalities of the cord
- • 2-Vessel cord
  - ○ The prevalence of a single umbilical artery is 0.6% of live births.[31]
  - ○ Associated anomalies include IUGR, chromosomal, renal, and cardiac.
  - ○ Current evidence suggests no further evaluation of renal system necessary unless other defects are recognized.[32]

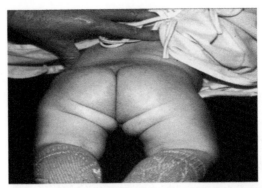

Fig. 15. Asymmetric gluteal folds. Unevenness of the gluteal folds is suggestive of congenital hip dislocation. Additional evaluation by ultrasound or radiograph needed to confirm. (*Courtesy of* International Hip Dysplasia Institute, Orlando, FL; with permission.)

- Umbilical hernia
    - Umbilical hernias are caused by a defect in the central fascia beneath the umbilicus. It is important to distinguish umbilical hernias from other pathologies, such as omphalocele, in which the defect in the anterior abdominal wall contains bowel. Incidence is highest in infants who are African American, are preterm, or have a congenital thyroid deficiency. Umbilical hernias are easily reducible and typically resolve without intervention over the first 5 years of life. Surgical repair is recommended for patients with incarcerated bowel, large defects (>1.5 cm in diameter) that fail to decrease, or persistent hernia beyond age 5.
- Umbilical granuloma
    - Granulomas are the most common umbilical mass
    - Granulomas are most frequently identified after cord separation due to persistant drainage from the umbilicus
    - Resolution of umbilical granulomas occur after treatment with topical silver nitrate

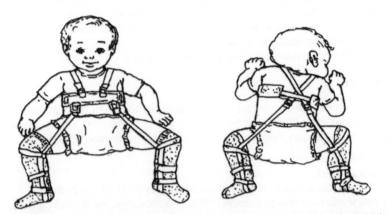

Fig. 16. Application of a Pavlik harness. Front and back views of a properly positioned Pavlik harness. (*Courtesy of* Nationwide Children's Hospital, Columbus, Ohio; with permission.)

CORD CARE

Recommendations for umbilical cord care depend on the type of health care setting. In a clinical setting of low resources where aseptic technique is not standard, the use of antiseptic agents, such as chlorhexidine, alcohol, triple dye, salicylic sugar powder, or green clay powder, for cord care is effective to reduce neonatal morbidity and mortality due to omphalitis. In developed countries, however, where aseptic care is routine in the clamping and cutting of the umbilical cord, additional topical care beyond dry cord care has not shown added benefit in the prevention of omphalitis.[33]

PLANNED HOME BIRTH

Another variation that has an impact on the assessment of normal newborns is delivery outside the health care system. Although the AAP and ACOG believe that a hospital or a birthing center is the safest setting for the delivery of a healthy term infant in the United States, they support the rights of a woman to make a medically informed decision about home delivery.[34] According to their joint policy statement, however, "every newborn infant deserves health care that adheres to the standards highlighted." Any infant born outside the safety standards of hospitals and birthing centers burdens primary care providers with the responsibility for assuring that all components of the assessment and care of the newborn are completed.[34] The joint statement regarding a planned home birth addresses 2 essential elements of newborn care: resuscitation and assessment. These elements are outlined by American Academy of Pediatrics in the Pediatrics article available at http://pediatrics.aappublications.org/content/131/5/1016.full. Readers are referred to this document for a detailed review of the elements.

SUMMARY

This article tries to focus on a few of the common variations that may be seen in otherwise healthy newborns. It is important for primary providers to recognize normal variations and reassure anxious parents when these common variants are present. When a newborn practitioner is not providing the subsequent follow-up care, communication with the infant's primary care provider regarding these findings as well as the pertinent perinatal history is critical. The after-visit or discharge summary provided to a parent may not be adequate to convey this information. A phone call, especially when an infant remains at risk for hyperbilirubinemia or group B streptococcal sepsis, is the most efficient means of communication.

REFERENCES

1. Desmond MM, Franklin RR, Vallvona C, et al. The clinical behavior of the newly born. I. The term baby. J Pediatr 1963;62:307–25.
2. Warren JB, Phillipi CA. Care of the well newborn. Pediatr Rev 2012;33(1):4–18.
3. American Academy of Pediatrics. Committee on Fetus and Newborn. Hospital stay for healthy term newborns. Pediatrics 2010;125(2):405–9.
4. Verani JR, McGee L, Schrag SJ. Prevention of perinatal group B streptococcal disease–revised guidelines from CDC, 2010. MMWR Recomm Rep 2010; 59(RR–10):1–36.
5. ACOG Committee Opinion No 579: Definition of term pregnancy. Obstet Gynecol 2013;122(5):1139–40.

6. Grummer-Strawn LM, Reinold C, Krebs NF. Use of World Health Organization and CDC growth charts for children aged 0-59 months in the United States. MMWR Recomm Rep 2010;59(RR-9):1–15.

7. Longo S, Bollani L, Decembrino L, et al. Short-term and long-term sequelae in intrauterine growth retardation (IUGR). J Matern Fetal Neonatal Med 2013;26(3):222–5.

8. Griffin IJ, editor. Fetal and postnatal growth, and the risks of metabolic syndrome in the AGA and SGA term infant. In: Perinatal growth nutrition. Boca Raton (FL): CRC Press; 2014. p. 65–118.

9. Paneth N, Susser M. Early origin of coronary heart disease (the "Barker hypothesis"). BMJ 1995;310(6977):411–2.

10. McCarton CM, Wallace IF, Divon M, et al. Cognitive and neurologic development of the premature, small for gestational age infant through age 6: comparison by birth weight and gestational age. Pediatrics 1996;98(6 Pt 1):1167–78.

11. Kramer MS, Morin I, Yang H, et al. Why are babies getting bigger? Temporal trends in fetal growth and its determinants. J Pediatr 2002;141(4):538–42.

12. Surkan PJ, Hsieh CC, Johansson AL, et al. Reasons for increasing trends in large for gestational age births. Obstet Gynecol 2004;104(4):720–6.

13. Schack-Nielsen L, Molgaard C, Sorensen TI, et al. Secular change in size at birth from 1973 to 2003: national data from Denmark. Obesity (Silver Spring) 2006;14(7):1257–63.

14. Crane JM, White J, Murphy P, et al. The effect of gestational weight gain by body mass index on maternal and neonatal outcomes. J Obstet Gynaecol Can 2009;31(1):28–35.

15. Rasmussen KM. The "fetal origins" hypothesis: challenges and opportunities for maternal and child nutrition. Annu Rev Nutr 2001;21:73–95.

16. Bofill JA, Rust OA, Devidas M, et al. Neonatal cephalohematoma from vacuum extraction. J Reprod Med 1997;42(9):565–9.

17. American Academy of Pediatrics Subcommittee on Hyperbilirubinemia. Management of hyperbilirubinemia in the newborn infant 35 or more weeks of gestation. Pediatrics 2004;114(1):297–316.

18. Bhutani VK, Johnson L, Sivieri EM. Predictive ability of a predischarge hour-specific serum bilirubin for subsequent significant hyperbilirubinemia in healthy term and near-term newborns. Pediatrics 1999;103(1):6–14.

19. Davis DJ. Neonatal subgaleal hemorrhage: diagnosis and management. CMAJ 2001;164(10):1452–3.

20. Kilani RA, Wetmore J. Neonatal subgaleal hematoma: presentation and outcome-radiological findings and factors associated with mortality. Am J Perinatol 2006;23(1):41–8.

21. Uchil D, Arulkumaran S. Neonatal subgaleal hemorrhage and its relationship to delivery by vacuum extraction. Obstet Gynecol Surv 2003;58(10):687–93.

22. Cheng JC, Tang SP, Chen TM, et al. The clinical presentation and outcome of treatment of congenital muscular torticollis in infants-a study of 1,086 cases. J Pediatr Surg 2000;35(7):1091–6.

23. Emami AJ, Brodsky L, Pizzuto M. Neonatal septoplasty: case report and review of the literature. Int J Pediatr Otorhinolaryngol 1996;35(3):271–5.

24. Wall LB, Mills JK, Leveno K, et al. Incidence and prognosis of neonatal brachial plexus palsy with and without clavicle fractures. Obstet Gynecol 2014;123(6):1288–93.

25. Bhat BV, Kumar A, Oumachigui A. Bone injuries during delivery. Indian J Pediatr 1994;61(4):401–5.

26. Donovan EF, Tyson JE, Ehrenkranz RA, et al. Inaccuracy of Ballard scores before 28 weeks' gestation. National Institute of Child Health and Human Development Neonatal Research Network. J Pediatr 1999;135(2 Pt 1):147–52.

27. Ballard JL, Khoury JC, Wedig K, et al. New Ballard Score, expanded to include extremely premature infants. J Pediatr 1991;119(3):417–23.

28. Sasidharan K, Dutta S, Narang A. Validity of New Ballard Score until 7th day of postnatal life in moderately preterm neonates. Arch Dis Child Fetal Neonatal Ed 2009;94(1):F39–44.

29. Volpe JJ. Neurologic examination: normal and abnormal features. In: Fletcher J, editor. Neurology of the newborn. 5th edition. Philadelphia: Saunders; 2008. p. 121–53.

30. Goldberg MJ. Early detection of developmental hip dysplasia: synopsis of the AAP Clinical Practice Guideline. Pediatr Rev 2001;22(4):131–4.

31. Hua M, Odibo AO, Macones GA, et al. Single umbilical artery and its associated findings. Obstet Gynecol 2010;115(5):930–4.

32. Thummala MR, Raju TN, Langenberg P. Isolated single umbilical artery anomaly and the risk for congenital malformations: a meta-analysis. J Pediatr Surg 1998; 33(4):580–5.

33. Imdad A, Bautista RM, Senen KA, et al. Umbilical cord antiseptics for preventing sepsis and death among newborns. Cochrane Database Syst Rev 2013;(5):CD008635.

34. Watterberg KL. Policy statement on planned home birth: upholding the best interests of children and families. Pediatrics 2013;132(5):924–6.

Sensory Development

Melinda B. Clark-Gambelunghe, MD, David A. Clark, MD*

KEYWORDS

- Neonate • Sensory • Vision • Hearing • Oral development • Taste • Smell

KEY POINTS

- Sensory development begins in early fetal life responding to in utero stimulation.
- Sound transmission from the mothers speech, heartbeat, and external noise stimulates fetal hearing development prior to birth.
- Color vision is absent in babies less than 34 weeks gestation and the first color perceived by newborns is red.
- Taste and smell in the newborn correlates with maternal dietary components in amniotic fluid.
- Primary care providers are poised to detect anatomic and sensory abnormalities and coordinate early intervention.

INTRODUCTION

Sensory development is complex, with both morphologic and neural components. The senses begin to develop well before birth based on in-utero stimuli. They all mature rapidly in the first year of life. This article focuses on the cranial senses of vision, hearing, smell, and taste. Tactile development and pain perception are not addressed. Sensory function, embryogenesis, external and genetic effects, and common malformations that may affect development are discussed, along with the corresponding sensory organ examination and evaluation.

VISION

Eye Development

The eye is derived from an outgrowth of neuroectoderm of the forebrain.[1,2] By the 32nd embryonic day, a distinct optic cup with a ventral groove is detectable. The optic cup further invaginates to form the globe with anterior and posterior chambers.

Disclosure: The authors have no conflicts of interest relevant to this article.
Department of Pediatrics, Albany Medical Center, MC88, 43 New Scotland Avenue, Albany, NY 12208, USA
* Corresponding author.
E-mail address: clarkd@mail.amc.edu

Pediatr Clin N Am 62 (2015) 367–384
http://dx.doi.org/10.1016/j.pcl.2014.11.003
0031-3955/15/$ – see front matter

Surface ectoderm is pulled in to form the lens, iris, and other associated structures to separate the 2 chambers. The cornea is formed from surface ectoderm and a fine layer of mesoderm between the neuroectoderm and surface ectoderm. The eyelids and lacrimal glands are formed from surface ectoderm. The retina forms from the internal walls of the optic cup. A thick neuroepithelium differentiates into rods and cones. Myelination is incomplete before birth at term but, after light exposure for approximately 10 weeks, myelination is complete. This process is markedly delayed in babies born prematurely and may be disrupted significantly in retinopathy of prematurity.[3]

Examination of the Eye

The eyelids meet and adhere by the tenth week of gestation.[2,4] They remain adherent until approximately 26 weeks' gestation. Although uncommon, babies born vaginally with a face presentation may have everted eyelids, which readily reduce with few complications and normal eyes otherwise (**Fig. 1**). An eyelid coloboma (notched lid) is a rare defect limited to the upper eyelid that requires surgery to protect the cornea and conjunctiva.

Conjunctival hemorrhage, often associated with a difficult delivery, is absorbed within several weeks. The sclera may be discolored yellow with significant jaundice and may appear bluish in inherited collagen vascular diseases because of scleral thinning and visualization of the underlying retina. Newborn eye prophylaxis to prevent bacterial infection often produces a transient chemical conjunctivitis. Conjunctival discharge may be caused by an infection, with gonorrhea and chlamydia being the most serious infections (**Fig. 2**). Obstruction of the nasolacrimal duct results in excessive tearing. Cloudy or protruding cornea indicates glaucoma (**Fig. 3**). The increased pressure of the aqueous humor in the anterior chamber is an emergency requiring immediate consultation and intervention by a pediatric ophthalmologist.

The iris color at birth is bluish in most infants. Pigmentation often progresses to a darker color, with the final iris color achieved by 4 months. Lack of pigmentation with a pink iris is a primary feature of albinism. Aniridia, complete lack of irises, is caused by an arrest of development of the rim of the optic cup at the eighth week. A failure of the ventral groove to fuse in early development leads to an iris coloboma, seen as a keyhole defect of the iris, which may extend into the ventral retina. The ciliary body is similarly affected, resulting in the inability to constrict the pupil and subsequent photophobia.

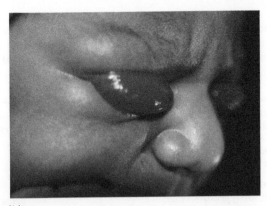

Fig. 1. Everted eyelids.

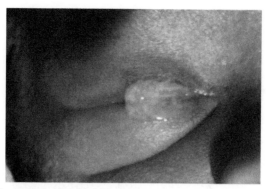

Fig. 2. Gonococcal purulent conjunctivitis.

The classic newborn eye test is the red reflex, elicited by shining a light into the eye, and the reflecting light off the highly vascular retina appears red. Any color but red may indicate anterior chamber disease (glaucoma), cataract, or retinal disorder such as detached retina or retinoblastoma (**Fig. 4**). Premature babies with immature retinas at birth may develop retinal scarring and detachment, a condition termed retinopathy of prematurity,[3] which can also cause abnormal red reflex.

Examination of the extraocular muscles is difficult at birth. It is common for newborns to have discordant muscle movement because their ability to focus and the resultant conjugate gaze take several months to mature. In addition, unusually long eyelashes can be an indication of a genetic syndrome, the foremost being Cornelia de Lange syndrome.

Early Vision

Neonatal vision is limited, such that term infants can only focus approximately 25 cm (10 inches) shortly after birth.[2,4–6] At less than 34 weeks' gestation, neonates do not have sufficient cone development to see color and can discriminate between dark and light only at a limited distance. The initial color humans see is red, presumably because of low light exposure from transillumination of the red color of maternal oxygenated hemoglobin into the uterus. With continued exposure to various

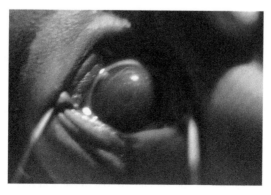

Fig. 3. Glaucoma.

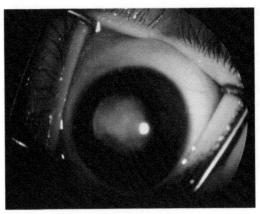

Fig. 4. Absent red reflex caused by retinoblastoma.

wavelengths of light, the retinal cones of other colors develop. The progression of eye function development is summarized in **Table 1**.

HEARING
Normal Development of Hearing

The most important aspects of the auditory system development take place during the second half of gestation.[7,8] Babies born prematurely and exposed during this period to multiple potential adverse effects of life-sustaining therapies are at great risk for hearing deficits and secondarily speech delay. Among neonatal intensive care unit (NICU) graduates, the incidence of hearing impairment is estimated to be at least 10-fold greater than in their term counterparts.[9,10]

Structure and Function

The auditory system comprises 3 related sets of structures: the peripheral components, including the outer, middle, and inner ears; the auditory nerves (cranial nerve VIII); and the auditory regions of the brain located primarily in the brainstem and left temporal lobe.

The outer ear of neonates features a narrow canal with thin cartilage, which is readily blocked and compressed. The shape, position, and peripheral tissue of the ear may provide clues to dysfunctional development. The classic low-set or malformed ear

Table 1 Visual development	
Characteristic	**Gestational Age (wk)**
Blink/squint in response to a bright light	26
Pupils constrict to light	30
Ability to fixate vision on a large object in close proximity	32
Track large moving objects	34
Color perception; red at first	34

Data from American Academy of Pediatrics, Section on Ophthalmology, American Academy of Ophthalmology. Screening examination of premature infants for retinopathy of prematurity. Pediatrics 2013;131:189–95; and Moore LM, Persaud TV. The developing human. Clinical oriented embryology. 8th edition. Philadelphia: Saunders; 2008. p. 429–32.

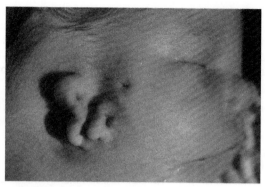

Fig. 5. Low-set, posteriorly rotated, malformed ear.

is found in more than 120 well-characterized syndromes.[11] For the ear to be considered low set, the entire ear must be below an extended line drawn from the inner canthus of the eye to the outer canthus (**Fig. 5**). A second criterion for low-set ear is the ear canal below an imaginary line drawn from the outer canthus to the base of the occiput. Posteriorly rotated ears or preauricular skin tags are more commonly seen in babies with syndromes.

The fluid-filled middle ear reaches adult size by 20 weeks' gestation, but the middle ear ossicles remain cartilaginous until 32 weeks' gestation. Cochlear structures, including inner and outer hair cells, are fully developed by 25 weeks' gestation. This process extends to myelination developing from the brainstem to higher level auditory pathways. The cochlea transduces acoustic wave energy into electrical impulses, which occurs in the inner hair cells. Outer hair cells adjust reflexively to sound input by producing frequency-specific echo sounds called otoacoustic emissions (OAE).

Hearing is the first sense exposed to stimulation that promotes development of the neural pathways. Functional hearing in human fetuses develops at 25 to 27 weeks' gestation. Low-frequency sounds, such as the mother's heartbeat and speech, elicit physiologic responses that are consistently detectable. Maturing fetuses respond to a wider range of sound frequencies progressing through the third trimester and shortly after birth. The functional maturation of hearing in the newborn is caused by structural changes in the outer and middle ears. Progressive myelination of auditory axons results in a maturing brainstem evoked response (auditory brainstem response [ABR]) test because of increased conduction velocities and wave amplitudes.

The incidence of permanent hearing loss in neonates ranges between 1.4 and 3 per 1000 births in the United States.[12–14] With progressive or new-onset hearing loss, the prevalence of permanent sensorineural hearing loss increases during childhood to estimated rates of about 2.7 per 1000 in 4-year-old children and 3.5 per 1000 in adolescents.[10,14]

Types and Causes of Hearing Impairment

Causes of hearing impairment

Based on the anatomic location of the hearing dysfunction, hearing loss can be classified as conductive, sensorineural, or neural[15–19]:

- Conductive hearing loss: blockage of sound transmission in the outer or middle ear caused by permanent conditions like anatomic malformations or transient problems such as fluid or debris.

- Sensorineural hearing loss: failure of sound transduction in the inner and outer hair cells of the cochlea, and of transmission through the auditory nerve.
- Neural hearing loss, also known as auditory neuropathy: dysfunction of the inner hair cells and auditory nerve, but OAE from the outer hair cells remain intact.
- Mixed hearing loss: combination of conductive and sensorineural hearing deficits.

In addition to the neurophysiologic classification described earlier, hearing loss can be further categorized according to severity (ie, mild, moderate, severe, or profound), based on the sound pressure level of the individual's hearing threshold. In addition, hearing loss can be unilateral or bilateral.[18,20]

About two-thirds of congenital hearing loss has an underlying genetic cause.[10,14] Mutations in the connexin 26 gene (*GJB2*), predominantly the 35delG point mutation, account for 20% of congenital deafness. An additional 44% of congenital deafness has other genetic causes; one-third of these being related to recognizable syndromes and two-thirds being nonsyndromic. Most nonsyndromic hearing loss cases follow an autosomal recessive inheritance pattern (*DFNB*), whereas a minority are autosomal dominant (*DFNA*); X-linked and mitochondrial inheritance is rare. Although many gene mutations have been associated with hearing loss, about 95% of congenitally deaf infants are born to parents with normal hearing, so a negative family history of deafness does not exclude the possibility of hereditary hearing loss. A newly diagnosed infant may serve as the index case to prompt genetic evaluation for the family.

The underlying pathophysiology of hearing dysfunction is complex. The 2007 Position Statement of the American Academy of Pediatrics Joint Committee on Infant Hearing[21] outlined causes of hearing loss that can be congenital, delayed onset, and/or progressive. These categories include:

- Infections
    Fetal: cytomegalovirus (CMV), varicella, syphilis, rubella, toxoplasmosis, and others
    Postnatal infections: meningitis, otitis media, encephalitis
- Environmental and therapeutic toxicity:
    Perinatal asphyxia, anoxia
    Ototoxic medications (aminoglycosides, loop diuretics)
    Mechanical ventilation, extracorporeal membrane oxygenation, sustained metabolic or respiratory acidosis
    Severe hyperbilirubinemia requiring exchange transfusion
- Trauma: perinatal, child abuse, temporal bone fracture
- Familial hearing loss
- Craniofacial anomalies/syndromes:
    Malformations of craniofacial structures derived from the first and second branchial arches, even without genetic associations, are embryologically related to the development of the inner ear, and are thus a risk factor for hearing loss. The many syndromes with craniofacial involvement include Waardenburg type I and II (white forelock), neurofibromatosis, and Alport.

Familial syndromes associated with progressive hearing loss include:

- Pendred syndrome accounts for only 3% of deafness diagnosed from birth, but comprises 12% of the cases of deafness in the preschool population.[10,11] Although deafness occurs early, the other clinically obvious component of the syndrome is goiter, which does not present until late childhood.

- Mitochondrial mutations or other neurodegenerative disorders, such as Friedrich ataxia, may first manifest beyond early infancy.
- Usher syndrome is a familial disorder characterized by progressive hearing loss and progressive retinitis pigmentosa leading to blindness.
- Jervell and Lange-Nielsen syndrome presents with cardiac dysrhythmias caused by a prolonged QT interval and should prompt reevaluation of hearing function.

Even if the newborn hearing screen is normal, a family history of hearing loss should trigger continued monitoring of the infant and formal audiologic assessment should be repeated by 24 to 30 months of age.

Medical screening systems cannot detect hearing loss in many children in a timely manner. Concerns by the family members regarding hearing, speech, language, or developmental delay must be addressed to improve early detection of hearing loss. Despite early hearing screening, more than two-thirds of children with subsequent hearing loss were diagnosed following parental concern and school hearing screens.[15,22,23]

Conditions with combined auditory and visual impairment, such as Usher syndrome, are particularly devastating to development of communication and psychosocial function. Increased association exists with autism spectrum disorder, which occurs in about 7% of 8-year-old children with visual or auditory impairment. The clinical diagnosis of hearing or visual deficits resulted in a substantial delay in the diagnosis of the coexisting autism spectrum disorder.[16]

Functional Consequences

Congenital or neonatally acquired permanent hearing loss adversely affects expressive and receptive language development, resulting in diminished academic achievement and social development. These sequelae can be mitigated by diagnosis and appropriate therapeutic intervention within the first 6 months of life.[10,18] Therefore, the age of 6 months represents a critical target for initial interventions in infants with hearing loss to optimize functional outcomes.[19]

The functional consequences of hearing loss depend on the age of onset and the specific subcategory of the hearing loss described earlier. Although bilateral deafness is most incapacitating, even unilateral hearing loss may affect language and educational performance.[20] Minimal information is available regarding the persistent effects of milder transient or reversible hearing dysfunction, such as that related to external ear debris in newborns, persistent otitis media with effusion, or auditory neuropathy in severe hyperbilirubinemia.

Screening in Newborns and Young Children

Intervention for hearing loss is most effective when initiated early to salvage speech and language development. Because of vigorous advocacy by the American Academy of Pediatrics, newborn hearing screening is performed in most individual birthing hospitals in the United States. There is great variability in accuracy because of multiple testers. **Table 2** summarizes the most useful hearing tests.

In newborn hearing screening, neither ABR nor OAE require an active response from the infant. The tests are more accurate when they are they performed on sleeping infants in a quiet environment. Both tests are cost-effective for early universal screening, given the high incidence and consequences of neonatal hearing loss.[22,23]

Automated auditory brainstem response screening uses scalp electrodes to detect the eight cranial nerve and auditory brainstem pathway responses to sound stimuli, applying automated algorithms to define hearing thresholds. ABR screening

Table 2		
Neonatal hearing tests		
Test	**Loss Detected**	**Significance**
Tympanometry	Conductive only	By changing pressure in the external ear canal, evaluates the intactness of the tympanic membrane and mobility with middle ear ossicles
Acoustic reflex	Conductive Sensorineural Neural	Measures stiffness of the middle ear Loud sounds trigger contraction of the tensor tympani and stapedius
ABR	Conductive Sensorineural Neural	Sound impulses of selected wavelengths generate electrical impulses that travel the auditory pathways to the brainstem and are reflected to the sensor

is sensitive to abnormalities in conductive, sensorineural, and purely neural hearing losses.

OAE tests detect the reflected echoes produced by the cochlear outer hair cells when stimulated by clicks across specified frequencies. These tests are abnormal in conductive and sensorineural hearing loss. However, they may be normal (ie, false-negative) in cases of purely auditory neuropathy. Because many of these cases are most likely to be found in the NICU setting, it is recommended that only ABR screening be used in NICUs.[21] Because OAE testing is easier and less expensive to perform, it is often used to screen healthy newborns. Some hospitals use a 2-stage protocol with ABR screening following OAE test failures to minimize the rate of false-positive screens.

The Joint Committee on Infant Hearing promotes the 1-3-6 principle of screening, diagnosis, and therapy for neonatal hearing loss, recommending that all infants undergo hearing screening by 1 month of age and those who fail their screens should have a diagnostic evaluation by an audiologist no later than 3 months of age. Infants whose hearing loss is confirmed should receive therapy appropriate to their diagnosis by age 6 months.[21] Neonatal hearing screening program failure rates range from 0.5% to 4%. Although false-negative neonatal hearing screens are exceedingly uncommon, such tests cannot detect progressive or later-onset hearing loss in childhood, which is as common as neonatal hearing loss.

The primary obstacle to neonatal hearing screening effectiveness in the United States is the 46% loss to follow-up of infants who fail their neonatal screen.[13] Primary care providers in the medical home have a critical role in ensuring that these infants receive the appropriate diagnostic testing in a timely manner. Major barriers to follow-up include ineffective communication of screening results, inadequate education of families regarding the importance of screening failures (which may have been deemed referrals), and lack of access to hearing diagnostic services for infants.

Early hearing detection and intervention (EHDI) programs, promoted and driven by professional organizations such as the American Academy of Pediatrics and supported by state and federal health agencies, have been implemented by many state health departments in association with early intervention programs. EHDI programs serve as coordinating centers for gathering data (shared with the Centers for Disease Control and Prevention), communicating with major stakeholders, and providing resources to maximize the success of the screening programs. A major focus of EHDI programs presently is the minimization of losses to follow-up in screening programs. Follow-up could be improved using currently available technological solutions, including documentation of hearing screening results in electronic medical records, and automated communication of test results from hospitals to the medical homes and EHDI programs (preferably coordinated with other neonatal screening test results); also, teleaudiology could expand the availability of diagnostic testing for infants and their families.[23]

The Joint Committee on Infant Hearing of the American Academy of Pediatrics has emphasized the need for a risk factor–based rescreening, even if the infants at risk passed the universal newborn screen.[17] Although the timing and number of hearing reevaluations should be individualized, infants with a risk factor should have at least 1 postnatal diagnostic audiologic evaluation by 24 to 30 months of age. Syndromic children or those infected with CMV may need more frequent reevaluation. Diagnostic services should be provided by audiologists with expertise and equipment appropriate for evaluating infants. When permanent hearing loss is confirmed, the primary care provider should coordinate further diagnostic evaluation, to define the cause of the hearing loss and possible comorbidities. This process should include consultation with genetics, an otolaryngologist experienced in pediatric hearing loss, and an ophthalmologist with expertise in evaluating infants.

Medical and Educational Interventions

Following diagnostic testing, the primary care provider needs to coordinate referrals for appropriate medical and surgical therapies, as well as community-based interventions. Input from multiple professionals, including audiology, speech-language pathology, and otolaryngology (ear, nose, and throat), as well as awareness of local community and school-based early intervention program resources, is needed to help families choose communication goals and interventions required to achieve them. Development of an individual family service plan is a first step in ensuring that the infant receives appropriate services no later than 6 months of age.[22] In addition to preventing loss to follow-up before diagnosis, the medical home must also promote timely therapeutic follow-up, given that only 39% of infants with hearing loss were fitted with hearing aids by 6 months.[23] It is important to establish appropriate initial therapy during the sensitive period for hearing development, to take advantage of plasticity of the auditory cortex, and to optimize cross-modal (eg, auditory and verbal) input of language acquisition. Aside from the coordinating functions, the medical home must provide continued surveillance for common conditions such as otitis media with effusion, which may affect hearing acuity and necessitate unplanned audiologic reevaluation, adjustments to existing amplification, or tympanostomy tubes. Close monitoring of developmental milestones is also essential.

Medical and Surgical Interventions

Ganciclovir
Detection of a CMV infection early allows the use of this antiviral medication to limit potential damage caused by the progressive CMV infection.

Surgical Implants

Bone-conducting miniature implants
SoundBite is a bone-conducting hearing aid inserted into the mouth.
BAHA Attract is a magnet-based bone-conduction device inserted behind the ear.

Cochlear Implant

Electric and acoustic stimulation
Cochlear implants transduce sound waves into frequency-specific electrical signals that are delivered to residual functioning auditory nerve fibers.[24] They can be placed

in children as young as 1 year of age with profound hearing loss and after 18 months of age in children with severe to profound bilateral sensorineural hearing loss, when amplification alone is inadequate. The device produces the greatest benefits in speech development when inserted by 7 years of age. Hearing loss caused by auditory neuropathy does not respond well to amplification alone, so early cochlear implantation may be advantageous in these situations.[24,25] Patients with cochlear implants are at increased risk for bacterial meningitis, particularly with *Streptococcus pneumoniae*, and should be immunized according to a high-risk schedule and monitored for early signs of meningitis associated with otitis media or other infections.

Modes of Communication

The family's choice of mode of communication may change over time, depending on the child's functional hearing, development, available interventions, and social environment factors.[26–30] Five options are currently available. The goal for the first 3 communication modes is spoken language, and the remaining 2 use sign language, with or without speech:

- Auditory verbal communication uses only optimized listening skills.
- Auditory-oral communication uses residual hearing with amplification, supported visually by speech reading.
- Cued speech combines listening with visual cues from 8 hand shapes near the face.
- American Sign Language (AMESLAN) can be learned by deaf children, with English or any other language as a second language.
- Total communication combines all modes of communication toward simultaneous use of speech and sign language.

Continued Interventions: Family and School

Parents and educators (including an expert in education of students with hearing loss) must develop an individualized education plan or section 504 plan to optimize student achievement, with support from the primary care medical home.[28,29] Adaptations in the learning environment may involve the student, teachers, modes of communication, physical design of the classroom, and curricular modifications, including supplemental instruction. Examples of such adaptations include an optimal amplification system, visual assistive devices (eg, telecommunication device for the deaf), optimal seating arrangements, individualized communication with the student, use of an interpreter, assistance with asynchronous learning (eg, new vocabulary provided in advance of the session or a buddy system for note taking), and alternative testing methods. In addition, there are various options for supplemental instruction, including sign language and support from a deaf or hard-of-hearing role model. Continuous evaluation is essential for optimal adjustment and coordination of the educational accommodations over time.

Because hearing disorders and related comorbidities have varied causes, the outcome of an individual child is difficult to predict. Children with isolated auditory neuropathy treated by cochlear implantation performed comparably with age-matched peers with sensorineural hearing loss, but those with auditory neuropathy associated with a cognitive or developmental disorder had significantly less benefit and continued to rely on nonauditory modes of communication.[25]

SMELL, TASTE, ORAL STRUCTURES, AND FUNCTION

The ability of a baby to smell is an important component of the early infant-mother interaction. Components of the maternal diet reach the amniotic fluid, are swallowed, and become familiar to the fetus. They may contribute to the scent of the mother, including her breast milk.[31] By 5 to 6 days of life, babies preferentially choose the breast pad of their mother rather than that from another mother or an unused pad.[32,33] Although the progressive development of smell is less well defined compared with vision and hearing, a few general observations have been made. Term babies prefer sweet odors such as lavender and vanilla and have a rapid avoidance response to foul odors like rotten eggs. Babies with choanal atresia or a tracheostomy have blunted development of smell, presumably caused by minimal airflow through the nose.[34]

Taste development is likewise poorly understood compared with the other senses.[35] Taste is supplied by the chorda tympani branch of the facial nerve (cranial nerve VII) on the anterior two-thirds of the tongue and by a branch of the glossopharyngeal (cranial nerve IX) over the posterior one-third of the tongue. Fetuses in the uterus continually swallow the components of amniotic fluid with proteins, carbohydrate, fat, and small molecules to initiate digestive enzymatic activity, so taste likely begins to develop in utero. Human neonates prefer sweet foods and can detect sour and bitter. Babies may not be able to detect salt until 3 to 4 months of age.[36] They prefer breast milk to infant formula because the bovine alpha casein protein is more bitter than human beta casein. Hydrolyzed protein formulas are less savory. Sucrose in soy formulas is sweeter than lactose, thus soy formula should not be used as an adjunct to breast feeding.

The structures of the oral cavity derive from the first branchial arch. By the end of the fourth week of development, the frontonasal, 2 maxillary, and 2 mandibular processes are discernible. These tissues eventually fuse midline to form the face and palate at between 6 and 12 weeks' gestation. Remnants of, and failure of, fusion can readily be detected on examination of newborns.

An appropriate neonatal oral examination includes both inspection and palpation. The provider should visually inspect the jaw and mouth size and shape, lips, gingiva, dentoalveolar ridge, palate, and mouth and tongue appearance and mobility. A gloved finger should be used to evaluate the sucking reflex and to palpate the hard and soft palates for a defect.

Drooping of the corner of the mouth at rest can result from facial nerve paralysis (**Fig. 6**). Normal appearance at rest, but failure of the affected side to move with crying, indicates hypoplasia or aplasia of the depressor anguli oris muscle. Facial nerve palsies are more like to occur with prolonged labor and compression of the facial nerve against the sacral bone or by use of forceps during delivery. The paralyzed side will have loss of the nasolabial fold, drooping of the mouth, and the mouth drawn to the normal side. It is important to determine whether there is branch 1 involvement of the facial nerve paralysis, because of the risk of corneal injury with improper eyelid closure. Most facial nerve palsies resolve spontaneously within days, but may persist weeks to months. Asymmetric crying facies caused by hypoplasia or aplasia of the depressor anguli oris muscle can be part of a genetic syndrome, the most significant association being congenital cardiac defects (Cayler syndrome).

Congenital soft tissue lesions of the oral cavity are common and practitioners must be able to distinguish normal findings from those that require intervention. There are 3 common types of oral inclusion cysts, which are epithelial tissue remnants. Inclusion cysts are small white or translucent papules or cysts[37] noted in 75% of newborns, although the prevalence of inclusion cysts in premature infants is less than that of their term counterparts.[38] Inclusion cysts are generally asymptomatic and require no further evaluation or management except for reassurance. Most cysts

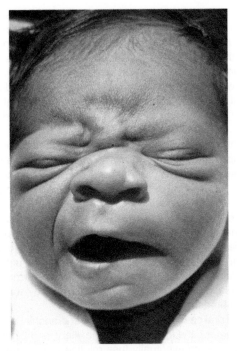

Fig. 6. Facial nerve palsy.

resolve spontaneously by 3 months of age. Three types of inclusion cysts can be seen in newborns:

1. Epstein pearls are the most common of the congenital inclusion cysts, occurring in 75% to 80% of all neonates.[37] They are found scattered along the midline raphe of the hard palate (**Fig. 7**).
2. Bohn nodules are heterotopic salivary gland remnants located on the buccal or lingual mucosal surface of the alveolar ridge (not the crest) or on the hard palate, away from the raphe (**Fig. 8**).
3. Dental lamina cysts are heterotopic salivary gland remnants located on the crest of the alveolar ridge.

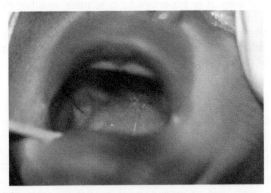

Fig. 7. Epstein pearls.

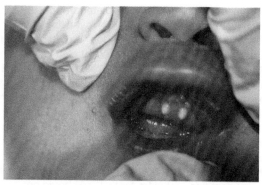

Fig. 8. Bohn nodules.

Failure of midline fusion during embryogenesis can result in the spectrum of cleft lip, cleft palate, cleft lip and palate, or submucosal cleft palate. Lip closure occurs during week 5 to 6 of embryonic development, the hard palate forms during week 6 to 10, and the soft palate fuses during week 10 to 12. Cleft lip and palate are among the common congenital abnormalities, with a prevalence of 17 in every 10,000 live births,[39] and cleft lip with palate is more common than isolated cleft palate (**Fig. 9**). Cleft lip can be unilateral, bilateral, or median, but midline lip cleft is rare.

The cause of clefts remains poorly understood, with genetic, syndromic, and environmental factors all being implicated. Teratogen exposures linked to cleft development include viral infections, metabolic abnormalities, medications, and drugs. Of inherited forms, the most common familial cleft lip and palate with no other anomalies is Van der Woude syndrome. Cleft lip and/or palate can be associated with genetic syndromes having other anomalies, including the spectrum of chromosome 22q11, oral-facial-digital syndrome, and Treacher-Collins syndrome. Micrognathia caused by mandibular hypoplasia can be isolated or associated with cleft palate, through the mechanical interference of the embryonic tongue with fusion of the 2 halves of the palate midline. This condition is termed the Robin sequence or Pierre Robin syndrome.

Care of neonates with cleft lip and/or palate requires aggressive feeding support and evaluation for airway concerns. Surgical primary lip repair is often undertaken at 3 months of age and primary palatal repair around 6 months. Management after discharge is often best coordinated through a multidisciplinary cleft and craniofacial team composed of experienced members of the medical, surgical, dental, and allied health disciplines.

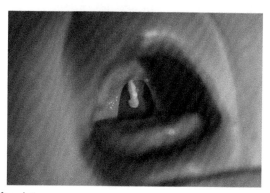

Fig. 9. Cleft of soft palate.

Submucosal cleft palate is a milder or incomplete form of cleft palate. Examination may reveal a bifid uvula, muscular defect with overlying membrane, or a bluish mucosal line the length of the soft palate. This form is often clinically challenging to detect in the neonatal period. However, submucosal clefts are often functionally significant, because the levator muscles do not interdigitate across the cleft to form the normal levator sling. If the levator muscle cannot elevate and retract the posterior soft palate to divide the nasal and oral pharynxes, the result is velopharyngeal incompetence, which can affect both feeding and speech development.

Humans are usually born edentulous, with the first primary teeth emerging between 6 and 8 months of age. However, tooth eruption occurs before birth (natal teeth) or within the first month of life (neonatal teeth) at a rate of 1 in 2000 to 1 in 3000 live births.[40] Central mandibular incisors are the most likely to erupt early and these are most often the primary dentition, not extra teeth,[41] so should not be extracted without cause. Natal teeth are most commonly an isolated finding (**Fig. 10**), but can be associated with genetic syndromes such as chondroectodermal dysplasia (Ellis–van Creveld syndrome) and oculomandibulofacial syndrome (Hallermann-Streiff syndrome).[42] Management is most often observation, although extraction may be considered if teeth are mobile and present an aspiration risk, interfere with breastfeeding, or lead to Riga-Fede ulceration.[40]

Ankyloglossia (tongue-tie) is anchoring of the tongue anteriorly causing limited tongue movement, which occurs in 4% to 10% of babies. Ankyloglossia varies in severity and clinical consequence with considerable debate regarding optimal management.[43] Restricted tongue movement can lead to a variety of problems in infants and children, such as inability to latch with breastfeeding, improper speech development, and compromised oral health.[44,45]

Initial symptoms of ankyloglossia include maternal nipple pain with breastfeeding, loss of suction or a clicking sound while feeding, and poor latch.[46,47] On examination, there is a frenulum inserted near the tip of the tongue, inability to extend the tongue to the lips or to the roof of the mouth, and notched or heart-shaped tongue on extension. Although interference with breastfeeding is the most common sequela, significant ankyloglossia is also associated with articulation difficulty,[45] but not delay in onset of speech.[46] Difficulty with oral hygiene increases the risk of dental caries and periodontal disease. Inability to lick and perform other activities that require tongue extension may have social consequences.

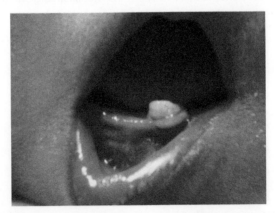

Fig. 10. Natal tooth.

Management of breastfeeding difficulties should include consultation with a lactation specialist, but frenectomy improves feeding for mother and baby significantly better than the intensive support of a lactation consultant.[44] Indications and timing of surgical division for ankyloglossia have been investigated and in 1 randomized, prospective, but unblinded trial of neonates with feeding concerns and ankyloglossia, and feeding improved in all of the infants who received immediate division of the frenulum, but in only 1 infant who received intensive lactation support. Frenotomy was then offered and performed for the infants in the control group and all but 1 baby improved and fed normally after the procedure.[48] Frenotomy (also called frenectomy) can be performed with blunt scissors, cautery, or laser if a simple membrane is present, but more complex anatomy should be referred for frenuloplasty. Absence of the inferior labial frenum is strongly correlated with infantile hypertrophic pyloric stenosis[49] and absence of the inferior labial frenum and lingual frenulum is commonly noted in Ehlers-Danlos syndrome.[50]

More recently, discussions have arisen around clinical consequence and management of a constricted maxillary frenum. The maxillary frenum normally extends over the alveolar ridge to form a raphe and persistence of this raphe during dental eruption may lead to widely spaced central incisors, termed a diastema. In addition to a cosmetic effect, there is concern that a prominent maxillary labial frenum can result in difficulty with plaque control and perhaps increased risk for dental caries caused by liquid trapping under the upper lip. Additional research is needed to better understand the appropriateness of performing preventive maxillary frenectomy on young children. At present, treatment is indicated in the rare cases in which the frenum attachment exerts tension on the gingiva of a permanent tooth or if the cosmetic appearance is unacceptable following orthodontic closure of the diastema.[51,52]

SUMMARY

The development of each sense is crucial to successful interaction of babies with their mothers, ranging from bonding to feeding and eventually to capacity to learn. Primary care physicians have the greatest opportunity to detect visual and hearing deficits, to intervene, and to improve lifelong development and intellectual achievement.

REFERENCES

1. Graven SN. Early visual development: implications for the neonatal intensive care unit and care. Clin Perinatol 2011;38:671–83.
2. Madan M, Good W. The eye. In: Taeusch HW, Ballard R, Gleason CA, editors. Avery's diseases of the newborn. Philadelphia: Elsevier Saunders; 2005. p. 1539–50.
3. American Academy of Pediatrics, Section on Ophthalmology, American Academy of Ophthalmology. Screening examination of premature infants for retinopathy of prematurity. Pediatrics 2013;131:189–95.
4. Braddick OJ, Atkinson J. Infants' sensitivity to motion and temporal change. Optom Vis Sci 2009;86(6):577–82.
5. Frank MC, Vul E, Johnson HP. Development of infants' attention to faces during the first year. Cognition 2009;110(2):160–70.
6. Moore LM, Persaud TV. The developing human. Clinical oriented embryology. 8th edition. Philadelphia: Saunders; 2008. p. 429–32.
7. Graven SN, Browne JV. Auditory development in the fetus and infant. Newborn Infant Nurs Rev 2008;8:187–93.

8. Lasky RE, Williams AL. The development of the auditory system from conception to term. NeoReviews 2005;6:e141–52.
9. Pineda RG, Neil J, Dierker D, et al. Alterations in brain structure and neurodevelopmental outcome in preterm infants hospitalized in different neonatal intensive care unit environments. J Pediatr 2014;164:52–60.
10. Pinheiro J. Hearing development and disorders. In: Ensher G, Clark D, editors. Working with families, infants, and toddlers with special needs: foundations for best practice. Washington, DC: Zero to Three; 2015. Chapter 7. p. 112–34.
11. Jones KL. Smith's recognizable patterns of human malformation. 6th edition. Philadelphia: Elsevier Saunders; 2006. p. 867–8, 897–9.
12. Dalzell L, Orlando M, MacDonald M, et al. The New York State Universal Newborn Hearing Screening Demonstration Project: ages of hearing loss. Ear Hear 2000; 21:118–30.
13. Gaffney M, Eichwald J, Grouse SD, et al. Identifying infants with hearing loss - United States, 1999-2007. MMWR Morb Mortal Wkly Rep 2010;59:220–3.
14. Morton CC, Nance WE. Newborn hearing screening – a silent revolution. N Engl J Med 2006;354:2151–64.
15. Dedhia K, Kitsko D, Sabo D, et al. Children with sensorineural hearing loss after passing the newborn hearing screen. JAMA Otolaryngol Head Neck Surg 2013; 139:1–5.
16. Kancherla V, Van Naarden Braun K, Yeargin-Allsopp M. Childhood vision impairment, hearing loss and co-occurring autism spectrum disorder. Disabil Health J 2013;6:333–42.
17. Harlor ADB, Bower C. Committee on Practice and Ambulatory Medicine, & the Section on Otolaryngology - Head and Neck Surgery Hearing assessment in infants and children: recommendations beyond neonatal screening. Pediatrics 2009;124:1252–63.
18. Yoshinaga-Itano C, Coulter D, Thomson V. The Colorado Newborn Hearing Screening Project: Effects on speech and language development for children with hearing loss. J Perinatol 2000;20:S132–7.
19. Moon C. The role of early auditory development in attachment and communication. Clin Perinatol 2011;38:657–69.
20. Lieu JE, Tye-Murray N, Karzon RK, et al. Unilateral hearing loss is associated with worse speech-language scores in children. Pediatrics 2010;125:e1348–55.
21. Joint Committee on Infant Hearing. Year 2007 position statement: principles and guidelines for early hearing detection and intervention programs. Pediatrics 2007;120:898–921.
22. Joint Committee on Infant Hearing of the American Academy of Pediatrics, Muse C, Harrison J, et al. Supplement to the JCIH 2007 position statement: principles and guidelines for early intervention after confirmation that a child is deaf or hard of hearing. Pediatrics 2013;131:e1324–49.
23. Spivak L, Sokol H, Auerbach C, et al. Newborn hearing screening follow-up: Factors affecting hearing aid fitting by 6 months of age. Am J Audiol 2009;18: 24–33.
24. McConkey RA, Koch DB, Osberger MJ, et al. Effect of age at cochlear implantation on auditory skill development in infants and toddlers. Arch Otolaryngol Head Neck Surg 2004;130:570–4.
25. Budenz CL, Telian SA, Ardent C, et al. Outcomes of cochlear implantation in children with isolated auditory neuropathy versus cochlear hearing loss. Otol Neurotol 2013;34:477–83.

26. Kennedy CR, McCann DC, Campbell MJ, et al. Language ability after early detection of permanent childhood hearing impairment. N Engl J Med 2006;354: 2131–41.
27. Kral A, O'Donoghue GM. Profound deafness in childhood. N Engl J Med 2010; 363:1438–50.
28. Mehl AL, Thomson V. The Colorado Newborn Hearing Screening Project, 1992-1999: on the threshold of effective population-based universal newborn hearing screening. Pediatrics 2002;109:e7.
29. Moeller MP. Early intervention and language development in children who are deaf and hard of hearing. Pediatrics 2000;106:E43.
30. White RD. Designing environments for developmental care. Clin Perinatol 2011; 38:745–9.
31. Varendi H, Porter RH, Winberg J. Does the newborn baby find the nipple by smell? Lancet 1994;344:989–90.
32. Varendi H, Porter RH, Winberg J. Attractiveness of amniotic fluid odor: evidence of prenatal olfactory learning? Acta Paediatr 1996;85(10):1223–7.
33. Delaunay El, Allam M, Marlier L, et al. Learning at the breast: preference formation for an artificial scent and its attraction against the odor of maternal milk. Infant Behav Dev 2006;29(3):308–21.
34. Romantshik O, Porter RH, Tillman V, et al. Evidence of a sensitive period for olfactory learning by human newborns. Acta Paediatr 1997;96(3):372–6.
35. Beauchamp GK, Pearson P. Human development and umami taste. Physiol Behav 1991;49(5):1009–12.
36. Beauchamp GK, Cowart BJ, Moran M. Developmental changes in salt acceptability in human infants. Dev Psychobiol 1986;19:17–25.
37. Hayes P. Hamartomas, eruption cyst, natal tooth and Epstein pearls in a newborn. ASDC J Dent Child 2000;67(5):365–8.
38. Donley CL, Nelson LP. Comparison of palatal and alveolar cysts of the newborn in premature and full term infants. Pediatr Dent 2000;22(4):321–4.
39. Canfield MA, Honein MA, Yuskiv N, et al. National estimates and race/ethnic-specific variation of selected birth defects in the United States, 1999-2001. Birth Defects Res A Clin Mol Teratol 2006;76(11):747.
40. Cunha RF, Boer FA, Torriani DD, et al. Natal and neonatal teeth: review of the literature. Pediatr Dent 2001;23(2):158–62.
41. Bodenhoff J, Gorlin RJ. Natal and neonatal teeth. Folklore and fact. Pediatrics 1963;32(6):1087–93.
42. Hattab FN, Yassin OM, Sasa IS. Oral manifestations of Ellis-van Creveld syndrome: report of two siblings with unusual dental anomalies. J Clin Pediatr Dent 1998;22(2):159–65.
43. Messner AH, Lalakea ML. Ankyloglossia: controversies in management. Int J Pediatr Otorhinolaryngol 2000;54(2–3):123.
44. Hogan M, Westcott C, Griffiths M. Randomized, controlled trial of division of tongue-tie in infants with feeding problems. J Paediatr Child Health 2005; 41(5–6):246.
45. Lalakea ML, Messner AH. Ankyloglossia: does it matter? Pediatr Clin North Am 2003;50(2):381.
46. Messner AH, Lalakea ML. The effect of ankyloglossia on speech in children. Otolaryngol Head Neck Surg 2002;127(6):539.
47. Ballard JL, Auer CE, Khoury JC. Ankyloglossia: assessment, incidence, and effect of frenuloplasty on the breastfeeding dyad. Pediatrics 2002;110(5):e63.

48. Buryk M, Bloom D, Shope T. Efficacy of neonatal release of ankyloglossia: a randomized trial. Pediatrics 2011;128:280.
49. De Felice C, Di Maggio G, Zagordo L, et al. Hypoplastic or absent mandibular frenulum: a new predictive sign of infantile hypertrophic pyloric stenosis. J Pediatr 2000;136(3):408.
50. De Felice C, Toti P, Di Maggio G, et al. Absence of the inferior labial and lingual frenula in Ehlers-Danlos syndrome. Lancet 2001;357(9267):1500.
51. Devishree, Gujjari SK, Shubhashini PV. Frenectomy: a review with the reports of surgical techniques. J Clin Diagn Res 2012;6(9):1587–92.
52. American Academy of Pediatric Dentistry, Council on Clinical Affairs. Guideline on Pediatric Oral Surgery. 2010; Revised 2014. Reference Manual 36(6):276–83.

Metabolic Screening and Postnatal Glucose Homeostasis in the Newborn

David H. Adamkin, MD

KEYWORDS

- Newborn metabolic screening • Tandem mass spectrometry
- Hypoglycemia screening and management

KEY POINTS

- Among 4 million newborns screened each year, approximately 12,500 are identified with heritable disorders, many of which are associated with severe effects if not identified before symptoms develop.
- Acute metabolic decompensation with inborn errors of metabolism occurs when there is an accumulation of the toxic metabolites associated with the newborn error.
- An acute clinical presentation of a multisystem decompensation strongly suggests an association with an inborn error of metabolism.
- There is no consensus for a specific value or range of glucose values in newborns that specifically defines hypoglycemia or when and how treatment should be provided.
- The American Academy of Pediatrics (AAP) guideline on postnatal glucose homeostasis aims to provide guidance where evidence is lacking.

Newborn screening has been among the most successful public health programs of the 21st century. The year 2013 was the 50th anniversary of newborn screening. Approximately 4 million infants are screened per year under newborn screening programs that are mandated in most states. About 12,500 infants are identified each year with heritable disorders. Many of these are associated with severe effects if not identified before the onset of symptoms.[1] Therefore, the goal of newborn screening programs is to detect these disorders that cause harm to life or threaten long-term health before they become symptomatic. Conditions like endocrine disorders, hemoglobinopathies, immunodeficiencies, cystic fibrosis, and critical congenital heart defects, as well as inborn errors of metabolism are among those that can

Disclosure Statement: D.H. Adamkin, MD, is a consultant and investor in Medolac Laboratories. He does not discuss any off-label use and/or investigational use in this article.
Division of Neonatal Medicine, Department of Pediatrics, University of Louisville, 571 South Floyd Street, Suite 342, Louisville, KY 40202, USA
E-mail address: david.adamkin@louisville.edu

Pediatr Clin N Am 62 (2015) 385–409
http://dx.doi.org/10.1016/j.pcl.2014.11.004   pediatric.theclinics.com
0031-3955/15/$ – see front matter © 2015 Elsevier Inc. All rights reserved.

be screened for. Early treatment may significantly improve outcome and improve survival.

Although individual metabolic diseases are relatively uncommon, inherited metabolic diseases collectively represent a more common cause of disease in the neonatal period than is generally appreciated. For example, the estimated incidence of inherited metabolic disease in the general population varies from 1 per 10,000 live births for phenylketonuria to as few as 1 per 200,000 live births with homocystinuria. Currently, there are approximately 100 such inheritable disorders that can be diagnosed in the neonatal period. The overall incidence for metabolic disease is about 1 per 2000 persons.[2] Newborn screening programs have found an incidence of about 1 in 4000 for a subset of these diseases.[2] It is also possible that this is an underestimate of the incidence of these disorders, because many with metabolic disease go undiagnosed.

New technologies have expanded the capabilities of newborn screening programs. Presently, 31 conditions are recommended to be screened on state newborn screening panels by the Discretionary Advisory Committee of Heritable Disorders in Newborns and Children. It all began in 1960 when Robert Guthrie developed a bacterial inhibition assay that detected elevated levels of phenylalanine after birth from infant's blood. Population studies for screening for phenylketonuria began in 1963 when Massachusetts became the first state to actually mandate newborn screening. This same technique, where a blood specimen contains greater than normal quantities of an amino acid or metabolite is associated with a large growth of bacteria, has been used to detect other conditions, including maple syrup urine disease, homocystinuria, tryosinemia, and histidinemia.

The new technologies that have expanded newborn screening included a radioimmunoassay for thyroxine, making possible screening for congenital hypothyroidism.[3] Isoelectric focusing and liquid chromatography have allowed for hemoglobinopathy screening. The polymerase chain reaction allowed screening for mutations in hemoglobin genes in DNA extracted from dried blood samples.[4,5] Tandem mass spectrometry (also known as MS/MS) as well as some other techniques now allow expanded possibilities for mass screening of many disorders.[6–9] This spectrometry detects molecules by measuring their weight and is a series of 2 mass spectrometers. They sort the samples and identify and weigh the molecules of interest in screening. It is best suited for inborn errors of organic acid, fatty acid, and amino acid metabolism. Newer methods have allowed this technique to also be used to detect lysosomal storage disorders.[10] New biochemical and genetic tests have recently allowed screening for cystic fibrosis[11] and severe combined immunodeficiency.[12] Tandem mass spectrometry because of its availability and its cost effectiveness has allowed expansion of newborn screening that can be provided and remains the strategy used to detect the majority of conditions that are screened for today.

PRINCIPLES OF SCREENING

Newborn screening tests are administered to healthy populations to detect infants who may have a serious disorder. They do not always provide definitive results, but they identify which infants require further testing.[13,14] The medical requirements of an acceptable mass screening program for a particular disease include the following, which are reviewed by Zinn[2]:

- The availability of a reliable screening test with a low false-negative rate;
- A test that is simple and inexpensive, because many tests will be performed for each case identified;

- A rapid screening test that can provide results quickly enough to permit effective intervention;
- A definitive follow-up test that is available for unambiguous identification of true positive results and elimination of false-positive results;
- A disorder of a sufficiently deleterious nature that, if untreated, would result in significant morbidity or death; and
- An effective therapy that significantly alters the natural history of the disease.

Unfortunately, few metabolic diseases satisfy all of these requirements. Certain principles also apply to all newborn screening programs and include the following[2]:

- Genetic heterogeneity, biologic variation, and error lead to false-positive results in any screening test. Thus, a definitive method must be available to confirm a positive screening result.
- Positive results must be acted upon on an emergent basis so that timely testing and intervention can be accomplished.
- Patients with positive screening tests should be referred to a pediatric specialist experienced in the diagnosis and management of the specific condition for definitive diagnosis and treatment, if needed.

TANDEM MASS SPECTROMETRY

The current MS/MS techniques allow analysis of large numbers of metabolites that may belong to a particular category of disease. Therefore, many disorders can be screened in every sample. Literally, hundreds of samples can be analyzed and studied each day. These devices are sensitive, accurate, and allow multiple metabolites to be identified simultaneously. Computerization allows pattern recognition using several related metabolites and thereby increases the reliability of the testing.

Normal ranges must be determined for the MS/MS screening programs for the different metabolites that are studied. Cut-offs are set, and values above or below those levels identify a potential case as an at-risk situation. It is important for these values to be accurate; if a cut-off is set too high, then there may be inordinately great number of false-negative results. Conversely, if cut-offs are set too low, there is an unacceptable rate of false-positive results. The onus is on the practitioner to decide whether a particular result is truly positive or is false positive as quickly as is possible. As mentioned, newborn screening programs have found that about 1 in 4000 newborns have a diagnosable error of metabolism.

It should also be appreciated that most programs do not screen for inborn errors that are associated with low concentrations of the specific amino acids. The organic acidemias and fatty acid oxidation disorders are detected by analyzing for increased blood concentrations of specific acylcarnitines, namely, the esters formed between carnitine and the acids that accumulate with the organic acidemias and fatty acid oxidation disorders. However, screening for the plasma membrane carnitine uptake defect looks for a reduced (rather than increased) concentration of free carnitine.

Table 1 provides the basics about inborn errors of metabolism that can be diagnosed by MS/MS used in newborn screening programs. The table from Zinn[2] names each disorder and provides information about the underlying enzymatic defect and the clinical features and natural history of the disorder. There is also an approach to treatment and what the prognosis may be. As discussed, some 4 million infants are screened each year in the United States and approximately 12,500 are diagnosed

Table 1
Inborn errors of metabolism diagnosable by tandem mass spectrometry

Disorder	Defect	Clinical Features and Natural History	Treatment	Prognosis with Treatment
Homocystinuria	Cystathionine β-synthetase deficiency	Generally asymptomatic at birth Developmental delay, dislocated lens, skeletal deformities, and thromboembolic episodes	Dietary protein restriction Selective amino acid restriction (methionine) vitamin B_6 supplementation plus betaine, folate, and vitamin B_{12}	Patients with vitamin B_6-responsive form of disease have fewer complications and later age onset of complications than do patients with vitamin B_6-nonresponsive form
Maple syrup urine disease	Branched-chain α-keto acid dehydrogenase deficiency	Patients might present before newborn screening results are available Difficulty feeding, vomiting, lethargy progressing to coma, opisthotonic posturing, and possibly death Ketoacidosis	Emergent treatment might be indicated for symptomatic neonates Chronic care includes dietary protein restriction, selective branched-chain amino acid restriction (leucine, isoleucine, valine), and thiamine supplementation for thiamine-responsive patients	Improved intellectual outcome can be expected if treatment is initiated before first crisis, but there is developmental delay in severe cases Recurrent episodes of ketoacidosis
Nonketotic hyperglycinemia	Glycine cleavage enzyme deficiency	Patients might present before newborn screening results are available Hypotonia, apnea, intractable seizures, and lethargy progressing to coma Burst-suppression electroencephalograph pattern Hiccups (characteristic) Transient forms very rare	Various drugs can lower plasma glycine, but none lower CSF glycine or improve clinical outcome Dextromethorphan for seizures	Intractable seizures and poor intellectual development in patients who survive the neonatal period, except in rare instances

Disorder	Clinical features	Treatment	Prognosis
Phenylketonuria / Phenylalanine hydroxylase deficiency	Generally asymptomatic at birth After a few months, microcephaly, seizures, and pale pigmentation develop, followed in later years by abnormal posturing, mental retardation, and behavioral or psychiatric disturbances	Dietary protein restriction Selective amino acid restriction (phenylalanine)	Normal development can be expected (although a mild decrease in IQ and behavioral difficulties relative to nonaffected siblings might be seen) if diet is instituted early
BH$_4$ biosynthesis or recycling defect	Patients with BH$_4$ defects have additional problems secondary to dopamine and serotonin deficiency	Biopterin defects require special care	Patients with biopterin defects have a more guarded prognosis
Tyrosinemia type I / Fumarylacetoacetate hydrolase deficiency	Patients might present before newborn screening results are available Severe liver failure associated with jaundice, ascites, and bleeding diathesis Peripheral neuropathy and seizures can develop Renal Fanconi syndrome leading to rickets Survivors develop chronic liver disease with increased risk of HCC	Emergency treatment might be indicated for symptomatic neonates Chronic care includes dietary protein restriction, selective amino acid restriction (phenylalanine and tyrosine), administration of selective enzyme inhibitor (NTBC), and liver transplantation when indicated to prevent HCC	Liver disease could progress despite dietary treatment NTBC treatment improves liver, kidney, and neurologic function, but it does not eliminate risk for HCC Liver transplantation might still be required
Tyrosinemia type II / Tyrosine aminotransferase	Corneal lesions and hyperkeratosis of the soles and palms	Selective amino acid restriction (tyrosine)	Good
Urea cycle disorders			
Argininosuccinic acidemia / Argininosuccinic acid lyase deficiency	Patients might present before newborn screening results are available Anorexia, vomiting, lethargy, seizures, and coma, possibly leading to death Hyperammonemia	Emergency treatment might be indicated for symptomatic neonates Chronic care includes dietary protein restriction, essential amino acid supplementation, arginine or citrulline supplementation, and alternative pathway drugs for removing NH$_3$ (sodium benzoate and phenylbutyrate)	Improved intellectual outcome could be expected if treatment is initiated early, but there is developmental delay in the severe cases Recurrent hyperammonemic episodes

(continued on next page)

Table 1
(continued)

Disorder	Defect	Clinical Features and Natural History	Treatment	Prognosis with Treatment
Arginemia	Arginase deficiency	Rarely symptomatic in neonatal period Progressive spastic diplegia or tetraplegia, opisthotonus, seizures Low risk of symptomatic hyperammonemia	Dietary protein restriction Selective amino acid restriction (arginine) Alternative pathway drugs for removing NH_3 (sodium benzoate and phenylbutyrate)	Uncertain but might improve neurologic outcome
Citrullinemia	Argininosuccinate synthetase deficiency	Patients might present before newborn screening results are available Anorexia, vomiting, lethargy, seizures, and coma, possibly leading to death Hyperammonemia	Emergency treatment might be indicated for symptomatic neonates Chronic care includes dietary protein restriction, essential amino acid supplementation, arginine or citrulline supplementation, and alternative pathways drugs for removing NH_3 (sodium benzoate and phenylbutyrate)	Improved intellectual outcome can be expected if treatment is initiated early, but there is developmental delay in the severe cases Recurrent hyperammonemic episodes
Organic acidemias				
Glutaric acidemia type I	Glutaryl-CoA dehydrogenase deficiency	Rarely symptomatic in neonatal period, although macrocephaly may be present Progressive macrocephaly, ataxia, dystonia and choreoathetosis, developmental regression, seizures, and stroke like episodes, possibly exacerbated by infection or fasting	Dietary protein restriction Selective amino acid restriction (lysine, tryptophan) Riboflavin and carnitine supplementation	Improved intellectual outcome if treatment is initiated early, but poor neurologic outcome if treatment is started after acute neurologic injury occurs Treatment might slow neurologic deterioration

Disorder	Enzyme deficiency	Clinical manifestations	Treatment	Outcome/Comments
Glutaric acidemia type II	ETF deficiency or ETF dehydrogenase deficiency	Commonly manifests in neonatal period Hypotonia, hepatomegaly, abnormal odor, with or without congenital anomalies, including facial dysmorphism and cystic kidney disease Metabolic acidosis and hypoglycemia Generally lethal Late-onset forms variable, rarely have structural birth defects	Emergency treatment might be indicated for symptomatic neonates Chronic care includes dietary protein restriction, selective amino acid restriction (isoleucine, methionine, threonine, and valine), and carnitine supplementation	Treatment for neonatal-onset forms invariably unsuccessful Dietary fat and protein restriction and riboflavin and carnitine supplementation might help patients with late-onset disease
3-Hydroxy-3-methylglutaric aciduria	3-Hydroxy-3-methylglutaryl-CoA lyase deficiency	Generally does not manifest in neonatal period Episodic hypoglycemia leading to developmental delay	Dietary protein restriction Selective amino acid restriction (leucine) Low-fat diet	Improved intellectual outcome may be expected if treatment is initiated early, but there is developmental delay in the severe cases Recurrent hypoglycemic episodes decrease in frequency and severity over time
Isobutyric acidemia	Isobutyryl-CoA dehydrogenase deficiency	Uncertain because number of cases is small	Dietary protein restriction Selective amino acid restriction (valine)	Unknown
Isovaleric acidemia	Isovaleryl-CoA dehydrogenase deficiency	Patients might present before newborn screening results are available Vomiting, lethargy and coma, possibly death Abnormal odor Thrombocytopenia, leukopenia, anemia Ketoacidosis Hyperammonemia	Emergency treatment might be indicated for symptomatic neonates Chronic care includes dietary protein restriction, selective amino acid restriction (leucine), and glycine and carnitine supplementation	Improved intellectual outcome if diagnosed and treated early If treated appropriately, most have normal development Recurrent metabolic episodes

(continued on next page)

Table 1
(continued)

Disorder	Defect	Clinical Features and Natural History	Treatment	Prognosis with Treatment
β-Ketothiolase deficiency	Mitochondrial acetoacetyl-CoA thiolase deficiency	Patients might present before newborn screening results are available Vomiting, lethargy, and coma, possibly death Abnormal odor Thrombocytopenia, leukopenia, anemia Possible basal ganglia damage Ketoacidosis Hyperammonemia	Dietary protein restriction Selected amino acid restriction (isoleucine) Avoidance of fasting Bicarbonate therapy and intravenous glucose in acute crises Carnitine supplementation	Highly variable clinical course Improved intellectual outcome if diagnosed and treated early If treated appropriately, some patients have normal development Recurrent metabolic episodes
2-Methylbutyric acidemia	2-Methylbutyryl-CoA dehydrogenase deficiency	Uncertain because number of cases is small	Dietary protein restriction Selected amino acid restriction	Uncertain
3-Methylcrotonyl-glycinuria	3-Methylbutyryrl-CoA-carboxylase deficiency	Neonatal form: Hypoglycemia and metabolic acidosis Maternal form: Transplacental transport of 3-methylcrotonyl glycine form generally asymptomatic mother to fetus	Neonatal form: Dietary protein restriction; selected amino acid restriction (leucine); carnitine and glycine supplementation Maternal form: Mother might benefit from carnitine supplementation if she has carnitine sufficiency	Neonatal form: Generally good Maternal form: Mother might benefit from carnitine supplementation
2-Methyl-3-hydroxybutyric academia	2-Methylbutyryl-CoA dehydrogenase deficiency	Uncertain because number of cases is small	Dietary protein restriction Selected amino acid restriction	Uncertain

Methylmalonic acidemia	Methylmalonyl-CoA mutase deficiency or vitamin B$_{12}$ (cobalamin) metabolism defect	Patients might present before newborn screening results are available Vomiting, lethargy and coma, possibly death Seizure and risk of basal ganglia infarcts Thrombocytopenia, leukopenia, anemia Ketoacidosis Hyperammonemia	Emergent treatment might be indicated for symptomatic neonates Chronic care includes dietary protein restriction (isoleucine, methionine, threonine, and valine), carnitine supplementation, antibiotic suppression of gut flora (metronidazole), liver and/or kidney transplantation might be considered Cobalamin defects require special treatment	Improved intellectual outcome if diagnosed and treated early If treated appropriately, most have normal development Recurrent metabolic episodes Renal failure often develops despite appropriate therapy
Propionic acidemia	Propionyl-CoA carboxylase deficiency	Patients might present before newborn screening results are available Vomiting, lethargy and coma, possibly death Seizures and risk of basal ganglia infarcts Thrombocytopenia, leukopenia, anemia Ketoacidosis Hyperammonemia	Emergency treatment might be indicated for symptomatic neonates Chronic care includes dietary protein restriction, selective amino acid restriction (isoleucine, methionine, threonine, and valine), carnitine supplementation, antibiotic suppression of gut flora (metronidazole and neomycin) Liver transplantation might be considered	Improved intellectual outcome if diagnosed and treated early If treated appropriately, most have normal development Recurrent metabolic episodes
Biotinidase deficiency	Biotinidase deficiency	Generally does not manifest in neonatal period Skin rash and alopecia, optic atrophy, hearing loss, seizures, and developmental delay Metabolic ketoacidosis	Biotin supplementation	Excellent if diagnosed and deficiency treated before irreversible neurologic damage occurs

(continued on next page)

Table 1
(continued)

Disorder	Defect	Clinical Features and Natural History	Treatment	Prognosis with Treatment
Multiple carboxylase	Holocarboxylase synthetase deficiency	Commonly manifests in neonatal period Lethargy leading to coma and possibly death Skin rash, impaired T-cell immunity, seizures, and developmental delay Metabolic ketoacidosis and hyperammonemia	Biotin supplementation	Most patients respond to some degree to biotin supplemental, but others show poor or no response to biotin supplementation and have significant residual neurologic impairment
Fatty acid oxidation				
Carnitine transporter deficiency	Carnitine transporter deficiency	Commonly manifests in neonatal period Cardiomyopathy, skeletal myopathy, and inability to tolerate prolonged fasting	Carnitine supplementation Avoid fasting Low-fat diet	Good response to treatment, often associated with reversal of cardiomyopathic changes
Carnitine/acylcarnitine translocase deficiency	Carnitine/acylcarnitine translocase deficiency	Commonly manifests in neonatal period Lethargy leading to coma, hepatomegaly Cardiomyopathy with ventricular arrhythmia, skeletal myopathy, and early death Hypoketotic hypoglycemia and hyperammonemia	Avoid fasting High-carbohydrate, low-fat diet Nightly cornstarch supplementation Carnitine supplementation	Severe neonatal cases generally have a poor outcome and early death Patients with later onset might respond to treatment, but they often succumb to chronic skeletal-muscle weakness or cardiac arrhythmias

CPT II deficiency	CPT II deficiency	Commonly manifests in neonatal period Coma, cardiomyopathy and ventricular arrhythmias, hepatic disease, and congenital malformation (brain and cystic renal disease) Hypoketotic hypoglycemia Late-onset forms (child or adult) characterized by weakness and exercise-induced rhabdomyolysis	Avoid fasting High-carbohydrate, low-fat diet supplemented with MCT oil Nightly cornstarch supplementation Carnitine supplementation	Severe neonatal cases generally have a poor outcome and early death Patients with late-onset disease generally do well
LCHAD deficiency	LCHAD deficiency	Sometimes manifests in neonatal period Cardiomyopathy, hypotonia, hepatic disease, and hypoketotic hypoglycemia Patients later develop rhabdomyolysis, peripheral neuropathy, and pigmentary retinopathy and are at risk for sudden death Heterozygous pregnant women are at risk for acute fatty liver of pregnancy if they are carrying a homozygous fetus	Avoid fasting High-carbohydrate, low-fat diet supplemented with MCT oil Nightly cornstarch supplementation Carnitine supplementation	Early diagnosis and treatment generally leads to improved outcome, but no change in risk of peripheral neuropathy and visual impairment

(continued on next page)

Table 1
(continued)

Disorder	Defect	Clinical Features and Natural History	Treatment	Prognosis with Treatment
MCAD deficiency	MCAD deficiency	Generally does not manifest in neonatal period Recurrent episodes of vomiting, coma, seizures, and possibly sudden death associated with prolonged period of fasting Cardiomyopathy not generally seen Hypoketotic or nonketotic hypoglycemia	Avoid fasting High-carbohydrate, low-fat diet (controversial) Nightly cornstarch supplementation Carnitine supplementation	Excellent intellectual and physical outcome generally seen if treatment is initiated before irreversible neurologic damage occurs
SCAD deficiency	SCAD deficiency	Generally does not manifest in neonatal period Highly variable presentation primarily associated with failure to thrive, developmental delay Hypoglycemia uncommon Many patients detected by newborn screening program have been asymptomatic	Avoid fasting High-carbohydrate, low-fat diet Nightly cornstarch supplementation Carnitine supplementation	Efficacy of treatment is unknown and metabolic acidosis

VLCAD deficiency	VLCAD deficiency	Commonly manifests in neonatal period Lethargy leading to coma, hepatomegaly, cardiomyopathy with ventricular arrhythmia, skeletal myopathy, and early death Hypoketotic hypoglycemia Later-onset forms (childhood or adult) characterized primarily by weakness and exercise-induced rhabdomyolysis	Avoid fasting High-carbohydrate, low-fat diet supplemented with MCT oil Nightly cornstarch supplementation Carnitine supplementation	Severe neonatal cases generally have poor outcome Patients with late-onset disease respond to treatment and do well
Galactosemia	Galactose-1-phosphate uridyltransferase deficiency	Early onset characterized by lethargy, poor feeding, jaundice, and possible sepsis (especially with *Escherichia coli*) Chronic problems include growth failure, cirrhosis, cataracts, seizures, mental retardation and (in females) ovarian failure	Strict dietary galactose restriction must be started immediately	Improved intellectual outcome and milder problems if diagnosed and treated early Ovarian failure develops despite appropriate therapy Recurrent metabolic episodes

This table does not provide a complete listing of all the inborn errors that have been identified or might be identified by tandem mass spectrometry. The last inborn error listed, galactosemia, is not detected currently using tandem mass spectrometry, but it is included in the table because it is part of current screening programs. All these disorders are characterized by considerable clinical variability and that treatment must be individualized for each patient.

Abbreviations: BH$_4$, tetrahydrobiopterin; CoA, coenzyme A; CPT II, carnitine palmitoyl-transferase type II; CSF, cerebrospinal fluid; ETF, electron transfer flavoprotein; HCC, hepatocellular carcinoma; LCHAD, long-chain-3 hydroxyacyl-CoA dehydrogenase; MCAD, medium-chain acyl-CoA dehydrogenase; MCT, medium chain triglycerides; NTBC, 2-(2-nitro-4-trifluoro-methylbenzoyl)-1,3-cyclohexanedione; SCAD, Short-chain acyl-CoA dehydrogenase; VLCAD, very-long-chain-acyl-CoA dehydrogenase.

Adapted from Zinn AB. Inborn errors of metabolism. In: Martin RJ, Fanaroff AA, Walsh MC, editors. Neonatal-perinatal medicine: diseases of the fetus and infant, vol. 2. 9th edition. St Louis (MO): Elsevier Mosby; 2011; with permission.

with 1 of the 29 core conditions on the screening panel. This means that 1 in 4000 live births are detected. The top 5 diagnosed conditions are:

- Hearing loss,
- Primary congenital hypothyroidism,
- Cystic fibrosis,
- Sickle cell disease, and
- Medium-chain acyl-coenzyme A dehydrogenase deficiency.

ACUTE METABOLIC DECOMPENSATION WITH INBORN ERRORS OF METABOLISM

Metabolic crises with inborn errors of metabolism occur when there is an accumulation of the toxic metabolites associated with the newborn error. Certain events, like infection, need for surgery, trauma, or even just being born, are triggers that cause increased catabolism or increase consumption of a food component (eg, protein intake when switching from human milk to cow milk) can all act as triggers. The acute metabolic deterioration typically follows a period of well-being. The period of being symptom free can range from as little as hours to months and even years. Acute metabolic decompensation requires prompt recognition and intervention to prevent death or a poor outcome. The acute clinical presentation of a multisystem decompensation strongly suggests that this may be associated with an inborn error of metabolism. The initial clinical picture may include[15]:

- Vomiting and anorexia,
- Lethargy that can progress to coma,
- Seizures, particularly intractable,
- Rapid deep breathing that can progress to apnea, and
- Hypothermia (related to illness, not specific to a particular metabolic pathway).

Of 53 patients who presented to the emergency department and then were subsequently diagnosed as having an inborn error of metabolism, 85% demonstrated neurologic symptoms and 58% with neurologic plus gastrointestinal signs.[16] Neurologic symptoms included hypotonia, lethargy, coma, seizures, and evidence of psychomotor delay. The gastrointestinal symptoms were vomiting, and evidence of liver disease.

METABOLIC ACIDOSIS

Acidosis is a frequent problem in critically ill neonates. Acid–base disorders may occur in most types of inborn errors of metabolism, with the exception of lysosomal storage diseases and peroxisomal disorders. Metabolic acidosis (low serum bicarbonate and low arterial pH) is usually present in organic acidemias. It may also be present with amino acid disorders, disorders of pyruvate metabolism, mitochondrial disorders, and disorders of carbohydrate metabolism.[17,18]

The metabolic acidosis in these disorders is usually accompanied by an increased anion gap. This gap results from the presence of abnormal metabolites that are unable to be metabolized, such as ketoacids, lactic acid, or the organic acid. Abnormal oxidative metabolism causes lactic acidosis in the mitochondrial disorders, glycogen storage disorders, and gluconeogenesis disorders.

A respiratory alkalosis (low arterial partial pressure of carbon dioxide Pco_2 and low arterial pH) is suggestive of hyperammonemia, which is a characteristic of the urea cycle disorders.[19] The respiratory alkalosis is caused by hyperpnea, which is induced by hyperammonemia. Respiratory alkalosis is also seen with Leigh syndrome (mitochondrial disorder) and other disorders associated with hyperammonemia. Hyperammonemia is characteristic of the urea acid cycle defects and organic acidemias (eg, propionic and methylmalonic acidemias).[20] There are other diseases that have hyperammonemia, including other amino acid disorders such as lysinuric protein intolerance and with the fatty acid oxidation defects. Lesser elevations of ammonia are less frequent in mitochondrial disorders or with hepatic dysfunction alone.

The highest levels of ammonia are with the urea cycle disorders and are only moderately elevated or even normal with organic acidemias. It should be noted that ammonia levels can even be normal in patients with the urea cycle disorders if they are not ill at the time of testing and other times be greater than 1000 μmol/L in organic acidemias. Finally, the ammonia level is usually normal in disorders of carbohydrate metabolism, lysosomal storage disorders, or peroxisomal disorders.[17]

Hypoglycemia is seen with disorders including ketogenesis, fatty acid oxidation (medium chain acyl-coenzyme A dehydrogenase deficiency), glycogen storage diseases, and disorders of gluconeogenesis and hereditary fructose intolerance. Hypoglycemia may also be seen with amino acid disorders, organic acidemias, and mitochondrial defects. Persistent hypoglycemic syndromes and hyperinsulinemc disorders are discussed in the section on Postnatal Glucose Homeostasis.

The detection of inborn errors of metabolism requires a high index of suspicion and "red flags" include patients who present with hypoglycemia and hyperammonemia. Those patients with extreme presentations should be evaluated for other conditions that are life threatening, such as sepsis or cardiac disease.

It is imperative to do testing when symptoms are most pronounced in such situations. Laboratory values may become normal when the same patient is well. Blood, urine, and cerebrospinal fluid in those patients who have persistent seizures, dystonia, or focal neurologic signs should be obtained at the time of initial presentation with symptoms. A list of basic tests that are routinely available can be obtained before more of the specialized metabolic investigations. These include the following in a patient with a suspected inborn error of metabolism[15]:

- Complete blood count: Helps to denote errors in any of the cell lines or provide clues about sepsis, which itself can be the reason for the crisis related to the metabolic disorder
- Arterial blood gas: Allows determination of acid–base problems. Looking for an increased anion gap suggesting organic acidemias or respiratory alkalosis seen with urea cycle disorders.
- Blood glucose: Hypoglycemia with ketogenesis associated with fatty acid oxidation abnormalities, or glycogen storage diseases and problems with carbohydrate metabolism.
- Ammonia: This sample must be obtained from an artery or vein without the aid of a tourniquet. It must be placed on ice for transport to the laboratory. It must also be analyzed immediately. Any level greater than 100 μmol/L should be repeated for confirmation immediately. As mentioned, these elevated levels may be diagnostic for urea cycle disorders and some of the organic acidemias. Levels greater than 120 μmol/L are neurotoxic for the newborn and those greater than 80 μmol/L are dangerous for older infants and children. These must be treated as a metabolic emergency.
- Electrolytes, blood urea nitrogen, and creatinine: Allows calculation of the anion gap. Metabolic acidosis with an increased anion gap is seen with organic acidemias.

- Uric acid: High in patients with glycogen storage diseases. It is decreased in patients with defects in purine metabolism, but increased in patients with Lesch–Nyhan disease.
- Examination of the urine: Including color, odor, dipstick, and presence of ketones are also helpful.

Optimal outcomes for children with inborn errors of metabolism depend on recognition of the signs and symptoms of these metabolic disorders. Prompt evaluation and referral to a center familiar with the evaluation of these disorders is important.[21] Delay in diagnosis may result in acute metabolic decompensation, progressive neurologic injury, or death.

POSTNATAL GLUCOSE HOMEOSTASIS

The definition of clinically significant hypoglycemia remains among of the most confused and contentious issues in neonatal medicine. Untoward long-term outcomes in infants with 1 or 2 low blood glucose levels have become grounds for litigation and for alleged malpractice, even though the causative relationship between the 2 is tenuous at best.[22] At birth, the normal newborn infant's plasma glucose concentration falls below levels that were prevalent in fetal life. This decrease is part of the normal transition to an extrauterine existence through a series of triggers and events that activate endocrine and metabolic responses associated with successful adaptation. When this adaptation fails, perhaps secondary to immaturity or illness, there may be a limitation of substrate supply, which may disturb cerebral function and potentially result in neurologic injury. A low plasma glucose may be indicative of this process, but is not diagnostic per se. These are the questions that remain without answers:

- What is meant by too low?
- How low is too low?
- At what glucose level does hypoglycemia result in irreversible changes in brain structure of function?

In 2009, a workshop with world experts in glucose metabolism and clinicians with expertise in management of hypoglycemia in newborns was convened by the Eunice Shriver National Institute of Child Health and Human Development and led to a publication of the proceedings in the *Journal of Pediatrics*.[23] The experts focused on gaps in knowledge and suggested areas of research needed for understanding and treating hypoglycemia. Conclusions from the workshop included the following:

- There is no evidence-based study to identify any specific plasma glucose concentration (or range of glucose values) to define pathologic hypoglycemia.
- Monitoring for and prevention and treatment of neonatal hypoglycemia remain largely empirical.
- At present, data are insufficient to produce definitive guidelines.

Maintenance of glucose homeostasis by initiation of glucose production is among the most critical transitional physiologic events that takes place for a fetus to adapt to extrauterine life. It is not usual for this transition to run into difficulties and result in alterations in glucose homeostasis and therefore an infant with a low plasma glucose level.[23]

The fetus depends on the maternal supply of glucose transplacentally as well as amino acids, free fatty acids, ketones, and glycerol for its energy supply from the placenta. For most of gestation, the lower limit of fetal glucose concentration is approximately 54 mg/dL (3 mmol/L). The fetus does not produce glucose under normal conditions.

The ratio of insulin to glucagon in the fetal circulation plays a critical role in regulating the balance between glucose consumption and energy storage. A high ratio results in activation of glycogen synthesis and a suppression of glycogenolysis through hepatic regulatory enzyme pathways (**Fig. 1**).[24] This system means that fetal glycogen synthesis and storage is promoted and glycogenolysis is minimized. This development is accompanied by a rapid increase in hepatic glycogen during the last 30% of gestation. There is also an increase in cortisol and circulating insulin. Finally, the high ratio of insulin to glucagon in the fetus suppresses lipolysis, which allows for energy to be stored subcutaneously. The subcutaneous and hepatic reservoir establishes a ready substrate supply for the fetus to transition metabolically and establish postnatal glucose homeostasis (see **Fig. 1**).

At birth, the dependence of the fetus on the maternal supply of glucose necessitates significant changes in regulation of glucose metabolism after the abrupt cessation of umbilical glucose delivery (**Fig. 2**).[24] A number of changes allow the newborn to maintain glucose homeostasis. These alterations include a surge in catecholamines, which stimulates glucagon secretion and reverses the insulin/glucagon ratio in favor of glucagon.

When glycogen synthase is inactivated and glycogen phosphorylase is activated, this leads to stimulation of glycogenolysis and inhibition of glycogen synthesis.[25] This shift is the exact opposite of the fetal environment. The release of glucose from the glycogen stores provides a rapidly and readily available source of glucose for the neonate for the first few hours of life. The estimates include that hepatic glycogen stores for the term infant provide enough glucose for the first 10 hours of life. Other mechanisms also come into play to maintain postnatal glucose homeostasis (see **Fig. 2**).

The next important pathway is the initiation of gluconeogenesis for maintaining postnatal glucose homeostasis. The glucagon predominance after delivery includes

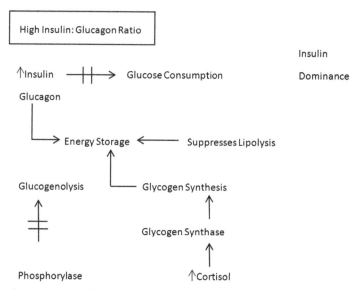

Fig. 1. Fetal maintenance of anabolic state promoting energy storage.

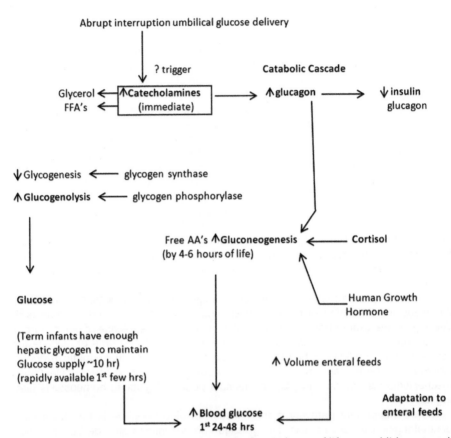

Fig. 2. Adaptations around delivery and over the first 24 hours of life to establish postnatal glucose homeostasis. AA, amino acid; FFA, free fatty acids.

enzymes required for gluconeogenesis.[25] Substrates available for gluconeogenesis that are associated with the surge in catecholamines at delivery include free fatty acids, glycerol, and amino acids from the circulation. By 4 to 6 hours of age, the term infant is capable of significant gluconeogenesis.

Therefore, until an exogenous supply of glucose is provided either enterally or intravenously, hepatic glucose production is the most significant source of glucose to meet the needs of postnatal glucose homeostasis. To maintain normal levels of hepatic glucose production, the infant must have the following:

- Adequate sources of glycogen and gluconeogenic precursors (fatty acids, glycerol, amino acids, and lactate);
- Concentrations of the hepatic enzymes necessary for glycogenolysis and gluconeogenesis; and
- A normally functioning endocrine system (counterregulatory hormones, human growth hormone, and cortisol).

If any of these systems are not in place, then there is a disruption of glucose homeostasis and increases the chances that a low plasma glucose will result. As for preterm infants, a long thought premise that they had lower levels of glucose the first days of life than term infants and were suited in some way to tolerate these lower levels is not true. This misconception came from observations of lower levels in these infants because they were commonly starved the first few days of life. These low levels are no longer observed in these infants because of early intravenous nutrition and/or enteral feedings. In fact, these preterm infants have a significantly greater decrease in glucose than term infants do the first hours of life. Also they have limited gluconeogenic ability because of limitations in there enzymatic pathways, which means that they are less able to adapt to the cessation of intrauterine nutrition.

DEFINITION OF HYPOGLYCEMIA

Around the time of birth, there is a transient increase in fetal glucose concentrations from glycogenolysis and gluconeogenesis. This increase is followed by a rapid decrease in neonatal glucose concentrations after birth and loss of the placenta to a nadir at 1 to 2 hours of age and then a low an increase to levels that are similar to late gestation fetal glucose levels (about two-thirds of normal values) by 2 to 4 hours of age. Neonatal glucose values remain less than adult levels until around 3 to 4 days of age. They do trend up slowly after the nadir.

A consistent definition of hypoglycemia does not exist for these first 2 days of life. When the first neonates were recognized as having significant hypoglycemia in the mid 1950s, the infants had striking clinical manifestations, often seizures, and the blood sugar values were consistently below 20 to 25 mg/dL (1.1–1.4 mm/L). The abnormal signs cleared quickly after increasing the blood glucose concentration to (>40 mg/dL [2.2 mmol/L]). Now, some 60 years later, after hypoglycemia was first described and "40" became a classic standard for defining hypoglycemia, our understanding of the metabolic disturbances and genetic disorders underlying alterations in postnatal glucose homeostasis has increased dramatically.[21,23,26] However, this growth of knowledge, if anything, has led us further from what we need to know about the blood glucose concentrations in the newborn: "How low is too low?"

At birth, the blood glucose concentration is about 70% of the maternal level. It falls rapidly to the nadir by 1 hour or so to as low as 25 to 30 mg/dL (1.8 mmol/L). These low levels are common in healthy neonates and are seen in all mammalian newborns. These levels are transient and the infants are asymptomatic. This decrease is considered to be part of the normal adaptation for postnatal life that helps to establish postnatal glucose homeostasis.[27–29] "Why" does this low blood glucose after birth happen in all mammals? Are there advantages to having a lower blood glucose concentration compared with adults for the first few days of life? There are some speculations[30]:

The decrease in glucose concentrations right after birth seem to be essential to stimulate physiologic processes that are required for postnatal survival, including promoting glucose production through gluconeogenesis.

The decrease in glucose concentration may stimulate appetite and help adapt to fast–feed cycles.

The decrease in glucose may enhance oxidative fat metabolism.

Persistently lower neonatal glucose concentrations might be the result of mechanisms that were vital for the fetus to allow maternal-to-fetal glucose transport and cannot be quickly reversed after birth.

There is little consensus regarding the significance of transient and asymptomatic low glucose concentrations. Most data suggest that adverse outcomes do not occur with such levels in asymptomatic infants.[30] However, transient asymptomatic low glucose concentrations may herald metabolic disorders that can cause serious neurologic injury. Therefore, vigilance to look for further low glucose levels is warranted and there must be careful scrutiny for the development of clinical signs of serious hypoglycemia and the clinician must be certain these infants with persistently low glucose levels not go home from the newborn nursery without proving that they can maintain glucose levels of greater than 65 to 70 mg/dL through several normal fast–feed cycles after 48 to 72 hours of life.[30]

Therefore, we have no consensus for a specific level or range of values that specifically define hypoglycemia or when and how much treatment should be provided. More important, a number of methods have attempted to identify the threshold blood glucose concentration at which there is substantial likelihood of functional impairment, particularly of the brain. These methods can be categorized as:

- Epidemiologic,
- Clinical,
- Metabolic–endocrinologic,
- Neurophysiologic, and
- Neurodevelopmental

The epidemiologic approach defines blood glucose concentrations in cohorts of healthy infants and uses either the mean or empirically derived cut-off such as less than 2 standard deviations below the mean. Any single value is unlikely to represent a threshold of abnormality, because the data represent a continuum from normal.[22,31] Most important is that a statistical abnormality does not imply a biologic impairment. This method reveals that the vast majority have blood glucose concentrations of greater than 40 mg/dL during the first 48 hours of life with actual mean values approximating 54 mg/dL (3.0 mmol/L) in healthy newborns.[22,23,31]

The clinical approach is based on the importance of glucose levels when signs of hypoglycemia manifest. However, jitteriness is just as likely among normoglycemic infants and those with a variety of other conditions. Also, equally low blood glucose levels are found in infants with no signs ("asymptomatic hypoglycemia"). Therefore, the presence of absence of signs and symptoms cannot be used to discriminate between normal and abnormal blood glucose levels.

The neurophysiologic approach has attempted to measure neurophysiologic changes in relation to various blood glucose concentrations. Studies used somatosensory evoked potentials. The studies have small numbers and have failed to show effects of hypoglycemia on evoked responses. Changes in cerebral blood flow with very low blood glucose levels have been studied in premature infants. However, the practicality of this technology and application remains unclear.

Two of the methods "competing" for the one that is best suited to be followed for screening and management of postnatal glucose homeostasis are the metabolic/endocrinologic, which analyzes data on transitional neonatal hypoglycemia with the goal of understanding the mechanisms underlying this transitional hypoglycemia. The second method is the neurodevelopmental approach, which has been used by the United Kingdom, Canada, and the United States to define significant hypoglycemia and produce algorithms for screening and management.[24]

The endocrine-based mechanism, which leads to critical levels of 55 to 65 mg/dL are based on observations that the low glucose concentrations in the first 48 hours are accompanied by evidence of hyperinsulinism, suppressed plasma levels of ketones (β-hydroxybutyrate and acetoacetate) and inappropriately large glycemic responses to glucagon or epinephrine.[32–34] The endocrinologists use reports providing information about fasting fuel and hormone responses to identify the common underlying mechanism of hypoglycemia. The endocrine approach focuses on mean levels of glucose being most representative of the group of normal newborns. The evaluation in this fashion suggests that the transitional neonatal hypoglycemia most closely resembles a known genetic form of congenital hyperinsulinism, which causes a lowering of the plasma glucose threshold for suppression of pancreatic insulin secretion.[32,33] This transitional neonatal hypoglycemia in normal newborns using this approach is a hypoketotic hypoglycemia.

Using mean values instead of nadir values this explanation describes the nadir value as 55 to 60 mg/dL, not 25 to 30 mg/dL at the 5th percentile at 1 to 2 hours of age. This value is followed by a steady increase over the first few days of life to return to the range of 70 to 100 mg/dL (3.0–5.6 mmol/L), which is normal for infants, children, and adults.[34] Therefore, the metabolic and endocrine profile of transitional hypoglycemia indicates that this is a form of physiologic hyperinsulinemic hypoglycemia in which the glucose set point for suppression of insulin secretion is set at 55 to 65 mg/dL (2.8–3.6 mmol/L). Using this method, endocrinologists conclude that this range is similar to the glucose thresholds for neuroendocrine responses to hypoglycemia found in adults and older children, and implies that this threshold for activating neuroendocrine defenses against hypoglycemia in newborns may be similar to the threshold in older ages.[35] Finally, studies in adults that are important in developing this strategy that the threshold is in the range of 55 to 65 mg/dL is that older children and adults develop neuroglycopenia (impaired brain function) at around 50 mg/dL (2.8 mmol/L).[35-37]

The neurodevelopmental approach was established by a very influential article in 1988 that reported an observational study among 543 infants weighing less than 1850 g enrolled in a nutritional study that reported seriously impaired motor and cognitive development at 18 months in those with recurrent, asymptomatic hypoglycemia (plasma glucose level <45 mg/dL [2.5 mmol/L] on more than 3 days).[38] This "threshold" of 47 mg/dL as alluded to in the paper profoundly influenced the neonatal care of the preterm infant across the developed world ever since. It was not long before clinicians were extrapolating from this single observational study on preterm infants and assuming that the healthy term infant could be equally at risk from similar blood glucose levels, even when the infant seemed normal on clinical examination.[39] Recently, and also from England, another study was initiated looking at all children born at less than 32 weeks in the north of England in 1990 and 1991 and had laboratory blood glucose levels measured daily for the first 10 days of life.[40] Those who survived to 2 years of age and had a blood glucose level of less than 45 mg/dL on more than 3 days were assessed at age 2. No differences in developmental progress or physical disability were detected versus hypoglycemia-free controls adjusting for appropriate confounders.[40]

The children were seen again at 15 years of age and 81% of the original children were studied. Findings in the 2 groups were nearly identical (mean full-scale IQ 80.7 versus 81.2). Nearly identical outcomes were also found for behavioral and emotional status and their adaptation to daily living.[40] The authors of this trial agree with the late Marvin Cornblath, who believed that the "adaptive fluctuations occurring the first days of life after birth...should not be designated as hypoglycemia with its connotation of disease.[41]

The English study, therefore, found no evidence to support the belief that recurrent low blood glucose levels (<45 mg/dL) in the first 10 days of life usually pose a hazard to preterm infants.[40] This study does not imply that low blood glucose levels cannot be damaging in the preterm infant, even in the absence of overt and recognizable signs. However, the data suggest that the danger threshold must be lower than many had come to think it was. Indeed and in fact, these data and the reviews by Cornblath were instrumental in the Screening and Management of Postnatal Glucose

Homeostasis that was published in *Pediatrics* in 2011 from the Committee on Fetus and Newborn of the AAP.[42]

As with normal infants with transient asymptomatic low glucose concentrations, there is no evidence that improved outcome follows identification and treatment of low glucose levels in infants of diabetic mothers, late preterm, small for gestational age, and large for gestational age screened infants.[29] The AAP recognized that screening and management of asymptomatic low glucose levels in these populations is a "controversial issue for which evidence is lacking but guidance is needed."[42] This led to the publication of the updated guidelines in 2011. The guideline recognized the normal 1- to 2-hour nadir in glucose concentration and proposed operational thresholds for action based on age (**Fig. 3**).[42]

The AAP guideline stresses the need to measure blood glucose levels as soon as possible (minutes not hours) in any infant who manifests clinical signs consistent with a low blood glucose concentration (ie, the symptomatic infant). The decision was to feed within 1 hour of birth and to screen after this feed. Making a decision to act on an early blood glucose concentration—in the first hour of life in an asymptomatic infant—did not seem appropriate, because "normal" cannot be distinguished from abnormal and no data suggested any untoward outcome associated with these lower values reached at the nadir in an asymptomatic infant.[31] Fortunately, even in the absence of any enteral nutrition intake, blood glucose concentrations increase by

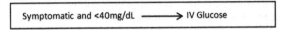

Symptomatic and <40mg/dL ⟶ IV Glucose

ASYMPTOMATIC

Birth tours of age 4 hours of age		4 to 24 hours of age	
INITIAL FEED WITHIN 1 Hour Screen glucose 30 minutes after 1st feed		Continue feeds q2-3 hours Screen glucose prior to each feed	
Initial screen <25 mg/dL		screen <35 mg/dL	
Feed and check in 1 hour		Feed and check in 1 hour	
<25 mg/dL	25-40 mg/dL	<35 mg/dL	35-45 mg/dL
IV Glucose[a]	Refeed/IV Glucose[a] as needed	IV Glucose[a]	Refeed/IV Glucose[a] as needed

Target Glucose screen ≥45 mg/dL prior to routine feeds

[a]Glucose dose = 200mg/dL (dextrose 10% at 2mL/kg) and/or IV infusion at 5 to 8 mg/kg/min (80-100 mL/kg/d) to achieve plasma glucose 40-50 mg/dL.

Symptoms of hypoglycemia include: irritability, tremors, jitteriness, exaggerated Moro reflex, high-pitched cry, seizures, lethargy, floppiness, cyanosis, apnea, poor feeding.

Fig. 3. Screening and management of postnatal glucose homeostasis from the American Academy of Pediatrics committee of fetus and newborn.

3 hours of age. Even in the infant at risk for hypoglycemia, blood glucose measurement is best avoided during the first 2 hours after birth.[31] Because the purpose of blood glucose monitoring is to identify the lowest blood glucose level, it makes sense to measure a value immediately before the next feeding.[24] Blood glucose concentrations show a cyclic response to an enteral feed, reaching a peak by about 1 hour after the feed, and the nadir just before the next feed is due.

The plasma glucose concentration at which intervention is indicated needs to be tailored to the clinical situation and the particular characteristics of the infant. The AAP clinical report on postnatal glucose homeostasis applies only to the first 24 hours after birth and should not be used beyond this period, and certainly not after 48 hours. It considers symptoms, mode of feeding, risk factors, and hours of feeding in a pragmatic approach for these infants (see **Fig. 3**).[42] Operational thresholds are an indication for action but not diagnostic for a disease. The 2 ranges in the guideline—25 to 35 mg/dL for the first 4 hours and 35 to 45 mg/dL for the next 20 hours—are the operational thresholds the clinician can use to make decisions about management suggested in the guideline (see **Fig. 3**).[42] One uses the available clinical and experimental data for these infants using conservative estimates for designating the lower level of normoglycemia. The belief is that the neonate can safely tolerate these levels at specific ages and under established conditions.[31] Values below the operational threshold level are an indication to increase the plasma glucose levels and do not imply neuroglycopenia or neurologic injury.[31]

It is not possible to define a plasma glucose level that requires intervention in every newborn infant because there is uncertainty regarding the level and duration of hypoglycemia that causes damage, and little is known of the vulnerability of the brain at various gestational ages for such injury.[30,31] Therefore, as reiterated in the AAP statement "significant hypoglycemia is not and can never be defined by a single number that can be applied universally to every individual patient. Rather it is characterized by a value(s) that is unique to each individual and varies with their state of physiologic maturity and the influence of pathology."[42] Treatment should be guided by clinical assessment and not by glucose concentration alone.[31]

A recent editorial addressing the continued controversy that is neonatal hypoglycemia states that, "what is clear is that the higher one's glucose threshold and the more often one tests for it, the more often asymptomatic patients with low glucose concentrations will be identified."[29] What clinicians do with this information depends on how they view any particular glucose concentration in an asymptomatic infant.[29] So, 50 years after Cornblath first proposed 40 mg/dL for defining hypoglycemia, the "questions remain the same."[43]

REFERENCES

1. Centers for Disease Control and Prevention (CDC). CDC grand rounds; newborn screening and improved outcomes. MMWR Morb Mortal Wkly Rep 2012;61(21): 390–3.
2. Zinn AB. Inborn errors of metabolism. In: Martin RJ, Fanaroff AA, Welsh MC, editors. Chapter 50 in neonatal-perinatal medicine disease of the fetus and infant, vol. 2, 9th edition. St Louis (MO): Elsevier Mosby; 2011.
3. Dussault JH, Laberge C. Thyroxine (T4) determination by radioimmunological method in dried blood eluate: new diagnostic method of neonatal hypothyroidism? Union Med Can 1973;102:2063 [in French].
4. Githens JH, Lane PA, McCurdy RS, et al. Newborn screening for hemoglobinopathies in Colorado. The first 10 years. Am J Dis Child 1990;144:466.

5. Shafer FE, Lorey F, Cunningham GC, et al. Newborn screening for sickle cell disease: 4 years of experience from California's newborn screening program. J Pediatr Hematol Oncol 1996;18:36.
6. Chace DH, DiPerna JC, Naylor EW. Laboratory integration and utilization of tandem mass spectrometry in neonatal screening: a model for clinical mass spectrometry in the next millennium. Acta Paediatr Suppl 1999;88:45.
7. Naylor EW, Cace DH. Automated tandem mass spectrometry for mass newborn screening for disorders in fatty acid, organic acid and amino acid metabolism. J Child Neurol 1999;14(Suppl 1):S4.
8. Bartlett K, Eaton SJ, Pourfarzam M. New developments in neonatal screening. Arch Dis Child Fetal Neonatal Ed 1997;77:F151.
9. Meikle PJ, Ranieri E, Simonsen H, et al. Newborn screening for lysosomal storage disorders: clinical evaluation of a two-tier strategy. Pediatrics 2004;114:909.
10. Scott CR, Elliot S, Buroker N, et al. Identification of infants at risk for developing Fabry, Pompe, or mucopolysaccharidosis-I from newborn blood spots by tandem mass spectrometry. J Pediatr 2013;163:498.
11. Gregg RG, Simantel A, Farrell PM, et al. Newborn screening for cystic fibrosis in Wisconsin: comparison of biochemical and molecular methods. Pediatrics 1997; 99:819.
12. Chan K, Puck JM. Development of population-based newborn screening for severe combined immunodeficiency. J Allergy Clin Immunol 2005;115:391.
13. Evans MI, Krivchenia EL. Principles of screening. Clin Perinatol 2001;28:273.
14. Khoury MJ, McCabe LL, McCabe ER. Population screening in the age of genomic medicine. N Engl J Med 2003;348:50.
15. Sutton VR. Up to date. Philadelphia: Wolters Kluwer; 2014. p. 1–27.
16. Calvo M, Artuch R, Macia E, et al. Diagnostic approach to inborn errors of metabolism in an emergency unit. Pediatr Emerg Care 2000;16:405.
17. Wappner RS. Biochemical diagnosis of genetic diseases. Pediatr Ann 1993; 22:282.
18. Gibson K, Halliday JL, Kirby DM, et al. Mitochondrial oxidative phosphorylation disorders presenting in neonates: clinical manifestations and enzymatic and molecular diagnosis. Pediatrics 2008;122:1003.
19. Maestri NE, Clissold D, Brusilow SW. Neonatal onset ornithine trandcarbamylase defiency: a retrospective analysis. J Pediatr 1999;134:268.
20. Broomfield A, Grunewald S. How to use serum ammonia. Arch Dis Child Educ Pract Ed 2012;97:72.
21. Champion MP. An approach to the diagnosis of inherited metabolic disease. Arch Dis Child Educ Pract Ed 2010;95:40.
22. Cornblath M, Ichord R. Hypoglycemia in the neonate. Semin Perinatol 2000;24(2): 136–49.
23. Hay W, Raju TN, Higgins RD, et al. Knowledge gaps and research needs for understanding and treating neonatal hypoglycemia: workshop report from Eunice Kennedy Shriver National Institute of Child Health and Human Development. J Pediatr 2009;155(5):612–7.
24. Adamkin DH. Glucose metabolism. In: Polin RA, Yoder MC, editors. Workbook in neonatology. Philadelphia: Elsevier; 2014.
25. McGowan JE. Neonatal hypoglycemia. Pediatr Rev 1988;20(7):6–15.
26. Heck LJ, Erenberg A. Serum glucose levels in term neonates during the first 48 hours of life. J Pediatr 1987;110:119–22.
27. Srinvasan G, Pildes RS, Cattamanchi G. Plasma glucose values in normal neonates: a new look. J Pediatr 1986;109:114–7.

28. Adamkin DH. Update on neonatal hypoglycemia. Arch Perinat Med 2005;11(3): 13–5.
29. Rozance P, Hay NW. Neonatal hypoglycemia answers but more questions. J Pediatr 2012;161(5):775–6.
30. Boluyt N, van KA, Offringa M. Neurodevelopment after neonatal hypoglycemia: a systematic review and design of an optimal future study. Pediatrics 2006;117: 2231–43.
31. Cornblath M, Hawdon JM, Williams AF, et al. Controversies regarding definition of neonatal hypoglycemia: suggested operational thresholds. Pediatrics 2000; 105(5):1141–5.
32. Stanley CA, Baker L. Hyperinsulinism in infants and children: diagnosis and therapy. Adv Pediatr 1976;23:315–55.
33. Glaser B, Kesavan P, Heyman M, et al. Familial hyperinsulinism caused by an activating glucokinase mutation. N Engl J Med 1998;338(4):226–30.
34. Hoe FM, Thornton PS, Wanner LA, et al. Clinical features and insulin hyperinsulinism. J Pediatr 2006;148(2):207–12.
35. Cryer PE. Hypoglycemia in diabetes: pathophysiology, prevalence, and prevention. Alexandria (VA): American Diabetes Association; 2009.
36. Amiel SA, Simonson DC, Sherwin RS, et al. Exaggerated epinephrine responses to hypoglycemia in normal and insulin-dependent diabetic children. J Pediatr 1987;110(6):832–7.
37. Jones TW, Boulware SD, Kraemer DT, et al. Independent effects of youth Diabetes and poor diabetes control on responses to hypoglycemia in children. Diabetes 1991;40(3):358–63.
38. Lucas A, Morley R, Cole TJ. Adverse neurodevelopmental outcome of moderate neonatal hypoglycemia. Br Med J 1988;297:1304–8.
39. Cornblath M, Schwartz R. Outcome of neonatal hypoglycemia in infancy: the need for a rational definition. A Ciba Foundation discussion meeting. Pediatrics 1990;85(5):834–7.
40. Tin W, Bruuskill G, Kelly T, et al. 15 year follow-up of recurrent "hypoglycemia" in preterm infant. Pediatrics 2012;130(6):e1497–503.
41. Cornblath M. Reminiscence of a 50-year adventure. Neoreviews 2006;90(2): 74–86.
42. Adamkin DH, Committee on Fetus and Newborn. Clinical report-postnatal glucose homeostasis in late-preterm and term infants. Pediatrics 2011;127:575.
43. Cornblath M, Odell GB, Levin EY. Symptomatic neonatal hypoglycemia associated with toxemia of pregnancy. J Pediatr 1959;55:545–62.

Common Genetic and Epigenetic Syndromes

 CrossMark

Darius J. Adams, MD[a,b],*, David A. Clark, MD[b]

KEYWORDS

- Syndrome • Genetic • Microdeletion • Epigenetic • Imprinting

KEY POINTS

- Cytogenetic anomalies should be considered in individuals with multiple congenital anomalies.
- DNA methylation analysis is the most sensitive initial test in evaluating for Prader-Willi and Angelman syndromes.
- The timely identification of cytogenetic anomalies allows for prompt initiation of early intervention services to maximize the potential of every individual as they grow older.
- Although many of these conditions are rare, keeping them in mind can have a profound impact on the clinical course of affected individuals.

Newborns with large genomic anomalies tend to have a pattern of malformations. If an isolated anomaly is noted, it is less likely a large genomic anomaly but could still be related to single gene mutations. There are exceptions as in the case of Turner syndrome; the only presenting sign at birth in some cases is lymphedema. The common large-scale chromosomal and genomic anomalies are reviewed.

LARGE-SCALE GENOMIC ANOMALIES
Down Syndrome

Down syndrome is one of the most common large-scale genomic anomalies with a prevalence of approximately 1 in 700 births.[1–5] Infants born with Down syndrome are typically hypotonic and consequently have feeding difficulties. Cardiac anomalies are present in approximately 40% of individuals with Down syndrome. Most commonly, an atrioventricular canal or endocardial cushion defect is noted; however, isolated ventricular septal defects, auricular septal defect, and aberrant subclavian arteries have also been noted less frequently. Additional findings include the following:

- Low-set ears
- Up-slanting palpebral fissures

Disclosure statement: Speakers Bureau/grants from BioMarin.
[a] Atlantic Health System, Morristown, NJ, USA; [b] Albany Medical Center, Albany, NY, USA
* Corresponding author. 100 Madison Avenue, Morristown, NJ 07690.
E-mail address: Darius.adams@atlantichealth.org

- Brushfield spots
- Flat facial profile
- Short neck
- Hypotonia/poor Moro reflex
- Mental retardation (**Figs. 1–4**)

Early intervention services can be beneficial and can help maximize potential. An increased risk of leukemia and Alzheimer disease has been noted in older individuals.

Trisomy 13 (Patau Syndrome)

Trisomy 13 has a prevalence of approximately 1 in 7000 births.[6] This condition can present on the holoprosencephaly spectrum, with some individuals having severe midline anomalies of the brain and other structures including a single nostril and pronounced hypotelorism (closely set eyes). Additional findings are as follows (**Figs. 5** and **6**):

- Cutis aplasia (usually of posterior scalp)
- Polydactyly
- Microphthalmia, coloboma of iris
- Cleft lip and/or palate
- Abnormal ears that are low set
- Cardiac anomalies
- Severe neurologic involvement

Life span is typically limited to weeks or months; however, there have been cases that have been described with individuals living years. Individuals with mosaicism can have milder manifestations and live much longer.

Trisomy 18 (Edwards Syndrome)

Trisomy 18 has a prevalence of approximately 1 in 4500 births.[6] Individuals with this syndrome have a characteristic clenched hand appearance with a tendency for overlapping of the index finger over the third digit and the fifth finger over the fourth digit. Additional findings include the following:

- Short sternum
- Low-set malformed ears
- Micrognathia
- Clenched hands with overlapping fingers (**Fig. 7**)

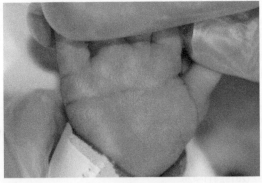

Fig. 1. Single transverse palmar crease noted in trisomy 21. (*Courtesy of* D. Clark, MD, Albany, NY.)

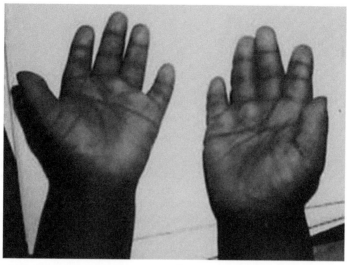

Fig. 2. Brachydactyly with single transverse palmar creases in Down syndrome.

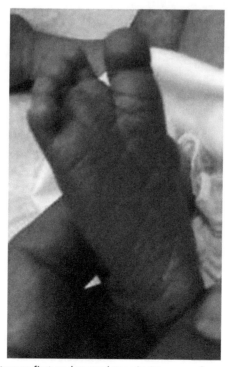

Fig. 3. Wide space between first and second toes in Down syndrome.

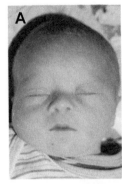
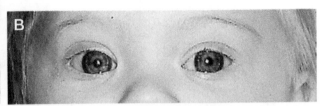

Fig. 4. (*A*). Typical facial features in Down syndrome with bilateral epicanthal folds, small mouth and depressed nasal root. (*B*). Brushfield spots, seen most often in individuals with lighter eye pigment in Down syndrome. ([*A*] *Courtesy of* D. Clark, MD, Albany, NY.)

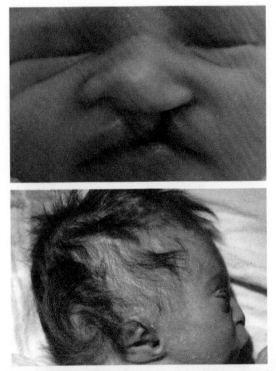

Fig. 5. Cleft lip/palate in trisomy 13 (*top*) and low-set ears in trisomy 13 (*bottom*). (*Courtesy of* D. Clark, MD, Albany, NY.)

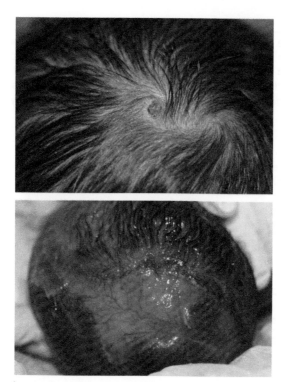

Fig. 6. Spectrum of posterior scalp cutis aplasia in trisomy 13. (*Courtesy of* D. Clark, MD, Albany, NY.)

- Short sternum
- Cardiac anomalies
- Severe mental retardation and neurologic dysfunction

Like trisomy 13, life span is typically limited to weeks or months; however, there have been cases that have been described with individuals living years. Individuals with mosaicism can have milder manifestations and live much longer.

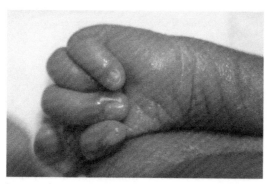

Fig. 7. Typical overlapping fingers in trisomy 18. (*Courtesy of* D. Clark, MD, Albany, NY.)

Turner Syndrome

Turner syndrome has a prevalence of approximately 1 in 3500 births.[7] The development of a cystic hygroma during fetal development can be pronounced. In many cases, the cystic hygroma interferes with the development of head and neck structures to such a degree that it results in a miscarriage. The fetuses that survive the cystic hygroma have the characteristic neck webbing seen in many individuals with Turner syndrome. Additional findings are as follows (**Fig. 8**):

- Lymphedema in the newborn period
- Neck webbing
- Short stature
- Subtle cognitive issues
- Shield chest
- Wide-spaced nipples
- Coarctation of the aorta

Individuals with Turner syndrome can have mild difficulties in school. Many are picked up when being evaluated for delayed menarche. Life span is normal. If a mosaic state is noted with some 46, XY cells, streak gonads may be present, which must be addressed immediately because of the high risk of gonadoblastoma formation.

Klinefelter Syndrome

Individuals with Klinefelter syndrome do not have any clinical findings in the newborn period. They tend to present with infertility and gynecomastia. Typical findings include the following:

- Hypogonadism
  - Small testes

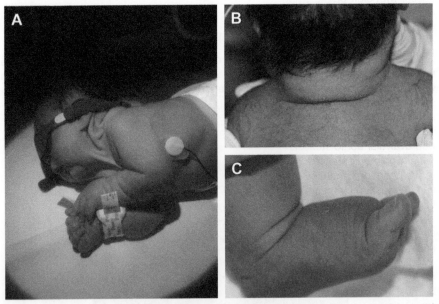

Fig. 8. (*A, B*) Neck webbing and (*C*) dorsal lymphedema in extremities in newborn with Turner syndrome. ([*B, C*] *Courtesy of* D. Clark, MD, Albany, NY.)

- ○ Azoospermia
- ○ Oligospermia
- Hyalinization and fibrosis of the seminiferous tubules
- Gynecomastia in late puberty
- Psychosocial problems

Endocrinologic findings include the following:

- Low serum testosterone levels
- High luteinizing hormone and follicle-stimulating hormone levels
- Frequently elevated estradiol levels
- Progressive decline in testosterone production during the life span, and not all men suffer from hypogonadism

MICRODELETION SYNDROMES

Several of the more common microdeletion syndromes that present with multisystem involvement are reviewed.

22q11.2 Syndrome (DiGeorge/Velocardiofacial Syndrome)

Velocardiofacial syndrome or 22q11.2 syndrome can present with a broad range of findings that can be primarily cardiac, which has been referred to as DiGeorge syndrome, or with learning delays and velopalatal insufficiency as the only findings. Dysmorphic facial features occur in greater than 90% of cases; however, they can be subtle and include a long, narrow face, a tubular nose with a bulbous tip, narrow palpebral fissures, ear anomalies, and a small mouth. Developmental and learning disabilities also occur in greater than 90% of cases, with math skills and social judgment the 2 areas most likely to be involved. Metal retardations can occur in 35% of cases. Hypernasal speech and velopalatal insufficiency are also seen in greater than 90% of cases, with cleft palate being a rare manifestation. Hypocalcemia and hypoparathyroidism occur in 65%, psychiatric disorders in 60%, recurrent seizures in 40%, and cardiac defects in 30% to 40% of cases.[8–10]

Williams Syndrome

Williams syndrome is the result of a microdeleted segment on chromosome 7q. It has been noted to involve multiple systems, including the cardiovascular, neurologic, and endocrine systems. The cardiovascular involvement is an elastin arteriopathy that can involve any artery. Manifestations include narrowing of the arteries, but the most clinically significant and most common cardiovascular finding is supravalvular aortic stenosis. Supravalvular aortic stenosis occurs in approximately 75% of affected individuals. Peripheral pulmonic stenosis is common in infancy but is not specific to Williams syndrome.

The neurologic manifestations can include cognitive deficits; however, these deficits can be masked by their exceptional language skills. Some have average intelligence. Strengths also include verbal short-term memory; extreme weakness in visuospatial construction is typical. The Williams syndrome cognitive profile is independent of the intelligence quotient (IQ). Their personality tends to include overfriendliness, empathy, generalized anxiety, and attention deficit disorder.

Individuals with Williams syndrome also have distinctive facial features: bitemporal narrowing, a broad brow, a stellate or lacy pattern to the iris, periorbital fullness, strabismus, a short nose, a full nasal tip, malar hypoplasia, long philtrum, full lips, wide mouth, malocclusion, a small jaw, and prominent earlobes can be observed at any age. Younger children have been noted to have transient findings that include epicanthal folds, full cheeks, and small and widely spaced teeth. Adults generally have a gaunt appearance with a long face and neck that tend to be more pronounced by sloping shoulders.

Endocrine manifestations include idiopathic hypercalcemia (15%), hypercalciuria (30%), hypothyroidism (10%), and early (but not precocious) puberty (50%). An increased frequency of subclinical hypothyroidism, abnormal results in oral glucose tolerance tests, and diabetes mellitus has been observed in adults with Williams syndrome.

Growth is characterized by prenatal growth deficiency, failure to thrive in infancy (70%), poor weight gain, and linear growth in the first 4 years; a rate of linear growth that is 75% of normal in childhood; and a brief pubertal growth spurt. The mean adult height is less than the third percentile.

They can also have connective tissue involvement that includes a hoarse voice, inguinal/umbilical hernias, bowel/bladder diverticulae, rectal prolapse, joint limitation or laxity, and soft, lax skin.

Wolf-Hirschhorn Syndrome

Wolf-Hirschhorn syndrome is associated with a microdeletion of the 4p region. The facial features tend to evolve over time. Early in life, patients tend to have a broad nasal root that gives a Greek warrior helmet appearance. As they approach puberty, this nasal root prominence tends to become less noticeable. Individuals with Wolf-Hirschhorn syndrome also have microcephaly, a high forehead, prominent glabella, ocular hypertelorism, epicanthal folds, highly arched eyebrows, a short philtrum, downturned mouth, micrognathia, and unusually formed ears with tags or pits.

Growth delays are typical and can be noted prenatally. The poor growth continues postnatally in all individuals.

Neurologic involvement includes developmental delays and cognitive deficiency of a variable degree but is present in all. Gross motor delays are also seen and are associated with hypotonia.

Cri du Chat Syndrome

Cri du chat syndrome is so named because of the characteristic finding of a high-pitched catlike cry. This sound leads one to strongly suspect cri du chat syndrome. The condition is the result of a microdeletion in 5p. There are some individuals who also have a catlike cry without any other findings. These individuals can have a smaller deletion in the 5p region, and it tends to be confined in the 5p15.3 region. Additional clinical features include microcephaly, a round face, ocular hypertelorism, micrognathia, epicanthal folds, low-set ears, hypotonia, and severe psychomotor and mental retardation.

Miller-Dieker Syndrome

Miller-Dieker syndrome is associated with a microdeletion in 17p. Lissencephaly is the characteristic MRI finding. Typical features include a characteristic furrowing of the forehead and microcephaly, and the pregnancy may be complicated by polyhydramnios. Life span is limited, with death occurring by 2 years of age in most children and a few reaching 10 years of age. The oldest known individual with Miller-Dieker syndrome lived to 17 years of age.

In lissencephaly, the cerebral gyri are absent or abnormally broad. The cerebral cortex is also thick, ranging from 12 to 20 mm, with a normal cerebral cortex being 3 to 4 mm thick. Classic lissencephaly findings also include the following:

- Cavum septi pellucidi et vergae
- Mild hypoplasia of the corpus callosum (the anterior portion often appears flattened)

- Mild vermis hypoplasia in some individuals with a normal brain stem and cerebellum
- The lateral ventricles are enlarged posteriorly

Subcortical band heterotopia can also be seen as a subcortical band of heterotopic gray matter, present just beneath the cortex. It is separated from the cortex by a thin zone of normal white matter. The subcortical bands are most often symmetric and diffuse, extending from the frontal to occipital regions; however, they may be asymmetric. Subcortical bands restricted to the frontal lobes are more typically associated with mutations of the *DCX* gene. Subcortical bands restricted to the posterior lobes are more typically associated with *LIS1* mutations. The gyral pattern is normal or demonstrates mildly simplified shallow sulci; a normal cortical ribbon is present.

Smith-Magenis Syndrome

Smith-Magenis syndrome is associated with a deletion of 17p11.2. In the infantile period, mild to moderate hypotonia that can result in feeding difficulties has been noted and this may result in failure to thrive. Minor skeletal anomalies, brachydactyly, and short stature can be seen. Congenital cardiac defects and structural renal anomalies have been reported. Hearing loss is variable, but speech delays are a more persistent finding. A peripheral neuropathy with decreased pain sensitivity, cognitive impairment (IQ 20–78), and developmental delays are also typical findings.

The most striking feature of Smith-Magenis syndrome is the distinct neurobehavioral phenotype, which includes a sleep disturbance whereby they tend to sleep during the day and remain awake at night. Abnormal melatonin regulation seems to be the cause. Patients also tend to engage in self-mutilation, pulling out fingernails and constantly picking at the skin. Insertion of foreign bodies into body orifices and eating nonfood items can also be typical manifestations. Many of the features may not be apparent in infants and young children, so a clinical diagnosis can be difficult in those age groups. Single-nucleotide polymorphism genomic microarray analysis detects 90% of cases. RAI1 gene sequencing and deletion/duplication analysis detects 5% to 10% of cases.

Wilms Tumor-Aniridia-Genital Anomalies-Retardation

Wilms tumor-aniridia-genital anomalies-retardation (WAGR) syndrome is associated with a deletion of the 11p13 region. There are 2 critical genes in the region, *PAX6* and *WT1*. There can be up to a 50% risk of developing a Wilms tumor with an increased incidence of bilateral involvement compared with those with isolated Wilms tumor. Those with WAGR also have an earlier age of diagnosis, but they have more favorable tumor histology and a better prognosis than those with isolated Wilms tumor.

Aniridia is almost always present in individuals with deletions encompassing the *PAX6* gene and is typically severe. There have been cases of deletions in the 11p13 region that do not include the *PAX6* gene and aniridia does not occur.

Up to 60% of male patients can have cryptorchidism. Additional genitourinary anomalies include uterine abnormalities, hypospadias, ambiguous genitalia, streak ovaries, urethral strictures, ureteral abnormalities, and gonadoblastoma.

Cognitive delays can be seen in 70% of individuals with IQ scores less than 74. Behavioral abnormalities can also be seen and include attention deficit hyperactivity disorder, autism spectrum disorders, anxiety, depression, and obsessive compulsive disorder. Up to one-third can have neurologic involvement, including hypertonia or hypotonia, epilepsy, enlarged ventricles, microcephaly, and agenesis of the corpus callosum.

End-stage renal disease risk is significant; Wilms tumor, focal segmental glomerulo-sclerosis, and occasional renal malformations can contribute to the increased risk. With unilateral Wilms tumor, the rate of end-stage renal disease is 36%, and it is 90% in those with bilateral Wilms tumor formation. Twenty-five percent of individuals can have variable proteinuria that can be overt nephritic syndrome in the more severe cases.

Obesity can also be a frequent manifestation of WAGR syndrome. Individuals can also have hemihypertrophy, facial dysmorphisms, growth delays, scoliosis, kyphosis, and, occasionally, polydactyly and diaphragmatic hernia.

A cytogenetically visible deletion can be observed in approximately 60% of affected individuals. An additional 14% have a microdeletion in the region, with an unknown percentage having smaller contiguous gene deletions of the PAX6 and WT1 genes.

Alagille Syndrome

Approximately 7% of individuals with Alagille syndrome have a deletion of the entire JAG1 gene detectable by genomic microarray analysis. Sequence analysis of JAG1 DNA detects mutations in about 88% of individuals with Alagille syndrome. Less than 1% of individuals have been noted to have mutations in the NOTCH2 gene. Clinical criteria have been established for the clinical diagnosis of Alagille syndrome. The histologic finding of bile duct paucity (an increased portal tract-to-bile duct ratio) on liver biopsy has been considered to be the most important and constant feature of Alagille syndrome; however, bile duct paucity is not present in infancy in many individuals ultimately shown to have Alagille syndrome. In the newborn, a normal ratio of portal tracts to bile ducts, bile duct proliferation, or a picture suggestive of neonatal hepatitis may be observed. Overall, bile duct paucity is present in about 90% of individuals.

Of the following 5 major clinical features, 3 features in addition to bile duct paucity establish a clinical diagnosis of Alagille syndrome:

- Cardiac defect (most commonly stenosis of the peripheral pulmonary artery and its branches)
- Characteristic facial features
- Cholestasis
- Ophthalmologic abnormalities (most commonly posterior embryotoxon)
- Skeletal abnormalities (most commonly butterfly vertebrae identified in antero-posterior chest radiographs)

In addition, abnormalities of the kidney, neurovasculature, and pancreas are important manifestations. The diagnosis of Alagille syndrome may be difficult due to the extreme range of expression of the clinical manifestations. The diagnosis of Alagille syndrome should be considered in individuals who do not meet the full clinical criteria but do have an affected first-degree relative. If an affected first-degree relative is identified, the presence of one or more features establishes a clinical diagnosis.

EPIGENETIC/IMPRINTING DISORDERS

- Imprinting (repression) is the determination of the expression of a gene by its parental origin.
- Imprinting results in monoallelic gene expression.
- Mechanism of imprinting is unclear.
- Methylation of DNA seems to play a major role in imprinting.
- For some genes, imprinting is confined to certain tissues or certain stages of development (see **Fig. 8**; **Fig. 9**).

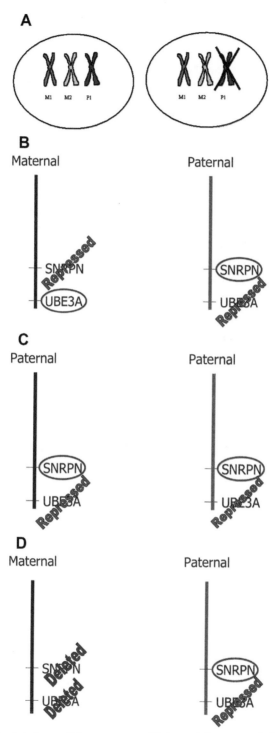

Fig. 9. (*A*) Uniparental disomy. Trisomy rescue with loss of the paternal chromosomes. The two maternal chromosomes with the same imprint results in uniparental disomy. (*B*) Normal germ line imprinting on chromosome 15. (*C*) Angelman syndrome—paternal UPD 15. (*D*) Angelman syndrome—maternal deletion 15q11q13.

Angelman Syndrome

Individuals with Angelman syndrome appear normal at birth but begin manifesting developmental delays by 6 to 12 months of age. This cognitive impairment progresses to severe mental retardation. One of the hallmark features of Angelman syndrome, in addition to microcephaly and seizures, is the absence of speech. Individuals with Angelman syndrome do not acquire more than 6 words throughout their life. The brain is generally structurally normal on MRI or computed tomography; however, they may have mild cortical atrophy or dysmyelination. Another significant feature is their ataxia and tremors of the limbs. Individuals with Angelman syndrome have a unique behavioral phenotype that includes frequent laughter and smiling, a happy demeanor, excitability with hand flapping, and other hypermotoric behaviors.

Most patients have microcephaly and seizures. The microcephaly is seen by 2 years of age and is acquired. Seizure also typically presents between 1 and 3 years of age. Some patients also have the following:

- Attraction to/fascination with water
- Feeding problems during infancy
- Hyperactive tendon reflexes
- Hypopigmentation of the skin and eyes
- Hypotonia
- Increased sensitivity to heat; sleep disturbance
- Strabismus
- Tongue thrusting, sucking and swallowing disorders, frequent drooling, excessive chewing and mouthing
- Uplifted, flexed arms during walking
- Wide mouth, wide-spaced teeth, prominent mandible

Those with hypopigmentation typically have a deletion of the *Pigment* gene (15q11.2-q13) The *Pigment* gene encodes a tyrosine transporter (P protein) important in melanin synthesis. In rare cases, the hypopigmentation can be so severe that a form of albinism is suspected.

Genetic counseling in Angelman syndrome

- The risk to sibs of an affected child who has a deletion or uniparental disomy (UPD) is typically less than 1%.
- A standard or high-resolution chromosome analysis should be offered to all sibs to detect a chromosomal rearrangement, which alters the recurrence risks.
- The risk to sibs of an affected child who has an imprinting defect with deletion of imprinting center (IC) or a mutation of a gene is as high as 50% (ie, *UBE3A*).
- Chromosome rearrangement depends on whether it is inherited or de novo.
- Mothers of patients with deletions should be tested for a possible balanced chromosomal rearrangement. Germ line mosaicism for large deletions has been described.
- Prenatal testing is possible when the underlying genetic mechanism is known.
- Unknown causes may be undetected mutations in the regulatory regions of gene (*UBE3A*) or other unidentified mechanisms or genes involved.

Prader-Willi Syndrome

Prader-Willi syndrome has characteristic neonatal manifestations that include severe neonatal hypotonia with poor feeding. In rare cases, the hypotonia may be mild and improves with age. Because of the feeding difficulties, failure to thrive is common in infancy. From 6 months to 6 years of age, there is a dramatic onset of weight gain and these individuals develop obesity. They also tend to have short stature; however, there have been cases of individuals who have been in the normal range for height.

The characteristic behavioral manifestation is an obsession with food. Patients break into refrigerators and cabinets to eat and wake up to eat overnight. Stealing food off the plate of other individuals is also commonly seen.

As individuals with Prader-Willi syndrome grow older, they have noticeably small hands and feet. Major findings include the following:

- Mild to moderate mental retardation (~90%)
- Learning disabilities
- Normal neuromuscular studies
- Seizures
- Poor gross motor coordination
- Poor fine motor coordination
- Global developmental delay
- Behavioral problems
- Sleep disturbances
- High pain threshold

Male patients have the following:
- Hypogonadotropic hypogonadism
- Small penis
- Scrotal hypoplasia
- Cryptorchidism

Even though the SNRPN gene has been used as a marker in the critical region for Prader-Willi syndrome, it is not thought to be causative for some forms of Prader-Willi syndrome, unlike the UBE3A gene in Angelman syndrome (**Table 1**).

Genetic counseling in Prader-Willi syndrome

- The risk to sibs of an affected child who has a deletion or UPD is typically less than 1%.
- A standard or high-resolution chromosome analysis should be offered to all to detect a chromosomal rearrangement, which alters the recurrence risks.
- The risk to sibs of an affected child who has an imprinting defect with deletion of IC is as high as 50%.
- Chromosome rearrangement depends on whether it is inherited or de novo.

Table 1
Testing for Prader-Willi syndrome

Test Methods	Mutations Detected	Percentage of Individuals
Methylation analysis	Methylation abnormality	99
FISH/Quantitative PCR	Deletion of PWCR[a]	70
Uniparental disomy studies	UPD of PWCR	25
Sequence analysis[b]	Imprinting center defect	<1

Abbreviations: FISH, fluorescent in situ hybridization; PCR, polymerase chain reaction; PWCR, Prader-Willi critical region.
[a] Deletion varies in size but always includes the PWCR.
[b] Sequence analysis detects small deletions that account for about 15% of imprinting center mutations. Most imprinting defects are epimutations (ie, alterations in the imprint, not the DNA).

- Fathers of patients with deletions should be tested for a possible balanced chromosomal rearrangement. Germ line mosaicism for large deletions has been described.
- Prenatal testing is possible when the underlying genetic mechanism is known.
- Unknown causes may be unknown genes or other unidentified mechanisms or genes involved (**Fig. 10**).

Beckwith-Wiedemann Syndrome

Beckwith-Wiedemann syndrome (BWS) is another disorder that has been associated with imprinting defects. A consensus for clinical criteria has not yet been established; however, having 3 criteria would be consistent with the diagnosis.

Criteria include the following:

- Positive family history (one or more family members with a clinical diagnosis of BWS or a history or features suggestive of BWS)
- Macrosomia (traditionally defined as height and weight >97th percentile)
- Anterior linear ear lobe creases/posterior helical ear pits
- Macroglossia
- Omphalocele (also called exomphalos)/umbilical hernia
- Visceromegaly involving one or more intra-abdominal organs including liver, spleen, kidneys, adrenal glands, and pancreas
- Embryonal tumor (eg, Wilms tumor, hepatoblastoma, neuroblastoma, rhabdomyosarcoma) in childhood

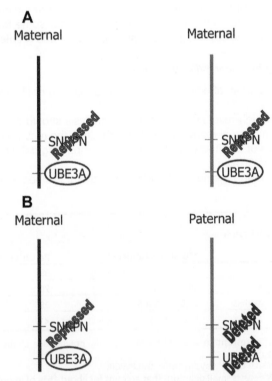

Fig. 10. Prader-Willi syndrome. (*A*) Maternal UPD 15. (*B*) Paternal deletion 15q11q13.

- Hemihyperplasia (asymmetric overgrowth of one or more regions of the body)
- Adrenocortical cytomegaly
- Renal abnormalities including structural abnormalities, nephromegaly, and nephrocalcinosis
- Cleft palate (rare)

In regards to management, up to 7.5% of individuals with BWS develop a tumor during the first 8 years of life and can include the following:

- Wilms tumor
- Hepatoblastoma
- Adrenal carcinoma
- Gonadoblastoma

Tumor incidence decreases after 8 years of age and is equivalent to population risk. BWS is primarily a syndrome of childhood. As they become older, the clinical findings disappear and they tend to "grow into" their macroglossia and macrosomia. Intelligence and development are normal. Molecular genetic testing can account for up to 75% of cases without a family history and up to 99% of cases with a family history.

Russell-Silver Syndrome

Individuals with Russell-Silver syndrome can be noted to have intrauterine growth retardation. Consequently, in the neonatal period, they are small for gestational age and have persistent failure to thrive. Additional findings include the following:

- Normal head circumference with height and weight less than 5th percentile
- Lateral asymmetries
- Fasting hypoglycemia
- Occasional growth hormone deficiency
- Frontal bossing and micrognathia resulting in triangular face
- Cardiac defects
- Hypospadias, posterior urethral valves
- Wilms and other tumors

Russell-Silver syndrome has multiple causes like many conditions associated with epigenetic causes. The following causes have been established:

- UPD7 7% to 10%
- H19 locus on chromosome 11% to 35%
- Genetic heterogeneity

As noted earlier, current testing is able to confirm a cause using molecular genetic testing in less than 50% of cases.

ETHICAL DILEMMAS—THE GENOMIC ERA

As the ease of genomic sequencing continues to increase, ethical challenges have arisen that are unique to the ability to sequence tens of thousands of genes on a single blood specimen. Specific challenges have arisen in regards to information that has been discovered that the patient or family may not have wanted to know about. For example, a pediatric patient could undergo genomic sequencing to determine a cause of developmental delay when it is discovered that the patient has a pathogenic mutation in the BRCA gene. This finding could have implications to the patient's mother who may have the same mutation noted in her child's sample. However, the patient's mother may not have wanted to know that she could be at increased risk for breast cancer. Many laboratories are now allowing families to opt out of certain gene categories if they feel that the information is not desirable. However, the American College of Medical Genetics has recommended that laboratories report medically actionable genetic information that can have a major impact on the health of the individual being tested. Panels of genes that are medically actionable are being reported unless the family specifically states that they do not want that information revealed to them during the consent process. These scenarios are starting to be encountered, which is why it is essential that families who choose to have genomic sequencing have genetic counseling so that issues like this can be discussed.

REFERENCES

1. Girard J. Metabolic adaptations to change of nutrition at birth. Biol Neonate 1990; 58(1):3–15.
2. Owen OE, Reichard GA Jr, Patel MS, et al. Energy metabolism in feasting and fasting. Adv Exp Med Biol 1979;111:169–88.
3. Ward Platt M, Deshpande S. Metabolic adaptation at birth. Semin Fetal Neonatal Med 2005;10:341–50.
4. Arnoux JB, Verkarre V, Saint-Martin C, et al. Congenital hyperinsulinism: current trends in diagnosis and therapy. Orphanet J Rare Dis 2011;6:63.
5. van Gameren-Oosterom HB, Buitendijk SE, Bilardo CM, et al. Unchanged prevalence of Down syndrome in the Netherlands: results from an 11-year nationwide birth cohort. Prenat Diagn 2012;32:1035–40.
6. Savva GM, Walker K, Morris JK. The maternal age-specific live birth prevalence of trisomies 13 and 18 compared to trisomy 21 (Down syndrome). Prenat Diagn 2010;30(1):57–64.
7. Gregor V, Sípek A, Sípek A Jr, et al. Prenatal diagnostics of chromosomal aberrations Czech Republic: 1994-2007. Ceska Gynekol 2009;74(1):44–54 [in Czech].
8. Kapadia RK, Bassett AS. Recognizing a common genetic syndrome: 22q11.2 deletion syndrome. CMAJ 2008;178(4):391–3.
9. Morris CA. Williams syndrome. In: Pagon RA, Bird TD, Dolan CR, et al, editors. GeneReviews. Seattle (WA): University of Washington, Seattle; 2006. Available at: http://www.ncbi.nlm.nih.gov/books/NBK1249/.
10. Dagli AI, Williams CA. Angelman syndrome. In: Pagon RA, Bird TD, Dolan CR, et al, editors. GeneReviews. Seattle (WA): University of Washington, Seattle; 2011. Available at: http://www.ncbi.nlm.nih.gov/books/NBK1144/.

Neonatal Nutrition

Scott C. Denne, MD

KEYWORDS

- Infant nutrition • Breastfeeding • Infant formula • Gastroesophageal reflux

KEY POINTS

- There is good evidence of the clinical benefit of breastfeeding to infants and mothers, and it should be the primary nutrition source for most infants.
- The breastfed infant is the normative model for infant growth, and the WHO growth curves should be used for all term infants.
- All standard term infant formulas are clinically equivalent and adequately support growth for the small proportion of infants who cannot breastfeed.
- Soy and other specialized formulas should be reserved for particular circumstances and conditions and should not be used routinely.
- Gastroesophageal reflux occurs in most infants and does not require intervention. Gastroesophageal reflux disease occurs in a small proportion of infants and an algorithm-based evaluation and management strategy should be used.

NEONATAL NUTRITION

There is accumulating evidence that nutrition and growth in early life can have substantial influences on adult health.[1] This article reviews the current knowledge, recommendations, and approaches to feeding the normal newborn. The current understanding and approach to the common and sometimes difficult problem of gastroesophageal reflux (GER) in normal infants is also discussed.

BREASTFEEDING

Based on the many demonstrated benefits for babies and mothers, the World Health Organization (WHO), the American Academy of Pediatrics (AAP), and Institute of Medicine recommend the exclusive use of human milk for healthy term infants for the first 6 months of life, and continued breastfeeding for at least 12 months.[2] The public health goal for Healthy People 2020 is for 82% of mothers to initiate breastfeeding, 60% of mothers to be breastfeeding at 6 months, and 34% to be breastfeeding at 1 year.[3] The Centers for Disease Control and Prevention (CDC) tracks these

Disclosure Statement: Nothing to disclose.
Department of Pediatrics, Indiana University, 699 Riley Hospital Dr, RR 208, Indianapolis, IN 46202, USA
E-mail address: sdenne@iu.edu

Pediatr Clin N Am 62 (2015) 427–438
http://dx.doi.org/10.1016/j.pcl.2014.11.006

breastfeeding rates and issues a breastfeeding report card yearly.[4] Significant progress has been made toward achieving these breastfeeding goals, and in 2011 79% of women initiated breastfeeding. However, additional progress is necessary in the duration and exclusivity of breastfeeding. The most recent data on breastfeeding rates and the goals of Healthy People 2020 are shown in **Fig. 1**.

To support higher breastfeeding rates, additional objectives of Healthy People 2020 include increasing the proportion of employers that have worksite lactation support programs, reducing the number of breastfed newborns who receive formula supplementation within the first 2 days of life, and increasing the proportion of live births that occur in facilities that provide recommended care for lactating mothers and their babies.[3]

Although there has been progress in overall breastfeeding rates, these gains have not been uniform across all populations and geographic regions.[5] Breastfeeding rates are lower for black infants, infants of mothers with lower incomes, and mothers with less education.[5–7] Breastfeeding rates are lower in the southern United States and in rural areas.[5,8] Health care workers should be aware of these disparities so that they can focus their attention on these groups to educate about and support breastfeeding, and help others overcome barriers to breastfeeding.

Breastfeeding and Clinical Outcomes

There is growing evidence that breastfeeding conveys important benefits during childhood and in later adult life, and to breastfeeding mothers.[9] However, the evidence for these benefits comes almost entirely from observational cohort studies and not randomized clinical trials; randomized controlled trials of breastfeeding are widely

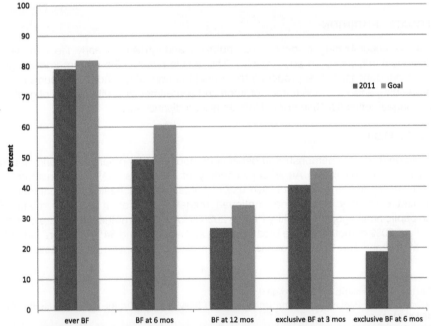

Fig. 1. US breastfeeding rates in 2011 (*red bars*) and Healthy People 2020 goals (*green bars*). BF, breastfed. (*Data from* National Center for Chronic Disease Prevention and Health Promotion. Breast feeding report card. Atlanta, GA: CDC, 2014. Available at: www.cdc.gov/pdf/2014breastfeedingreportcard.pdf. Accessed November 3, 2014.)

considered to be impractical and unethical.[2,9] Observational trials of clinical benefit have not always been consistent and can be subject to bias and contain multiple confounders. However, careful evaluation of multiple studies evaluating breastfeeding effects in clinical outcomes has been conducted, and meta-analyses performed.[9] Based on these meta-analyses, there is convincing evidence of the beneficial effects of breastfeeding on a variety of infant and maternal clinical outcomes. A list of those significant outcomes is provided in **Box 1**.

Several other benefits associated with breastfeeding have also been reported, but the evidence has been inconsistent and/or less convincing. This includes associations between breastfeeding and cognitive development, obesity in later life, cardiovascular mortality in adulthood, and postpartum depression.[9]

Composition of Human Milk

Human milk is a complex and dynamic fluid that supports ideal infant growth and immune function development.[10] The composition of human milk changes over time, and contains live cells along with macronutrients and micronutrients and bioactive factors.

Colostrum is the first fluid secreted by the breast following delivery, and has an intense yellow color because of the high concentration of carotenoids. Colostrum is produced in low quantities for the first few days, and contains bioactive components including secretory IgA, lactoferrin, leucocytes, and epidermal growth factor. Compared with later milk, colostrum contains relatively low concentrations of lactose, potassium, and calcium and higher levels of sodium chloride and magnesium.[10] As lactose secretion becomes more efficient and milk lactose concentration increases, the colostrum/milk sodium concentration decreases proportionally.

Transitional milk appears at 5 to 14 days and contains increased amounts of lactose, fat, and total calories along with lower concentrations of immunoglobulins and total proteins. At 2 to 4 weeks, human milk is considered mature and the

---

Box 1
Reduction in disease/condition associated with breastfeeding

Infant

Otitis media

Recurrent otitis media

Respiratory tract infection

Asthma

Atopic dermatitis

Gastroenteritis

Type 1 and 2 diabetes

Leukemia

Sudden infant death syndrome

Mother

Breast cancer

Ovarian cancer

Data from Ip S, Chung M, Raman G, et al. A summary of the Agency for Healthcare Research and Quality's evidence report on breastfeeding in developed countries. Breastfeed Med 2009;4 Suppl 1:S17–30.

composition remains stable for the next several months.[11] The change in macronutrient concentration in human milk over time is shown in **Fig. 2**.

The macronutrient mineral, vitamin, and micronutrient concentration of mature human milk is shown in **Table 1**. It must be pointed out that **Table 1** lists average composition values; there is substantial variability in the nutrient content of human milk across individual mothers. Furthermore, aliquots of milk from one mother can also be quite different in composition. However, the mother-infant dyad seems to successfully adapt to these variations, and successful breastfeeding and normal infant growth is achieved for most mothers and infants.

Human milk contains live cells and a large variety of bioactive substances.[5,10] Macrophages, T cells, and lymphocytes are all found in human milk, with macrophages being the predominant cell type. These cells most likely perform an important host defense function for the infant. Multiple bioactive factors are present in human milk including immunoglobulins, growth factors, cytokines, and other small molecules. A partial list of bioactive substances contained in human milk along with their proposed function is shown in **Table 2**.

Growth and Growth Standards

The WHO conducted a well-designed, longitudinal study of healthy term breastfed infants accurately measuring growth from birth to 2 years of age.[12] Data were obtained from 903 infants who were exclusively or predominantly breastfed for 4 to 6 months and who continued breastfeeding for at least 12 months. The study was conducted in six diverse geographic areas (Brazil, India, Ghana, Norway, Oman, and the United States). The resulting growth charts contain extensive information including weight for age, length for age, head circumference for age, and weight for length and body mass index for age. These WHO growth curves are considered the normative model for growth and development regardless of infant ethnicity or geography, and reflects optimal growth of the breastfed infant. The CDC and AAP recommend the use of the

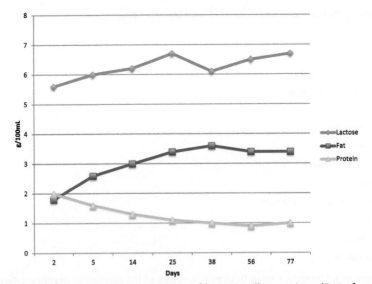

Fig. 2. Change in macronutrient composition of human milk over time. (*Data from* Gidrewicz DA, Fenton TR. A systematic review and meta-analysis of the nutrient content of preterm and term breast milk. BMC Pediatr 2014;14(1):216.)

Table 1
Concentrations of selected nutrients in mature (2 wk) human milk

Energy	66 ± 9 kcal
Protein	1.3 ± 0.2 g
Fat	3.0 ± 0.9 g
Lactose	6.2 ± 0.6 g
Calcium	28 ± 7 mg
Phosphorus	15 ± 4 mg
Sodium	18 ± 4 mg
Potassium	53 ± 4 mg
Chloride	42 ± 6 mg
Iron	0.03 ± 0.01 mg
Vitamin D	2.2 ± 0.4 IU/100 mL

All concentrations per 100 mL; mean ± SD.
Data from Kleinman R. Pediatric Nutrition Handbook. 7th edition. Elk Grove Village (IL): American Academy of Pediatrics; 2014; and Gidrewicz DA, Fenton TR. A systematic review and meta-analysis of the nutrient content of preterm and term breast milk. BMC Pediatr 2014;14(1):216.

WHO growth curves for all children younger than 24 months. These growth charts are readily available on the CDC Web site (www.cdc.gove/growthcharts/who_charts.htm).

Supplements for Breastfed Infants

Although human milk is uniquely suited to support normal infant growth, human milk is low in vitamin D and iron, and deficiency can occur. Therefore, the AAP recommends 400 IU/day vitamin D supplementation for all breastfed infants.[5] Vitamin D supplementation should begin in the first few days of life and continue until the infant is weaned to at least 1 L/day or 1 quart/day of vitamin D–fortified formula or whole milk. Supplementation of 1 mg/kg/day of oral iron should start at 4 months of age and continue until the infant consumes adequate oral iron from foods.

Table 2
Selected bioactive compounds in human milk

Compound	Proposed Function
Immunoglobulins (IgA, IgM, IgG)	Infection prevention
Cytokines	Infection prevention, reduce inflammation
Oligosaccharides	Promote beneficial flora
Nucleotides	Promote beneficial flora
Lactoferrin	Intestinal growth, immunomodulation
Epidermal growth factor	Intestinal maturation and repair
Insulin-like growth factor 1 and 2	Tissue growth
Erythropoietin	Prevention of anemia, intestinal development
Vascular endothelial growth factor	Regulation of angiogenesis

Data from Kleinman R. Pediatric nutrition handbook. 7th edition. Elk Grove Village (IL): American Academy of Pediatrics; 2014; and Ballard O, Morrow AL. Human milk composition: nutrients and bioactive factors. Pediatr Clin North Am 2013;60(1):49–74.

Duration of Breastfeeding

The AAP, WHO, and Institute of Medicine recommend exclusive breastfeeding for about 6 months, with continuation after complementary foods have been introduced for at least the first year of life.[2,5] Breastfeeding can be extended beyond the first year of life as mutually desired by the mother and child. It is important to point out that the definition of exclusive breastfeeding includes the administration of vitamin D and iron.

Contraindications to Breastfeeding

There are a limited number of medical circumstances where breastfeeding is contra-indicated. These include some maternal infections, particular inborn errors of metabolism in infants, and a few maternal medications.

Maternal medical conditions that preclude breastfeeding include human T-cell lymphotropic virus (type 1 and 2), untreated brucellosis, active pulmonary tuberculosis without 2 weeks of completed treatment, and active herpes simplex lesions on the breast.[2,5] In the industrialized world, breastfeeding is also contraindicated for HIV-positive mothers. Because the primary carbohydrate of breast milk is lactose, a disaccharide composed of glucose and galactose, infants with the inborn error of metabolism of galactosemia should not be breastfed. Although most maternal medications are compatible with breastfeeding, certain medications are a contraindication to breastfeeding, such as mothers receiving antineoplastic drug therapy. Because of the rapidly changing information on medications relative to breastfeeding, it is advisable to consult the drugs and lactation database (LacMed) before making a determination. LacMed is easily accessible from the US National Library of Medicine Web site (http://docsnet.nlm.nih.gov).

Supporting Breastfeeding

Providing support to the breastfeeding mother requires appropriate institutional policies and the knowledge and attention of health care providers. To ensure that breastfeeding is supported in the hospital, the World Health Organization has provided 10 steps to successful breastfeeding (**Box 2**). The 10-step program has been effective in increasing rates of breastfeeding initiation, exclusivity, and duration.[13]

Following hospital discharge, the primary care physician should see all breastfeeding newborns at 3 to 5 days of age or within 48 to 72 hours after discharge from the hospital.[2] At this visit, the physician should evaluate body weight and establish that weight loss is no more than 7% from birth, and that there is no further weight loss by Day 5. If weight loss is of concern, feeding should be assessed and more frequent follow-up should be scheduled. Infant elimination patterns should be discussed and hydration evaluated. One feeding should be observed and any other maternal and infant issues discussed.

Common Breastfeeding Problems

Common problems of breastfeeding mothers include nipple pain, engorgement, and mastitis.[14] Nipple pain is common in the first few days of breastfeeding. This can usually be addressed with good positioning, optimal attachment of the infant at the breast, and removal from the breast when the infant is satisfied. A lactation expert may be useful in helping mothers achieve proper attachment and removal.

Breast engorgement and tenderness often occurs at 3 to 5 days. More frequent breastfeeding and breast massage after feeds are helpful. Mastitis is characterized by a painful red swollen and hard area of the breast, fever, and malaise; mastitis

---

Box 2
World Health Organization ten steps to successful breastfeeding

1. Have a written breastfeeding policy that is routinely communicated to all health care staff.

2. Train all health care staff in the skills necessary to implement this policy.

3. Inform all pregnant women about the benefits and management of breastfeeding.

4. Help mothers initiate breastfeeding within the first hour of birth.

5. Show mothers how to breastfeed and how to maintain lactation even if they are separated from their infants.

6. Give newborn infants no food or drink other than breast milk, unless medically indicated.

7. Practice rooming-in (allow mothers and infants to remain together) 24 hours a day.

8. Encourage breastfeeding on demand.

9. Give no artificial nipples or pacifiers to breastfeeding infants.[a]

10. Foster the establishment of breastfeeding support groups and refer mothers to them on discharge from hospital.

[a] The AAP does not support a categorical ban on pacifiers because of their role in sudden infant death syndrome risk reduction and their analgesic benefit during painful procedures.
From World Health Organization. Evidence for the Ten Steps to Successful Breastfeeding. Geneva, Switzerland, 1998. Available at: www.who.int/nutrition/publications/evidence_ten_step_eng.pdf. Accessed November 3, 2014.

---

can occur in 10% to 20% of mothers. Treatment consists of frequent and effective milk removal and sometimes antibiotics.

FORMULA FEEDING: INDICATIONS

Although breastfeeding is preferred for most normal healthy term infants, formula feeding can support nutrition and growth. The indications for the use of infant formulas include (1) as a substitute (or as a supplement) for human milk in infants whose mothers choose not to breastfeed or not to do so exclusively, (2) as a substitute for human milk in infants where breastfeeding is medically contraindicated, and (3) as a supplement for breastfed infants who's intake of human milk does not support adequate weight gain.[5] It must be noted that the supplementation should be instituted only after interventions to increase milk supply have been ineffective.

Infant Formulas

Infant formulas are regulated by the Food and Drug Administration and manufacturers must ensure by analysis the amount of 29 essential nutrients in each batch of formula.[15] All commercially available standard term infant formulas in the United States support normal growth and development of healthy term infants. Although products from different manufacturers may vary slightly in their nutrient composition, the products are much more similar than different. At present, there is no clinical evidence that differences in term infant formulas have any important measurable clinical effects, and there is no medical reason to prefer one brand over another.

Infant formulas are available in ready to feed, in concentrated liquid, and in powder. Proper preparation of the liquid concentrate and the powder forms is essential, and detailed instructions are found on each manufacturer's Web site. Standard infant formula contains 19 or 20 calories per ounce, which is similar to the average caloric content of breast milk (recognizing the previously discussed variability of human milk).

However, infant formula contains about a 50% higher amount of protein than human milk (approximately 1.4 g/100 mL protein in infant formula). The amount of fat in infant formula is similar to human milk (approximately 3.6 g/100 mL); the fat is provided primarily by mixtures of vegetable oils. Most infant formula manufacturers have added very long chain polyunsaturated fatty acids (arachidonic acid and docosahexaenoic acid) to their formulas. These compounds may help to promote brain and visual development, although the long-term benefit of these additives seems to be minimal or nonexistent.[16] There are, however, no safety concerns by the addition of docosahexaenoic acid and arachidonic acid to infant formulas. The carbohydrate concentration in infant formula (approximately 7.5 g/100 mL) and composition (predominantly lactose) is similar to human milk.

All standard infant formulas contain iron, ideally at a concentration of 12 mg/L. This concentration of iron prevents development of iron deficiency and anemia. However, low-iron infant formulas continue to be available based on a perception of gastrointestinal (GI) symptoms (colic, constipation) with the use of higher-iron formulas. However, multiple well-controlled studies have consistently failed to demonstrate any difference in GI symptoms between higher and lower iron-containing formulas. It is the position of the AAP that there is no role for low-iron formulas in the feeding of healthy term infants.[5]

Other Nutrients in Infant Formulas

The composition of infant formulas is constantly changing, often with the intent to become closer in composition to human milk. Many available commercial infant formulas now contain nucleotides and oligosaccharides (prebiotics). Although there are no concerns about the safety of these additions, there is currently no compelling clinical evidence demonstrating benefit.

Several infant formulas contain probiotics, nonpathogenic microorganisms that may promote "healthy" colonic microflora. Although these probiotics seem to be safe for use in healthy term infants, there is currently insufficient evidence to recommend routine use of these formulas.[5]

Soy Formulas

Although the routine use of soy formulas is not recommended, current commercially available soy formulas adequately support growth and bone mineralization of healthy term infants.[17,18] All soy formulas are lactose free, and can be used to feed infants who cannot tolerate milk protein or lactose. The specific conditions where soy formula is recommended and not recommended by the AAP is shown in **Box 3**.[5,19]

Infant Formulas with Extensively Hydrolyzed Protein

These specialized infant formulas are expensive and have a bitter taste, and should not be used for healthy term infants. The extensively hydrolyzed protein formulas are lactose free and often contain a large amount of medium chain triglycerides, and can sometimes be useful in selected infants with malabsorption syndromes (eg, cystic fibrosis, short gut syndrome, biliary atresia, cholestasis, and protracted diarrhea). These formulas can also be useful for infants who are severely intolerant to intact cow milk protein. The use of extensively hydrolyzed protein formulas should be limited to these indications.[5]

GASTROESOPHAGEAL REFLUX AND GASTROESOPHAGEAL DISEASE

GER occurs in most infants (70%–85% within the first 2 months of life), and is often seen as a problem by parents and physicians. However, it is clear that GER is part

---

Box 3
AAP recommendations for the use of soy formula in term infants

Recommended for the following conditions or situations:

1. Galactosemia or hereditary lactase deficiency

2. Documented transient lactase deficiency

3. Documented IgE-associated allergy to cow milk without allergy to soy protein

4. Desired vegetarian diet

Not recommended for:

1. Preterm infants with birth weights less than 1800 g

2. Prevention treatment of colic

3. Prevention of atopic disease

4. Infants with cow milk protein–induced enteropathy or enterocolitis

Data from Kleinman R. Pediatric nutrition handbook. 7th edition. Elk Grove Village (IL): American Academy of Pediatrics; 2014; and Bhatia J, Greer F. Use of soy protein-based formulas in infant feeding. Pediatrics 2008;121(5):1062–8.

---

of normal physiology and occurs multiple times a day in healthy infants, children, and adults. Most infants have uncomplicated GER ("happy spitters") and require no more than parental education and reassurance. However, it is important to identify the small portion of infants who have gastroesophageal reflux disease (GERD) who require additional evaluation, monitoring, and sometimes treatment. These issues are briefly discussed here; a variety of excellent and comprehensive recent reviews of GER and GERD are available.[19–24]

Symptoms of Gastroesophageal Reflux Disease

Distinguishing between GER and GERD can be difficult in infants. Symptoms associated with GERD include feeding refusal, poor weight gain, irritability, dysphasia, arching of the back during feedings, sleep disturbance, and respiratory symptoms. However, no single symptom or group of symptoms can reliably diagnose GERD in infants, or predict which infants will respond to therapy.[23] However, there is a validated questionnaire for documenting and monitoring of parent report of GERD symptoms in infants that may be useful to clinicians.[25]

Evaluation and Management of Gastroesophageal Reflux/Gastroesophageal Reflux Disease

Evaluation of GER/GERD in infants primarily consists of a comprehensive history and physical examination. In addition to eliciting a history of GERD-associated symptoms, it is important to ensure the absence of other concerning symptoms: bilious vomiting, GI bleeding, forceful vomiting, abdominal tenderness or distention, bulging fontanel, macrocephaly and microcephaly, and seizures.[20,23] The presence of any of these symptoms should prompt additional evaluation based on the particular symptom. With a normal physical examination, appropriate weight gain, and the absence of GERD-associated and other concerning symptoms, no additional diagnostic evaluation is necessary. Education and reassurance should be provided to the parents. In some cases, thickened feedings could be considered. If thickened feedings are to be used, they can be provided by adding up to 1 tablespoon of dry rice cereal to 1 ounce of formula or by using a commercially thickened full term infant formula.[23] Thickened feedings are likely to have little effect on the actual number of reflux episodes but rather reduce the number of observed regurgitations. There is no information on the long-term effects of thickened infant feedings. There is a possible association between thickened feedings and necrotizing entercolitis in preterm infants, and therefore commercial thickened infant formula should not be used in infants born before 37 weeks gestation who have been discharged from the hospital in the past 30 days.

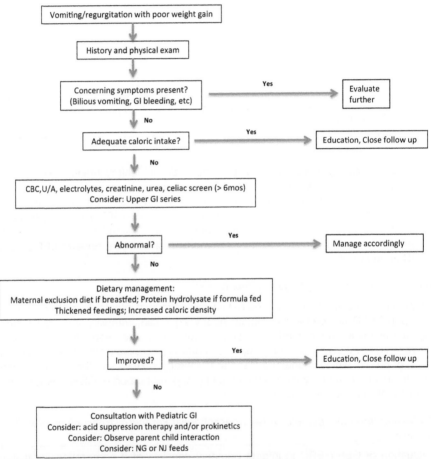

Fig. 3. Algorithm for the evaluation and management of infants with vomiting/regurgitation and poor weight gain as developed by the North American Society for Pediatric Gastroenterology, Hepatology, and Nutrition and endorsed by the AAP. CBC, complete blood count; GI, gastrointestinal; NG, nasogastric; NJ, nasojejunal; U/A, urinalysis. (*Adapted from* Vandenplas Y, Rudolph CD, Di Lorenzo C, et al. Pediatric gastroesophageal reflux clinical practice guidelines: joint recommendations of the North American Society for Pediatric Gastroenterology, Hepatology, and Nutrition (NASPGHAN) and the European Society for Pediatric Gastroenterology, Hepatology, and Nutrition (ESPGHAN). J Pediatr Gastroenterol Nutr 2009;49(4):498–547, with permission; and Lightdale JR, Gremse DA. Gastroesophageal reflux: management guidance for the pediatrician. Pediatrics 2013;131(5): e1684–95.)

Although most infants with GER need only routine evaluation and minimal if any intervention, infants with poor weight gain along with regurgitation and/or vomiting require additional evaluation and possible treatment. An approach to the infant with recurrent regurgitation and poor weight gain, as proposed by the North American Society for Gastroenterology, Hepatology and Nutrition, is shown in **Fig. 3**.[20] After ensuring that there are no significant concerning other symptoms and caloric intake is adequate, evaluation consists of some screening blood work along with possibly an upper GI tract series. An upper GI series is useful for evaluating a possible malrotation or duodenal web. If there is persistent or forced vomiting in the first few months of life, pyloric ultrasonography should be performed to evaluate for pyloric stenosis. If these screening tests are normal, a trial of dietary management can be initiated. For breastfeeding mothers, a 2- to 4-week trial of a diet that restricts milk and egg is recommended; this is to address a potential milk protein allergy. For formula-fed infants, some extensively hydrolyzed protein formula may be appropriate. In addition, thickened feedings may also be useful.

If these interventions result in clinical improvement, they should be continued with additional close follow-up. If there is no improvement, consultation with a pediatric gastroenterologist should be strongly considered. Some consideration may be given to acid-suppression therapy. Although treatment with a prokinetic (eg, metoclopramide) may be considered, the risks of this therapy may outweigh the benefits.[26] Indeed, metoclopramide carries a Food and Drug Administration black box warning regarding its adverse effects. In general, use of pharmacologic therapy for infants with GERD should be uncommon and likely requires comanagement with a pediatric gastroenterologist.

REFERENCES

1. Robinson S, Fall C. Infant nutrition and later health: a review of current evidence. Nutrients 2012;4(8):859–74.
2. Breastfeeding and the use of human milk. Pediatrics 2012;129(3):e827–41.
3. Healthy People 2020. Gov. Available at: http://www.healthypeople.gov/2020/topics. Accessed November 3, 2014.
4. Centers for Disease Control and Prevention. Breastfeeding Report Card, United States, 2014. Available at: www.cdc.gov/pdf/2014breastfeedingreportcard.pdf. Accessed November 3, 2014.
5. Kleinman R. Pediatric nutrition handbook. 7th edition. Elk Grove Village (IL): American Academy of Pediatrics; 2014.
6. Fein SB, Labiner-Wolfe J, Shealy KR, et al. Infant feeding practices study II: study methods. Pediatrics 2008;122(Suppl 2):S28–35.
7. Ryan AS, Wenjun Z, Acosta A. Breastfeeding continues to increase into the new millennium. Pediatrics 2002;110(6):1103–9.
8. U.S. Department of Health and Human Services. The Surgeon General's Call to Action to Support Breastfeeding. Washington (DC): U.S. Department of Health and Human Services, Office of the Surgeon General; 2011.
9. Ip S, Chung M, Raman G, et al. A summary of the Agency for Healthcare Research and Quality's evidence report on breastfeeding in developed countries. Breastfeed Med 2009;4(Suppl 1):S17–30.
10. Ballard O, Morrow AL. Human milk composition: nutrients and bioactive factors. Pediatr Clin North Am 2013;60(1):49–74.
11. Gidrewicz DA, Fenton TR. A systematic review and meta-analysis of the nutrient content of preterm and term breast milk. BMC Pediatr 2014;14(1):216.

12. de Onis M, Garza C, Onyango AW, et al. Comparison of the WHO child growth standards and the CDC 2000 growth charts. J Nutr 2007;137(1):144–8.
13. World Health Organization. Evidence for the Ten Steps to Successful Breastfeeding. Geneva, Switzerland, 1998. Available at: www.who.int/nutrition/publications/evidence_ten_step_eng.pdf. Accessed November 3, 2014.
14. Bergmann RL, Bergmann KE, von Weizsacker K, et al. Breastfeeding is natural but not always easy: intervention for common medical problems of breastfeeding mothers. A review of the scientific evidence. J Perinat Med 2014;42(1):9–18.
15. Drugs Fa. 21 CFR 107. 2009. Available at: http://www.gpo.gov/fdsys/pkg/CFR-2009-title21-vol1/content-detail.html. Accessed November 3, 2014.
16. Simmer K, Patole SK, Rao SC. Long-chain polyunsaturated fatty acid supplementation in infants born at term. Cochrane Database Syst Rev 2011;(12):CD000376.
17. Lasekan JB, Ostrom KM, Jacobs JR, et al. Growth of newborn, term infants fed soy formulas for 1 year. Clin Pediatr 1999;38(10):563–71.
18. Venkataraman PS, Luhar H, Neylan MJ. Bone mineral metabolism in full-term infants fed human milk, cow milk-based, and soy-based formulas. Am J Dis Child 1992;146(11):1302–5.
19. Bhatia J, Greer F. Use of soy protein-based formulas in infant feeding. Pediatrics 2008;121(5):1062–8.
20. Vandenplas Y, Rudolph CD, Di Lorenzo C, et al. Pediatric gastroesophageal reflux clinical practice guidelines: joint recommendations of the North American Society for Pediatric Gastroenterology, Hepatology, and Nutrition (NASPGHAN) and the European Society for Pediatric Gastroenterology, Hepatology, and Nutrition (ESPGHAN). J Pediatr Gastroenterol Nutr 2009;49(4):498–547.
21. Forbes D. Mewling and puking: infantile gastroesophageal reflux in the 21st century. J Paediatr Child Health 2013;49(4):259–63.
22. Czinn SJ, Blanchard S. Gastroesophageal reflux disease in neonates and infants: when and how to treat. Paediatr Drugs 2013;15(1):19–27.
23. Lightdale JR, Gremse DA. Gastroesophageal reflux: management guidance for the pediatrician. Pediatrics 2013;131(5):e1684–95.
24. Rosen R. Gastroesophageal reflux in infants: more than just a phenomenon. JAMA Pediatr 2014;168(1):83–9.
25. Kleinman L, Revicki DA, Flood E. Validation issues in questionnaires for diagnosis and monitoring of gastroesophageal reflux disease in children. Curr Gastroenterol Rep 2006;8(3):230–6.
26. Craig WR, Hanlon-Dearman A, Sinclair C, et al. Metoclopramide, thickened feedings, and positioning for gastro-oesophageal reflux in children under two years. Cochrane Database Syst Rev 2004;(4):CD003502.

Management of the Late Preterm Infant

Not Quite Ready for Prime Time

Michael J. Horgan, MD

KEYWORDS

- Late preterm • Near term • Respiratory immaturity • Feeding difficulties
- Hypoglycemia • Body temperature regulation

KEY POINTS

- Appropriate resources and personnel should be available to manage the late preterm infant.
- Late preterm infants are increasingly at risk for disorders of prematurity with decreasing gestational age.
- Parents, staff, and providers need to be aware that feeding problems are common and related to immaturity and gestational age.

DEFINITION

Late preterm or early term infants are those that are born between 34 0/7 to 36 6/7 weeks of gestation. The now accepted term is late preterm infant and is the result of a consensus workshop convened by the National Institute of Health in 2005.[1] This definition better reflects the problems and outcomes of infants born prior to term compared with the term infant.

EPIDEMIOLOGY

There has been a steady increase in the rate of preterm births in the United States over the last several decades. Preterm births account for approximately 12.5% of all births, and late preterm births account for 72% of the preterm births (**Fig. 1**).[2] This problem is not limited to the United States alone; emerging data suggest that the rate and number of preterm births are increasing in all races and in countries around the world.[3]

Disclosure: None.
Division of Neonatology, Department of Pediatrics, Children's Hospital at Albany Medical Center, Albany Medical College, MC-101, Albany, NY 12208, USA
E-mail address: horganm@mail.amc.edu

Pediatr Clin N Am 62 (2015) 439–451
http://dx.doi.org/10.1016/j.pcl.2014.11.007   pediatric.theclinics.com
0031-3955/15/$ – see front matter © 2015 Elsevier Inc. All rights reserved.

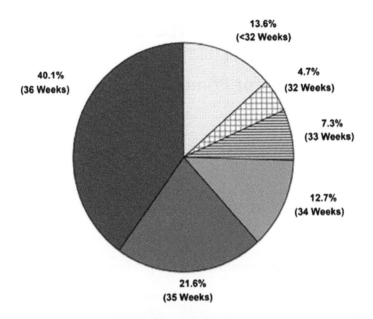

N= 394,996 Preterm Singletons

Fig. 1. Gestational age distribution of singleton premature births in the United States 2002. (*From* Davidoff MJ, Dias T, Damus K, et al. Changes in the gestational age distribution among U.S. singleton births: impact on rates of late preterm birth, 1992 to 2002. Semin Perinatol 2006;30(1):8–15; with permission.)

The reason for the increase in late preterm births is not clearly understood; however, several causes have been theorized. These include better risk assessment of maternal/fetal disorders, increase in elective inductions, increased elective caesarian sections, increasing maternal age, and increasing rates of multiple gestations (**Figs. 2** and **3**).[4] The increase in inductions and caesarean sections has been described as a significant factor in the downward shift in gestational age at birth. As a result, both the American Congress of Obstetricians and Gynecologists (ACOG) and the March of Dimes have begun campaigns to raise awareness in both patients and providers on the importance preventing nonindicated preterm deliveries ("No infant before 39 weeks and Healthy babies are worth the wait").[5] This effort appears to have stopped the increase in late preterm births and brought the late preterm birth percentage of all births back to 2003 levels (**Fig. 4**).

Multiple gestations have elevated the rates of late preterm births compared with singletons (**Fig. 5**). The increase in multiples is believed to be related to the delay in first pregnancies and the increased use of assisted reproductive technologies (ARTs).[6] The contribution of ART to multiples is approximately 50%, but the effect on national preterm birth rates is more limited.[6]

Maternal age plays a significant role in late preterm births, with the highest rates in women younger than 20 and older than 35 years of age (see **Fig. 3**). Maternal comorbidities are also age related, with hypertension, diabetes, and use of or need for ART being associated with advanced maternal age, and lower socioeconomic status and behavioral risk factors higher in the younger women.[4]

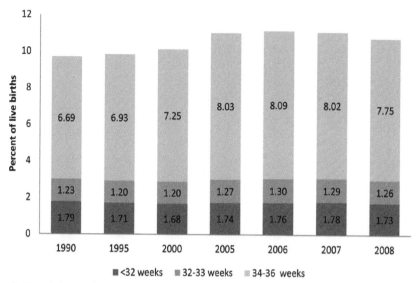

Fig. 2. Trends in singleton preterm birth rates, United States. Centers for Disease Control and Disease Prevention, National Center for Health Statistics 2011.

CONSEQUENCES OF LATE PRETERM BIRTH
Hospital Course

Neonatal intensive care unit admission

The incidence of neonatal intensive care unit (NICU) admission for the late preterm infants depends on gestational age, comorbidities, and each institution's organization of care (well baby, intermediate care, special care, and intensive care nurseries).[7] It has been estimated that 33% of NICU admissions each year are greater than 34 weeks of

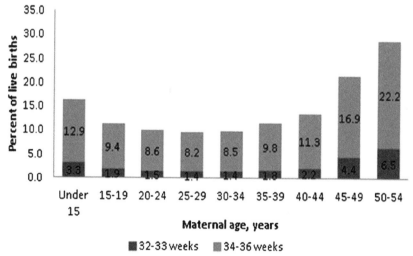

Fig. 3. Percent of live births born moderate and late preterm by maternal age. Centers for Disease Control and Prevention, National Center for Health Statistics 2011.

Percent of live births

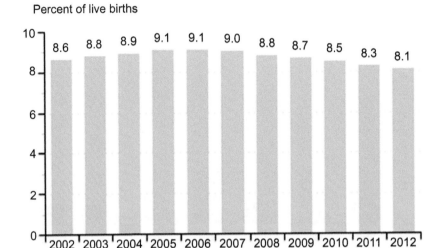

Fig. 4. Incidence of late preterm births: United States 2002–2012 National Center for Health Statistics 2012.

gestational age.[8] Infants born at 34 weeks gestation require NICU admission more than 50% of the time, with a decline in admission rates with increasing gestational age at birth (**Fig. 6**). Admission to the NICU should be for infants requiring supplemental heat, cardiorespiratory monitoring, care giver assessment of transition adaptation, and management of the complications of prematurity. Associated with the increased need for NICU admission is the increased overall morbidity and mortality associated with late preterm birth compared with term births (**Box 1** and **Table 1**). The appropriate placement of these late preterm infants should be according to specific admission criteria for each type of nursery. An understanding of the issues of prematurity in late preterm infants is essential to the determination of the resources needed to take care of these infants.

Percent of live births

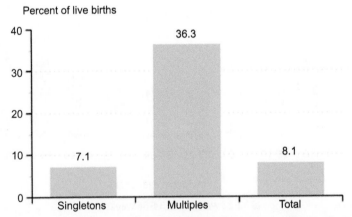

Fig. 5. Late preterm births by plurality: United States 2012. National Center for Health Statistics 2012.

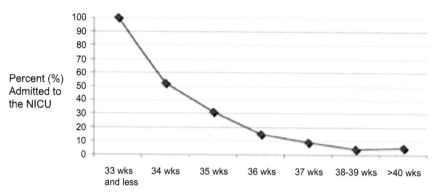

Fig. 6. Incidence of neonatal intensive care unit admission: late preterm versus term neonates. (*From* Pradeep VM, Bailey S, Hendricks-Munoz KD. Clinical issues in the management of late preterm infants. Curr Probl Pediatr Adolesc Health Care 2010;40:218–33; with permission.)

Hospital length of stay

A recent report suggests that 66% of the late preterm infants are discharged 4 or more days after birth. A report from Kaiser noted that the mean length of stay for a 34-week gestational age infant was 5.9 days compared with 1.8 days for term infants.[9] The increased length of stay is also associated with higher birth hospitalization costs compared with term infants (5–6 fold higher).

Respiratory

Respiratory distress syndrome/transient tachypnea of the newborn

Preterm infants are at higher risk for respiratory morbidities (respiratory distress syndrome [RDS] and transient tachypnea of the newborn [TTN]) than term infants. These diagnoses account for a significant portion of the reason that late preterm infants are admitted to the NICU.[10,11] Fetal lungs are filled with fluid, and that fluid must be absorbed. Traditional explanations such as vaginal squeezing and starling forces account for only some of the fluid reabsorption needed. Epithelial sodium channels (ENaCs) play a significant role in the transepithelial fluid movement in the lung (**Fig. 7**). ENaC expression is gestational age dependent, with the highest expression in term gestations.[12] Late preterm infants therefore have lower levels of ENaC expression, and this limits their ability to clear lung fluid at birth.

Birth in the absence of labor contributes to the pulmonary dysfunction seen in late preterm infants. Labor is associated with surges in steroids and catecholamine secretion, which is related to the maturation of the pulmonary system at birth. With the increase in caesarean deliveries in late preterm births and its depressive effect on neonatal pulmonary transition at birth, late preterm infants are at increased risk for acute respiratory issues in the immediate newborn period.

The incidence of respiratory distress increases with decreasing gestational age (**Fig. 8**). Recent studies report a eight- to nine-fold increase in respiratory distress occurring in late preterm infants compared with term infants (**Table 2**). Respiratory support is needed in 23% to 30% of late preterm infants, and 3% to 4% require some form of mechanical ventilation (**Fig. 9**).[13] Respiratory distress therefore is one of the most common adverse outcomes of late preterm infants. Recognition of the increased risk of respiratory compromise in late preterm births is an important factor in planning both the place and timing of their delivery (**Table 3**). Appropriate resources and personnel need to be available for the birth and during the initial hospitalization.

Box 1
Management of late preterm and early term infants: guidelines from a single institution

Admission criteria

Infants born at 35 weeks completed gestation or greater with a birth weight of at least 1800 g can be admitted to regular nursery.

Infants born at <35 weeks completed gestation or less than 1800 g will be admitted to the special care nursery.

Temperature regulation

Late preterm infants have a higher risk of hypothermia in the first days after birth.

Temperature maintenance is improved with use of a hat.

Temperature should be taken and recorded every hour for the first 6 hours after birth, then every 6 hours until discharge.

If the temperature is found to be <36.0°C, the infant should be swaddled, and a hat should be placed on the head. If at 30 minutes the temperature remains <36.0°C, the infant should be placed under a radiant warmer for rewarming. A second failure of maintaining temperature >36.0°C will necessitate transfer to the special care nursery.

Feeding

Late preterm infants are at a greater risk of poor feeding and subsequent dehydration during the first days after birth. Therefore, they require close observation and documentation of their feeding skills.

Intake and output should be recorded for all newborns. Weights should be recorded daily. Obtain special care nursery consultation for weight loss of greater than 3% daily or total of 7% of birth weight

At least 1 feeding every 12 hours for the first 2 days after birth should be observed by a trained caregiver to document feeding ability. If the infant is breast-feeding, a lactation specialist should observe the feeding for position, latch, and milk transfer.

If the infant is not capable of adequate feeding, consultation with the special care nursery staff is warranted before beginning a supplementation strategy.

Glycemic control

Late preterm infants born to mothers who are on medication for diabetes (type 1, type 2, or gestational) will follow the policy for infants of diabetic mothers.

Late preterm infants are at higher risk of hypoglycemia because of immature glycogenolysis, immature gluconeogenesis, and hormonal dysregulation.

Blood glucose levels should be checked at 1 hour after birth and every 4 hours until greater than 50 mg/dL twice consecutively.

If blood glucose levels are less than 50 mg/dL, refer to hypoglycemia protocol.

Jaundice

Late preterm infants are at higher risk of jaundice requiring intervention because of hepatic immaturity and potential feeding difficulties.

Transcutaneous bilirubin measurements should be obtained and documented daily. Refer to American Academy of Pediatrics guidelines on treatment of hyperbilirubinemia for the threshold for intervention.

Adapted from Engle WA. Morbidity and mortality in late preterm and early term newborns—a continuum. Clin Perinatol 2011;38:493–56; with permission.

Table 1
Neonatal mortality versus gestational age in a 2001 cohort from the United States

Weeks of Gestation	Neonatal Mortality per 1000 Live Births	
	Rate	Relative Risk (RR) (95% CI)
34	7.1	9.5 (8.4–10.8)
35	4.8	6.4 (5.6–7.2)
36	2.8	3.7 (3.3–4.2)
37	1.7	2.3 (2.1–2.6)
38	1.0	1.4 (1.3–1.5)
39	0.8	1.00 (reference)
40	0.8	1.0 (0.9–1.1)
41	0.8	1.1 (0.9–1.2)

Adapted from Engle WA. Morbidity and mortality in late preterm and early term newborns—a continuum. Clin Perinatol 2011;38:493–56; with permission.

Metabolic Concerns

Temperature regulation

Late preterm infants have decreased brown adipose tissue and the hormones necessary for its breakdown.[14] They are at increased risk for heat loss because of an increased body surface area to body weight ratio and decreased insulation from white adipose tissue. Hypothermia is one of the leading reasons for admission to the NICU.[15]

Cold stress

Cold stress is an important stressor that can potentially hinder a successful transition to the extrauterine environment. Late preterm infants are especially prone to cold stress because of their immature epidermal barrier, increased surface area to weight ratio and the more frequent need for interventions following delivery.[15] Cold stress can lead to poor respiratory transition and exacerbate hypoglycemia. Recognition of the increased risk of cold stress in late preterm infants following birth can lead to

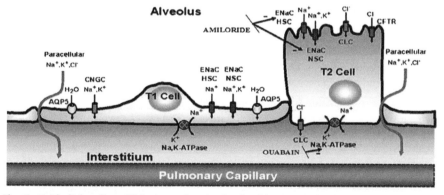

Fig. 7. Epithelial sodium (Na) absorption in the fetal lung near birth. CFTR, cystic fibrosis transmembrane conductance regulator; CLC, chloride channels; ENaC, epithelial Na channels; HSC, highly selective channels; NSC, nonselective channels. (*From* Jain L. Respiratory morbidity in late-preterm infants: prevention is better than cure! Am J Perinatol 2008;25:75–8; with permission.)

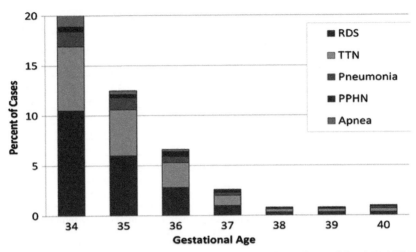

Fig. 8. Respiratory morbidity according to gestational age. (*Data from* Hibbard JU, Wilkins I, Sun L, et al. Consortium on safe labor, respiratory morbidity in late preterm births. JAMA 2010;304:419–25.)

prevention strategies such as plastic wrap, warm blankets, and skin-to-skin contact with the mother (even following caesarean deliveries).

Hypoglycemia

The incidence of hypoglycemia in late preterm infants is 2 to 3 times greater than that seen in term infants. Postnatal decreases in plasma glucose concentrations are much greater than those seen in term infants, implying a poor adaptation to extrauterine life.[8] Most late preterm infants who develop hypoglycemia require dextrose infusions to maintain normal plasma glucose concentrations.[11] The reason for the increased risk of hypoglycemia in late preterm infants is likely due to a delay in activity of hepatic glucose-6-phosphate coupled with poor enteral intake due to gastrointestinal imma-turity and poor suck–swallow coordination.

The increased risks for cold stress and hypoglycemia are not limited to the immedi-ate newborn but continue into the first 1 to 2 days of life. The presence of additional transitional problems, such as respiratory compromise, increases the likelihood that

Table 2	
Late preterm infants and neonatal morbidities	
Morbidity	**Late Preterm vs Term Infants**
Respiratory issues	Higher incidence of transient tachypnea of newborn, respiratory distress syndrome, pulmonary hypertension, and respiratory failure
Resuscitation at birth	Almost twice the chance of need for any resuscitation at birth
Jaundice	2–4 times likely to develop severe jaundice
Metabolic	Greater susceptibility to cold stress, more often requires phototherapy for jaundice, more likely to have feeding problems
Cognitive development	Higher risk for developmental delay and school readiness issues

Adapted from Mally PV, Bailey S, Hendricks-Muñoz KD. Clinical issues in the management of late preterm infants. Curr Probl Pediatr Adolesc Health Care 2010;40(9):218–33.

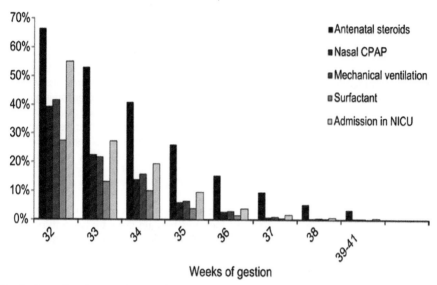

Fig. 9. Gestational age and rates of respiratory treatments and admission to neonatal intensive care unit. (*From* Gouyon JB, Iacobelli S, Ferdynus C, et al. Neonatal problems of late and moderate preterm infants. Semin Fetal Neonatal Med 2012;17(3):146–52; with permission.)

hypoglycemia may extend beyond the initial few hours of life. Standardized clinical management guidelines for the transitioning late preterm infant should address these issues. **Box 1** is an example of such a set of guidelines from a single institution.

Gastrointestinal and Feeding Maturation

Suck/swallow

Late preterm infants have a poor suck and swallow coordination because of neuronal immaturity and decreased tone overall but especially oromotor tone compared with term infants. This leads to improper latch-on for the breast-feeding infant and inadequate intake in the bottle-fed infant. Sucking, swallowing, and breathing must all be synchronized and coordinated to allow safe and efficient oral feeding. Feeding difficulties occur in 30% to 40% of late preterm infants and decrease with increasing

Table 3			
Risk of respiratory morbidities in late preterm and term neonates			
Diagnosis/Intervention	**Late Preterm (n = 138)**	**Term (n = 303)**	**Odds Ratio (95% Confidence Interval [CI])**
RDS	23%	4%	8.0 (3.9–16.5)
TTN	20%	15%	1.3 (0.8–2.2)
Nasal cannula	35%	31%	1.2 (0.8–1.9)
NCPAP	35%	6%	9.0 (4.9–16.4)
Ventilator	13%	3%	4.9 (2.1–11.2)
Surfactant	12%	0.3%	42.2 (5–322)

Adapted from Mally PV, Bailey S, Hendricks-Muñoz KD. Clinical issues in the management of late preterm infants. Curr Probl Pediatr Adolesc Health Care 2010;40(9):218–33.

gestational age (**Fig. 10**).[16] Using feeding readiness cues that are gestational age-derived will improve the feeding success of the late preterm infant (**Box 2**).

Gastrointestinal motility

Feeding intolerance is common in late preterm infants due because of several aspects of intestinal motor function. Suck–swallow incoordination as noted previously is not fully developed until after 34 weeks of gestation. Motility and gastric emptying maturation are also gestational age dependent. Deglutition, peristaltic function, and sphincter tone in the esophagus, stomach, and intestines are less mature compared with the term infant.[17,18] This may result in a significantly longer time period to achieve normal feeding patterns and a potential prolonged hospital stay and delayed discharge.

Hyperbilirubinemia

Jaundice in the late preterm infant results from an increased bilirubin load and decreased bilirubin elimination. The exaggerated hepatic immaturity contributes to the greater prevalence, severity, and duration of neonatal jaundice in the late preterm infant.[8] Hyperbilirubinemia in late preterm infants is often more prevalent, severe and prolonged than that observed in term infants. The suck–swallow immaturity noted previously also plays a role in the increased risk for hyperbilirubinemia. Inadequate breast milk intake resulting in varying degrees of dehydration can increase the enterohepatic circulation of bilirubin leading to an increased bilirubin load. One of the consequences of this increase in bilirubin load is an increased risk for developing bilirubin neurotoxicity or kernicterus.[19]

Breast-feeding issues

Breast-feeding the late preterm infant presents a significant challenge not found in term infants. Fewer awake periods, less stamina, and less efficient sucking all lead

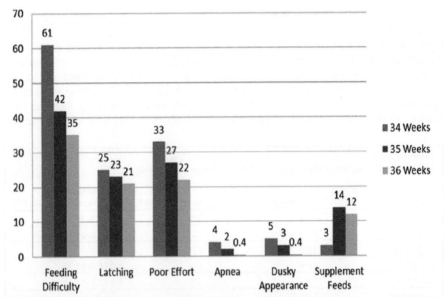

Fig. 10. Feeding difficulties by gestational age. (*From* Cooper BM, Holditch-Davis D, Verklan MT, et al. Newborn clinical outcomes of the AWHONN late preterm infant research-based practice project. J Obstet Gynecol Neonatal Nurs 2012;41:774–85; with permission.)

Box 2
Feeding issues for the late preterm infant

Feeding challenges

Late preterm neonates may have immature suck and swallow reflexes.

These infants may have altered sleep–wake cycles and decreased endurance, which can inhibit breast-feeding.

Inadequate nutritional intake is a risk factor for hypoglycemia.

Determine gestational age to assess risk for poor suck and swallow.

Obtain assistance of lactation consultant to assess infant's ability to latch; also discuss the benefits of breast-feeding and breast milk for preterm newborns.

Assess adequacy of feedings, including weight loss, dehydration, and hypoglycemia.

If the infant is stable, arrange for mother to initiate breast-feeding within the first hour of life, as well as unlimited skin-to-skin contact.

Teach mother early feeding cues.

Obtain blood glucose levels according to hospital guidelines.

Signs of feeding readiness and infant cues include alertness and rooting.

Parents must learn how to assess their infant's feeding adequacy.

Stress the importance of frequent follow-up with pediatrician or infant care provider after discharge.

Nursing, the lactation consultant, and the infant care provider should create a feeding plan for the late preterm neonate.

From Cleaveland K. Feeding challenges in the late preterm infant. Neonatal Network 2010;29(1):37–41; with permission.

---

to an inadequate job of stimulating and emptying the breast.[20] This results in poor milk production and an increased risk for inadequate nutrition. Poor feeding places these infants at increased risk for dehydration and delayed discharge. Parents and nurses may assume that when the late preterm infant falls asleep at the breast, they have ingested an adequate volume of milk. However, in reality, the infant may have exceeded his or her energy stores and stopped feeding well short of adequate caloric intake. There are few published guidelines addressing the specific problems with feeding late premature infants. Generally they are fed on the basis of institution protocols or prescribers' orders without any regard to the readiness of the infant. One such guideline from the Academy of Breastfeeding Medicine counsels parents and caregivers on the need to use the infant's cues in determining the need for and duration of breastfeeding.[21]

Central Nervous System Maturation

Brain development
Late preterm infants have many risks that are associated with less mature neuronal control compared with term infants. Brain development continues through gestation and beyond. There is, however, a critical period of brain growth that occurs in late gestation, which allows for the development of various neural structures and pathways. Nearly 50% of the increase in cortical volume occurs between 34 and 40 weeks (See Late Preterm Brain Development Card. Available at: www.marchofdimes.org),

and the growth is linear. The late preterm brain at 34 weeks of gestation weighs only 65% of the term infant's brain.[22] This immaturity of the late preterm brain and its rapid growth between 34 and 40 weeks underscores its vulnerability to the extrauterine environment. The volume of the cerebellum constitutes a larger relative percentage of the total brain volume with increasing gestational age. Approximately 25% of the cerebellum volume develops after the late term birth.[23] The late preterm period is one of proliferation and migration of the cerebellar granule cells. Impairments in blood flow during this time as the result of the problems associated with late preterm birth can lead to cerebellar injury and subsequent neurologic sequelae (cognitive, motor, and behavioral).[8]

SUMMARY

The numbers of late preterm births are increasing throughout the world and account for more than 70% of preterm births. Late preterm infants have increased risks for the development of respiratory morbidities including RDS and transient TTN. Due to their developmental immaturity, these infants are prone to disorders of adaptation–cold stress and hypoglycemia. Feeding difficulties present early, persist, and impact on the discharge readiness of the infant.

A comprehensive understanding of these issues by primary care providers (physicians and nurses) is essential in determining the resources necessary to care for this group of infants in whom the risks of significant morbidities are often overlooked. As many as 1 in 5 late preterm births can be avoided by implementing guidelines and strategies to limit the number of births less than 39 weeks gestation while maintaining a safe fetal, maternal, and neonatal environment. Families need to be involved in the discussion of the proper placement of the infants (NICU vs regular nursery), what adaption issues these infants may have, and the risks associated with late preterm birth. Just because these infants are born near term and admitted to a regular nursery does not mean that they act like term infants or have the risk of neonatal morbidities similar to those of infants born at term.

PRACTICE POINTS

- Appropriate resources and personnel should be available to manage the late preterm infant
- Late preterm infants are increasingly at risk for disorders of prematurity with decreasing gestational age
- An individualized approach to care (expecting different infants to respond differently)
- Standardized admission and initial evaluation guidelines based on gestational age and not birth weight
- Individual review of metabolic maturation should be used to maximize nutrient intake and weight gain
- Healthy late preterm infants should be fed using feeding readiness cues
- Parents, staff, and providers need to be aware that feeding problems are common and related to immaturity and gestational age

REFERENCES

1. Raju TN. The problem of late preterm (near term) births: a workshop summary. Pediatr Res 2006;60:775–6.

2. Martin JA, Hamilton BE, Sutton PD, et al. Births: final data for 2006. In: National vital statistics reports, vol. 57. Hyattsville (MD): National Center for Health Statistics; 2009. p. 1–8.
3. Ramachandrappa A, Jain L. Health issues of the late preterm infant. Pediatr Clin North Am 2009;56:565–77.
4. National Center for Health Statistics. Final natality data. 2012. Available at: http://www.marchofdimes.com/peristats. Accessed October 1, 2014.
5. March of Dimes. Healthy babies worth the wait. 2010. Available at: http://www.marchofdimes.com. Accessed October 1, 2014.
6. Lee YM, Cleary-Goldman J, D'Alton ME. Multiple gestations and late preterm deliveries. Semin Perinatol 2006;30:103–12.
7. Whyte RK. Neonatal management and safe discharge of late preterm infants. Semin Fetal Neonatal Med 2012;17:153–8.
8. Pradeep VM, Bailey S, Hendicks-Munoz KD. Clinical issues in the management of late preterm infants. Curr Probl Pediatr Adolesc Health Care 2010;40:218–33.
9. Darcy AE. Complications of the late preterm infant. J Perinat Neonatal Nurs 2009;23:78–86.
10. Colin AA, McEvoy C, Castle RG. Respiratory morbidity and lung function in preterm infants of 32-36 weeks gestational age. Pediatrics 2010;126:115–28.
11. Wang ML, Dorer DJ, Fleming MO, et al. Clinical outcomes of near-term infants. Pediatrics 2004;114:372–6.
12. Jain L. Respiratory morbidity in late-preterm infants: prevention is better than the cure. Am J Perinatol 2008;25:75–8.
13. Gilbert WM, Nesbitt TS, Danielsen B. The cost of prematurity: quantification by gestational age and birth weight. Obstet Gynecol 2003;102:488–92.
14. Sedin G. The thermal environment of the newborn infant. In: Martin JA, Fanaroff AA, Walsh MC, editors. Fanaroff and Martin's neonatal–perinatal medicine: diseases of the fetus and infant, vol. 1, 9th edition. Philadelphia: Mosby; 2011. p. 555–70.
15. Vachharajani AJ, Dawson JG. Short-term outcomes of late preterm infants. Clin Pediatr (Phila) 2009;48:383–8.
16. Cooper BM, Holditch-Davis D, Verklan MT, et al. Newborn clinical outcomes of the AWHONN late preterm infant research-based practice project. JOGN Nurs 2012;41:774–85.
17. Berseth CL. Gastrointestinal motility in the neonate. Clin Perinatol 1996;23:179–90.
18. Adamkin D. Feeding problems in the late preterm infant. Clin Perinatol 2006;33:831–7.
19. Newman TB, Escobar GJ, Gonzales VM, et al. Frequency of neonatal bilirubin testing and hyperbilirubinemia in a large health maintenance organization. Pediatrics 1999;104:1198–203.
20. Cleaveland K. Feeding challenges in the late preterm infant. Neonatal Netw 2010;29:37–41.
21. Academy of Breastfeeding Medicine. Protocol 10: breastfeeding the near term infant (35-37 weeks gestation). 2008. Available at: www.bfmed.org/resources/protocols.aspx. Accessed October 1, 2014.
22. Huppi PS, Warfield S, Kikinis R, et al. Quantitative MRI of brain development in premature and mature brain. Ann Neurol 1998;43:224–35.
23. Limperopoulos C, Soul JS, Gauvreau K, et al. Late gestation cerebellar growth is rapid and impeded by premature birth. Pediatrics 2005;115:685–95.

Neonatal Respiratory Distress

A Practical Approach to Its Diagnosis and Management

Arun K. Pramanik, MD[a],*, Nandeesh Rangaswamy, MD[b],
Thomas Gates, MD[a]

KEYWORDS

- Respiratory distress syndrome • Transient tachypnea of newborn
- Meconium aspiration syndrome • Bronchopulmonary disease
- Interstitial lung disease • Congenital lung disorders

KEY POINTS

- Respiratory disorders are the most frequent cause of admission to the special care nursery both in term and preterm infants.
- In critically ill infants or when the diagnosis in unclear, a neonatologist, cardiologist, pulmonologist, or ear, nose, and throat (ENT) surgeon must be promptly consulted.
- The need for referral to a tertiary perinatal-neonatal center for fetal intervention or early neonatal intervention, such as congenital diaphragmatic hernia, other congenital malformations, or delivery of very low-birth-weight (BW) infants is of paramount importance.

Respiratory disorders are the most frequent cause of admission to the special care nursery both in term and preterm infants. Pediatricians and primary care providers may encounter newborn infants with respiratory distress in their office, emergency room, delivery room, or during physical assessment in the newborn nursery. Often these infants may be in distress because of the failure of transition from fetal to extra-uterine environment due to retained lung fluid commonly seen in neonates born by cesarean delivery, being immature with relative surfactant deficiency, or having meconium aspiration syndrome (MAS).[1–4] In some instances, the cause of respiratory distress may pose a diagnostic challenge, especially in differentiating from cardiac diseases.[5] Significant advances have been made in fetal diagnosis, pathophysiology,

Disclosures: none.
[a] LSU Health, 1501 Kings Highway, Shreveport, LA 71130, USA; [b] University of Texas Southwestern, Dallas, TX, USA
* Corresponding author.
E-mail address: aprama1998@yahoo.com

and early management of these diseases.[6–8] Therefore, referral to a tertiary perinatal-neonatal center for fetal intervention or early neonatal intervention for congenital diaphragmatic hernia, other congenital malformations, or delivery of a very low-BW infant is of paramount importance.

In this article, the authors have proposed a practical approach to diagnose and manage such infants with suggestions for consulting a neonatologist at a regional center (**Box 1**). For an in-depth review, the reader is encouraged to preview a text on the subject.[9] The authors' objective is that practicing pediatricians should be able to asses and stabilize a newborn infant with respiratory distress, and transfer to or consult a neonatologist, cardiologist, or pulmonologist after reading this article.

PHYSIOLOGIC CHANGES AT BIRTH

Before birth, the lung is fluid filled, receiving less than 10% to 15% of the total cardiac output, and fetal oxygenation occurs by the placenta. The transition from intrauterine to extrauterine life requires establishment of effective pulmonary gas exchange.[2,10] This complex process entails rapid removal of fetal lung fluid controlled by ion transport across the airway and pulmonary epithelium with varying roles of catecholamines, glucocorticosteroids, and oxygen-regulating sodium uptake in alveolar fluid clearance.[10] During fetal life, the high pulmonary vascular resistance directs most of the blood from the right side of the heart through the ductus arteriosus into the aorta. At birth, clamping the umbilical vessels removes the low-resistance placental circuit with increase in systemic blood pressure and relaxation of the pulmonary vasculature.[2,10,11] Adequate expansion of the lungs and increase in Pao_2 values results in an 8- to 10-fold increase in pulmonary blood flow and constriction of the ductus arteriosus. The cardiopulmonary transition takes approximately 6 hours, resulting in rise in Pao_2 values and decrease in Pco_2 values as the intrapulmonary shunt decreases, and the functional residual capacity (FRC) after crying establishes adequate lung volume. Initially the respiratory pattern may be irregular but soon becomes rhythmic modulated by chemoreceptors and stretch receptors, with rates of 40 to 60 breaths per minute.[12] Respiratory distress is common in preterm infants because of poor respiratory drive, weak muscles, compliant chest wall, and surfactant deficiency.[3,9,12]

Clinical presentation involves tachypnea (rate>60 breaths per minute), cyanosis, expiratory grunting with chest retractions, and nasal flaring. The underlying disease may be due to pulmonary, cardiac, infectious, metabolic, or other systemic disorders. Peripheral cyanosis or acrocyanosis is often observed in normal newborn infants or in ill infants with poor cardiac output. Central cyanosis is assessed by examining the oral mucosa and suggests inadequate gas exchange signifying more than 3 to 5 g/dL of desaturated hemoglobin. Clinical determination of central cyanosis may be unreliable

---

Box 1
When to call a neonatologist for respiratory distress in an infant

- Inability to stabilize or ventilate infant, or requiring vasopressors
- Suspect cardiac disease
- Meconium aspiration with and without pulmonary hypertension
- Sepsis with pneumonia
- Pulmonary hemorrhage
- Pneumothorax or pneumomediastinum

(ie, not observed) in severely anemic patients despite low Pao_2 values; in contrast, polycythemic infants may appear cyanotic despite normal values of Pao_2. Hence, oxygen saturation measured by pulse oximetry (arterial oxygen saturation [Sao_2]) is recommended by the American Academy of Pediatrics to screen infants for hypoxemia, and Sao_2 values less than 90% after 15 minutes of age are considered abnormal.[11] Decrease in O_2 saturation, apnea, or both may be present in infants with respiratory distress.[5,11-13] Irregular (seesaw) or slow respiratory rates of less than 30 breaths per minute if associated with gasping may be an ominous sign.

Chest retractions occur because the neonatal chest wall is compliant making it susceptible to alterations in lung function resulting in substernal, subcostal, or intercostal retractions. The retractions result from negative intrapleural pressure generated by the contraction of diaphragm and accessory chest wall muscles along with impaired mechanical properties of the lungs and chest wall. Retractions are observed in lung parenchymal diseases such as respiratory distress syndrome (RDS), pneumonia, airway disorders, pneumothorax, atelectasis, or bronchopulmonary dysplasia (BPD).

Nasal flaring is caused by contraction of alae nasi muscles decreasing the resistance in the nares with resultant reduced work of breathing. Neonates primarily breathe through the nose, hence nasal resistance contributes significantly to total lung resistance, which occurs in choanal atresia or obstruction due to secretions. During resuscitation, suction of mouth is followed by suctioning the nose to prevent aspiration of secretions, blood, or meconium. Occasionally, nasal flaring is observed during feeding or active sleep in normal infants.

Grunting is a compensatory effort made during expiration by closure of the glottis, increasing the airway pressure and lung volume with resultant increased ventilation perfusion (V/Q) ratio. Unlike normal breathing, wherein the vocal cords abduct to enhance inspiratory flow, expiration through partially closed vocal cords in some respiratory disorders produces a grunting sound. Depending on the severity of lung disease, grunting may be either intermittent or continuous. Grunting can maintain FRC and values of Pao_2 equivalent to those during the application of 2 or 3 cm H_2O of continuous distending pressure.

Accessory respiratory muscles also assist in optimizing upper airway functions. The genioglossus muscle protrudes the tongue and maintains pharyngeal patency, whereas the laryngeal muscles move the vocal cords regulating airflow during expiration.

Assessing a Neonate with Respiratory Distress

It is not surprising that incomplete cardiopulmonary transition results in respiratory distress with approximately 10% of neonates requiring respiratory support immediately after delivery and up to 1% requiring intensive resuscitation.[11] Therefore, the American Heart Association and the American Academy of Pediatrics recommend that the personnel attending to the newborn in the delivery room should be Neonatal Resuscitation Program (NRP) certified.[11] The cause of respiratory distress can be either pulmonary or nonpulmonary in origin.

The initial approach in assessing an infant with respiratory distress involves physical examination and rapid assessment to identify any life-threatening conditions such as tension pneumothorax, chylothorax, congenital diaphragmatic hernia, or upper airway anomalies. Infants with significant respiratory distress and hypoxia should be initially stabilized. When attending a high-risk delivery, antenatal history of oligohydramnios suggests hypoplastic lungs, whereas polyhydramnios may be present in infants with tracheoesophageal fistula (TEF). Infants of diabetic mothers are at risk for RDS, transient tachypnea of newborn (TTN), or cardiac anomalies causing respiratory distress; fetus in distress with meconium-stained amniotic fluid are at risk for developing meconium aspiration pneumonia, pneumothorax, and persistent pulmonary hypertension (**Box 2**). History of chorioamnionitis may give a clue to the infant developing pneumonia or sepsis. Repeating physical examinations after initial stabilization for temperature instability with worsening clinical status suggests infection; tachycardia may indicate sepsis or hypovolemia. Stridor is often associated with upper airway obstruction. A scaphoid abdomen with bowel sounds auscultated in the left side of chest indicates congenital diaphragmatic hernia. Asymmetric breath sounds suggest tension pneumothorax or inadvertent placement of endotracheal tube in the main stem bronchus.

DIFFERENTIAL DIAGNOSIS

Breathing occurs because of movement of air in and out of the lungs. Impairment of airflow because of disease states leads to respiratory distress (**Box 3**). However, it is important to remember that parenchymal lung disease may also lead to obstruction as seen in pneumonia, where the obstruction of airways can be due to increased secretions requiring suctioning. The signs and symptoms of airway obstruction in the neonates are characteristic of the site. Irrespective of the cause of the obstruction, respiratory distress results in hypoventilation with an increase in the Pco_2 value and a decrease in the Po_2 value. Differentiation from congenital cyanotic heart disease can be challenging. By placing the infant on fraction of inspired oxygen (Fio_2) equal to 1.0 (hyperoxia test), in lung diseases the Pao_2 value usually increases over 150 torr, whereas in cyanotic congenital heart disease, it is below 120 torr. If the patient has ductal-dependent cyanotic heart disease, intravenous prostaglandin may have to be administered to keep the ductus arteriosus patent and the patient has to be transferred to a tertiary center (preferably where a cardiac surgery can be performed) to confirm the diagnosis by echocardiogram and manage the cardiac diseases.

UPPER AIRWAY ANOMALIES

Some neonates diagnosed with choanal atresia may require consultation from a geneticist to rule out anomalies, such as CHARGE (Coloboma, Heart defect, Atresia choanae, Retarded growth and development, Genital abnormality and Ear

---

Box 2
Maternal history giving a clue to neonatal respiratory distress

- Diabetes mellitus: RDS, cardiomyopathy, CHD, hypoglycemia, polycythemia
- Polyhdramnios: tracheoesophageal fistula
- Oligohydramnios: hypoplastic lungs
- Drug withdrawal
- Anesthesia causing neonatal depression
- Antepartum hemorrhage: anemia
- Meconium-stained amniotic fluid: aspiration syndrome
- Hydrops fetalis: pleural effusion
- Premature labor: RDS
- PROM and chorioamnionitis: pneumonia, sepsis

Abbreviations: CHD, congenital heart disease; PROM, prolonged rupture of membranes.

> **Box 3**
> **Differential diagnosis of respiratory distress in the newborn**
>
> - Upper airway obstruction: choanal atresia, nasal stenosis, nasal stuffiness (? congenital syphilis), Pierre Robin anomaly, cleft palate, glossoptosis, laryngeal stenosis or atresia, hemangioma, vocal cord paralysis, vascular rings, tracheobronchial stenosis, cystic hygroma.
> - Pulmonary diseases
>   a. Congenital: hypoplasia, congenital diaphragmatic hernia, chylothorax, pulmonary sequestration, congenital cystic adenomatous malformation of lung, arteriovenous malformation, congenital lobar emphysema, congenital alveolar proteinosis.
>   b. Acquired: TTN, RDS, aspiration pneumonia, other pneumonia (bacterial, viral, fungal, syphilis), air leak syndrome (pneumothorax, pneumomediastinum), atelectasis, hemorrhage, BPD, PPHN, diaphragmatic paralysis.
> - Chest wall deformities: asphyxiating thoracic dystrophy.
> - Cardiac diseases: cyanotic and acyanotic heart diseases, congestive heart failure, cardiomyopathies, pneumopericardium.
> - Metabolic: hypoglycemia, inborn errors of metabolism.
> - Hematologic: polycythemia, severe anemia, hypovolemia.
> - Neuromuscular diseases: hypoxic-ischemic encephalopathy, hemorrhage, hydrocephalus, seizure, narcotic withdrawal, muscle and spinal cord disorders.
> - Miscellaneous: asphyxia, acidosis, hypothermia or hyperthermia.
>
> *Abbreviation:* PPHN, persistent pulmonary hypertension of the newborn.

abnormality) association. Regardless of the cause of obstruction, establishing a secure airway is paramount. In the absence of underlying lung disease or laryngotracheal abnormalities, placement of an oral airway may be sufficient, along with supplemental oxygen. Alternatively, oral endotracheal intubation with ventilator support may be required. In any infant with airway obstruction, failure to maintain adequate ventilation and/or oxygenation with an endotracheal tube in place may signify progressive pulmonary disease, hence neonatology consultation should be obtained (see **Box 1**). Although the larynx is the most common site of stridor, neonates with supraglottic or glottis laryngeal abnormalities often present with a combination of problems involving respiration, phonation, and/or deglutition. The clinical presentation of the abnormalities is variable and includes stridor, abnormal cry, snorting during sleep, retractions and coarse inspiration. These symptoms could be due to laryngomalacia, cysts, hemangioma, stenosis, stricture due to prolonged intubation in premature infants, or laryngeal web. In severe cases, suprasternal and intercostal retractions may be seen. Aspiration may occur, and feeding may be difficult in patients with a mass lesion or severe obstruction. Laryngomalacia is the most frequent cause of stridor and often worsens in the supine position, with feeding, or due to agitation. Rarely, laryngospasm may occur secondary to gastroesophageal reflux disease (GERD), sometimes leading to apnea, bradycardia, or desaturation, and it should be considered when the cause of obstruction is obscure.[3,14] In addition, GERD has been identified frequently in patients with apnea, chronic cough, laryngomalacia, recurrent croup, and subglottic stenosis, although 1 study did not find a temporal relationship between gastroesophageal reflux and apnea of prematurity.[14] Examination of the oropharynx may reveal macroglossia, glossoptosis, retrognathia, cleft palate (Pierre Robin anomaly), or cyst. Flexible endoscopy may be required to diagnose lingual thyroid, dermoid, hemangiomas, or lymphangioma. Computed tomography (CT) or magnetic resonance imaging has been used to confirm the diagnosis of complex upper airway anomalies in some patients. If no obvious anatomic abnormality can be identified by examination, video fluoroscopy may be used to diagnose glossoptosis, pharyngeal wall collapse, or laryngomalacia. All infants should have cardiorespiratory monitoring including pulse oxymetry. Tracheobronchial abnormalities causing respiratory distress in the neonates include tracheal rings, tracheomalacia, tracheal stenosis, hemangioma, and tracheo-esophaeal fistula. The clinical presentation of these abnormalities may be expiratory stridor, wheezing, or brassy cough. Anterolateral radiograph of the chest and barium esophagogram may be used for diagnosis in addition to endoscopy. Endotracheal intubation with assisted ventilation is used in severe cases to stabilize them. A pediatric ENT surgeon should be consulted if upper airway disease is suspected, and the parents should be informed that severe cases may require tracheostomy.

Transient Tachypnea of Neonate

This condition occurs in near-term, term, or late preterm infants, affecting 3.6 to 5.7 per 1000 term infants and up to 10 per 1000 preterm infants. Risk factors include cesarean delivery, and it may occur in mothers with diabetes, asthma, prolonged labor, and fetal distress requiring anesthesia or analgesia. Clinical presentation is rapid shallow breathing with occasional grunting and rarely respiratory failure.[1,15,16] Arterial blood gases show varying degrees of hypoxemia with normocarbia or hypercarbia. The chest radiograph shows perihilar streaking, patchy infiltrates, increased interstitial markings, and fluid in interlobar fissures (**Fig. 1**). It can be difficult to differentiate TTN from neonatal pneumonia or meconium aspiration in the presence of risk factors for these disorders. There may be a wet silhouette around the heart as well as signs of alveolar edema.[17] Treatment of TTN is supportive.[1,15,16] However, a definitive diagnosis of TTN is usually made on retrospection once the symptoms resolve within 1 to 5 days after minimal therapeutic intervention. Hence, it takes time to differentiate TTN from other causes of neonatal respiratory distress. Until then, the overall management of the neonates with respiratory distress should cover all the diagnostic possibilities. The disorder usually responds to oxygen therapy, but maintaining appropriate oxygen saturation may require continuous positive airway pressure (CPAP), which increases the distending pressure of the alveoli and aids the absorption of the extra lung fluid. Very rarely is mechanical ventilation necessary.[14]

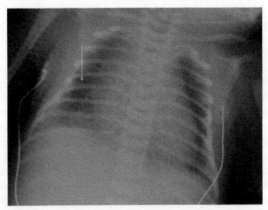

Fig. 1. Radiograph of chest showing transient tachypnea of newborn; note patchy densities and fluid in the horizontal fissure (*arrow*).

Although TTN is a common pathologic diagnosis designated to the neonates presenting with respiratory distress due to delayed clearance of fetal lung fluid, these neonates almost invariably show complete recovery with no long-term sequelae.[15] Differential diagnosis includes pneumonia and cerebral hyperventilation in patients with perinatal asphyxia. The neonates are tachypneic without changes in chest radiograph apart from mild cardiomegaly related to asphyxia.

Pneumonia

Pneumonia is a significant cause of respiratory distress in newborns and may be classified as either early-onset ($\leq$7 days of age) or late-onset pneumonia (>7 days of age). The routes of acquiring infection and the pathogens commonly associated with them are listed in **Table 1**.

Congenital pneumonia is a severe disease that frequently results in either stillbirth or death within the first 24 hours after birth. Signs typically present in the first several hours after birth unless the pneumonia is acquired postnatally.[1,9] Pneumonias that are acquired later present most often as systemic disease.[9] The clinical signs in neonatal pneumonia mimic other conditions like TTN, RDS, or MAS, thus making it difficult to distinguish from them. Nonrespiratory signs and symptoms may include lethargy, poor feeding, jaundice, apnea, and temperature instability. If pneumonia is suspected, initial screening tests, including complete blood cell with differential count and blood culture, should be obtained before beginning antibiotic therapy. Ampicillin and gentamicin, or amikacin, are the antibiotics used most frequently in the neonatal period for treating infection. Findings from chest radiograph are variable, depending on the cause.[17] In utero infection typically manifests as bilateral consolidation or whiteout. Other pneumonias can manifest as lobar consolidations on chest radiograph (**Fig. 2**). It should be borne in mind that 50% of infants who have group B beta Streptococcus pneumonia have radiographic findings indistinguishable from those of RDS or TTN.[17] When present, pleural effusion or mild heart enlargement in the absence of cardiac anomalies suggests the diagnosis of pneumonia. Treatment of pneumonia focuses on supportive care of the infant and administration of antibiotic medications that target the causative organism. Oxygen therapy, mechanical ventilation, and vasopressor administration may be necessary. Oxygen should be used to maintain saturations in the normal ranges for gestational age.

Table 1
Modes of transmission and the pathogens causing neonatal pneumonia

Intrauterine	Perinatal	Postnatal
Rubella	Group B streptococcus	Respiratory viruses
Herpes simplex virus	Escherichia coli	(adenovirus, respiratory
Cytomegalovirus	Klebsiella	syncytial virus)
Adenovirus	Syphilis	Gram-positive bacteria (Groups
Mumps	Neisseria gonorrhoeae	A, B, and G streptococci or
Toxoplasma gondii	Chlamydia trachomatis	Staphylococcus aureus)
Varicella zoster virus	(usually occurs for >2 wk)	Gram-negative enteric bacteria
Treponema pallidum		(Klebsiella, Proteus,
Mycobacterium tuberculosis		Pseudomonas aeruginosa,
Listeria monocytogenes		flavobacteria, Serratia
Human immunodeficiency		marcescens, and E coli)
virus		

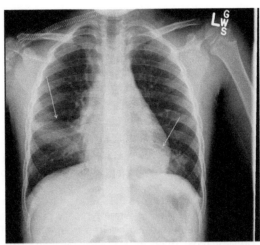

Fig. 2. Radiograph of chest showing pneumonia of right middle lobe and left lower lobe (*arrows*).

Respiratory Distress Syndrome

RDS is seen soon after birth and worsens over the next few hours. RDS is commonly seen in premature infants and occurs because of surfactant deficiency. The risk of RDS increases with decreasing gestational age with approximately 5% of near-term infants affected, 30% of infants of gestational age less than 30 weeks affected, and 60% of premature infants of gestational age less than 28 weeks affected.[3,9,18] Surfactant is a complex mixture of 6 phospholipids and 4 apoproteins produced by the type II pneumocytes in the lung epithelium. Functionally, dipalmitoyl phosphocholine or lecithin is the principal phospholipid, which along with surfactant protein A and B lowers the surface tension at the air-liquid interface in vivo.[3,9,18] With decrease in surfactant or its function, alveolar surface tension increases and collapses at the end of expiration. The disease progresses rapidly with increase in work of breathing, intrapulmonary shunting, V/Q mismatch, and hypoxia with eventual respiratory failure. Factors contributing to RDS are male sex in Caucasians, infants of mothers with diabetes, perinatal asphyxia, hypothermia and multiple gestations, born via cesarean delivery without labor, or presence of RDS in a previous sibling.

On physical examination, infants have grunting, retraction, cyanosis, and tachypnea. Radiograph of the chest shows reticulogranular appearance, air bronchogram, or ground glass appearance of the lungs because of microatelectasis and poor expansion (**Fig. 3**). Arterial blood gases show respiratory acidosis, hypoxia, and eventually metabolic acidosis. Mothers with extremely premature infants should be managed at a perinatal center if not in labor. Amniocentesis should be performed to assess lung maturity for elective cesarean delivery and in mothers with diabetes. Management involves antenatal corticosteroids to increase fetal lung maturity, preventing preterm labor with use of tocolytic agents, and use of antibiotics for chorioamnionitis.[19] At birth, after resuscitation by skilled personnel, avoiding hypothermia and stabilizing the infant, intratracheal surfactant is administered.[11] Babies that do not have significant chest retraction and require Fio_2 values less than 40% may be placed on nasal CPAP of 6 to 7 cm H_2O. If infant has labored breathing, assisted ventilation is provided. Surfactant is administered via endotracheal tube, umbilical vessels are catheterized, and the ventilator and Fio_2 values are adjusted to keep the pH between

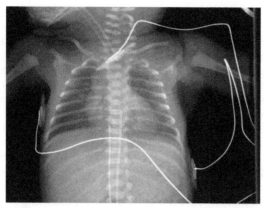

Fig. 3. Radiograph of chest showing respiratory distress syndrome. Note diffuse granularity of lung fields, air bronchogram, and decreased lung volume.

7.25 and 7.40, Pao_2 value between 50 and 70 torr, Pco_2 value at 45 to 65 torr, and base deficit less than 10.[3,9,18,20,21] Studies comparing use of various types of surfactant preparations, timing of administration, and various modalities of ventilation are discussed in several publications.[3,9,17,19,20] Care should be taken to optimize V/Q by using minimally invasive ventilation and optimal positive end-expiratory pressure. Supportive therapy involves maintaining fluid and electrolyte balance and avoiding hypoglycemia and hypothermia.[3,9,18,20] Blood cultures are obtained along with total white blood cell and differential count along with C-reactive protein estimation. Antibiotics (ampicillin and gentamicin or amikacin) are administered and withdrawn after 48 hours if the infant is stable. Nutrition is provided and trophic feeding commenced as soon as possible, preferably using mother's milk. Blood gases and chest radiographs are repeated as clinically indicated. The neonatal intensive care unit (NICU) staff should encourage maternal-infant bonding and family support.

Complications seen early in the course of RDS are air leaks, apnea, intraventricular hemorrhages, anemia, hypoglycemia, hypernatremia, patent ductus arteriosus, necrotizing enterocolitis, as well as renal and growth failure.[9,22,23] Outcome is improved by avoiding complications.

Late complications include gastroesophageal reflux, feeding intolerance, growth failure, apnea, sudden death, BPD, as well as developmental and neurologic deficits including visual and auditory handicaps.[14,22] After discharge, they are followed up by a team composed of developmental pediatrician, nutritionists, social worker, physical therapist, and other medical and surgical consultants.[9,18,24]

Meconium Aspiration Syndrome

Most infants born to mothers with meconium-stained amniotic fluid are asymptomatic. MAS occurs in term or postterm infants born through meconium-stained amniotic fluid; these infants have in utero hypoxia and are at increased risk for respiratory distress.[1,4,15] Although meconium-stained amniotic fluid occurs in 10% to 15% of deliveries, MAS is seen in 4% to 5% of them. Passage of meconium in utero is a sign of fetal distress occurring because of relaxation of anal sphincter. The resultant hypoxia and gasping breathing leads to aspiration of meconium before birth. Maternal risk factors include preeclampsia, diabetes, chorioamnionitis, and illicit substance abuse. Evidence suggests that patients with severe MAS have chronic in utero hypoxia. Severe MAS is associated with alterations in the pulmonary vasculature, including remodeling and thickening of the muscle walls. This process results in pulmonary vascular hyperreactivity, vasoconstriction, and high resistance and pressure. Meconium consists of desquamated cells from the gastrointestinal tract, skin, lanugo, hair, bile salts, pancreatic enzymes, lipids, mucopolysaccharides, and water. Chemical pneumonitis occurs from the bile salts and other components deactivating pulmonary surfactant. This phenomenon along with particulate matter in the meconium results in atelectasis. Meconium also activates the complement cascade, which leads to inflammation and constriction of pulmonary veins.

Infants with MAS develop respiratory distress within a few hours of birth. On clinical examination, they may have staining of nails and umbilical cord, barrel-shaped chest on inspection, and signs of respiratory distress along with crackles (rales) and rhonchi on auscultation.[4] The chest radiographic findings are variable and are composed of patchy atelectasis due to terminal airway obstruction, areas of overinflation due to air trapping; in severe cases, widespread involvement of all lung fields are seen with whiteout lung fields (**Fig. 4**).[17] There may also be evidence of air leak, such as pneumothorax, pneumomediastinum, or interstitial or subcutaneous air (**Fig. 5**). The last of these is uncommon because of improved resuscitation techniques at birth.

Management: Although in the past amnioinfusion and suctioning of oropharynx before delivery at birth was practiced widely, it has been abandoned because meta-analysis of randomized controlled studies did not show their benefit. At present, the *Neonatal Resuscitation Textbook* of the American Academy of Pediatrics recommends to suction the trachea after intubation only in apneic infants, even though no controlled studies have confirmed its benefit. It is recommended that if there is no meconium after 1 attempt to suction the trachea in apneic infants, they should be intubated, ventilated, oxygenated, and stabilized immediately.[4] If the infant is vigorous as defined by strong respiratory effort, heart rate greater than 100 beats per minute, and good muscle tone, bulb syringe suctioning should be done, followed by standard procedures described in the NRP manual. Cord blood gases should be obtained to determine the degree of acidosis, and if the pulse oximeter shows Sao_2 values less than 90% after 10 minutes, arterial blood gases should be obtained, particularly if the infant requires resuscitation. Management in most patients is supportive. Infants who develop respiratory distress should be admitted to the NICU. Oxygen therapy may be delivered via oxygen hood, and arterial blood gases are monitored after placing umbilical vessel catheters. CPAP at 5 to 6 cm of H_2O should be provided if oxygen requirement exceeds 0.4 to 0.5.[4,25] In patients with respiratory acidosis, assisted

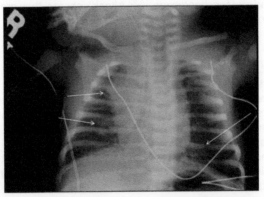

Fig. 4. Radiograph of chest showing meconium aspiration syndrome; note bilateral patchy infiltrates (*arrows*).

A   **B**

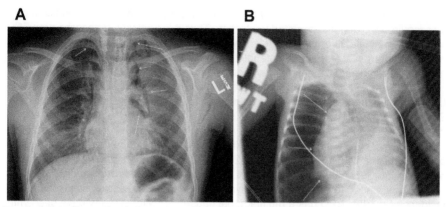

Fig. 5. (A) Radiograph of chest showing pneumomediastinum borders shown by arrows. Note thymic silhouette. (B) Radiograph of chest showing tension pneumothorax (arrows). Marked collapse of the right lung with large lucency peripherally. Depression of the right hemidiaphragm and shift of the cardiothymic silhouette to the left.

ventilation may be required to maintain pH between 7.3 and 7.5, Pco_2 values at 30 to 50 torr, and Pao_2 values above 100 torr.[4] Infants developing severe MAS should be cared for at a tertiary center with the ability to administer surfactant, high-frequency ventilation, inhaled nitric oxide (iNO), and extracorporeal membrane oxygenation (ECMO), because of their predilection to suddenly develop hypoxia due to their labile pulmonary vasculature. Surfactant therapy should be administered cautiously in infants and requires moderately high settings and oxygen on conventional ventilator because the surfactant is inactivated by the aspirated meconium, and this is considered a standard therapy. Recent studies have suggested that early use of high-frequency ventilation to optimize V/Q along with early use iNO therapy may decrease the use of ECMO and improve outcome.[4] These infants should be followed up longitudinally, and despite appropriate interventions, they may have sequelae, such as learning disability or neurodevelopmental or hearing handicaps due to perinatal asphyxia and their NICU course, hence, should be followed up.[4,24]

Bronchopulmonary Dysplasia

BPD develops in low-birth-weight infants weighing less than 1500 g, particularly those weighing less than 1000 g. In 2001, a National Institutes of Health workshop developed a consensus on definition of BPD based on gestational age at birth, time of assessment, and severity of disease.[26]

In 1967, Northway and his colleagues described BPD classifying it into 4 stages in infants with RDS. The form that occurs in neonates receiving high inspired oxygen and developing ventilator-induced injury is termed old or classical BPD and is rarely seen these days. With the use of antenatal steroid, surfactant therapy, caffeine therapy, and gentler modes of ventilation as the new standard of care for RDS, smaller infants who survive develop a milder form of BPD that is termed by Jobe as new BPD, and this is associated with disruption of lung development, specifically an arrest of alveolar septation and vascular development in the distal part of the lung and impaired pulmonary function in later years of life.[3,9,26–29] Some extremely preterm infants develop lung disease after an initial period without oxygen or mechanical ventilation, and this form has been labeled as chronic lung disease (CLD) of prematurity. CLD is similar to what Dr Peter Auld described as "chronic pulmonary insufficiency of prematurity," which usually developed after the second week of life in premature infants after apnea and/or bradycardia for which the infant required oxygen and assisted ventilation. Thus it is unclear whether the new BPD represents a single different disease entity or is a group of entities with complex epigenetic, environmental (especially antenatal and postnatal infections), and inflammatory-mediated dysregulation of lung maturation or other factors.

The incidence of BPD varies with gestational age, respiratory illness severity, duration of oxygen, and ventilator support requirement, the Fio_2 value required to maintain Sao_2 value greater than 90%. In a 2007 study by Fanaroff and colleagues,[9] the incidence of BPD when defined as oxygen requirement at 28 days was 42% (BW 501–750 g), 25% (BW 751–1000 g), and 11% (BW 1251–1500 g), respectively, with majority occurring in infants with BW less than 1250 g. Application of a definition to asses the adequacy of oxygenation and ventilation at 36 weeks postmenstrual age and the level of the infant's need for supplemental oxygen and/or ventilator assistance reduces the incidence by 10%. BPD has a multifactorial cause.[26–29] Within a few days of premature birth, inflammatory biomarkers (chemokines, adhesion molecules, proinflammatory and antiinflammatory cytokines, proteases, and growth factors) have complex interactions that alter subsequent lung maturation. An imbalance between proinflammatory and antiinflammatory cytokines released because of various factors leads to apoptosis in the lung with varying degrees of repair. This condition leads to impaired alveolaraization and angiogenesis, which lead to larger, more simplified alveoli and a dysmorphic pulmonary vasculature, the pathologic hallmark of BPD.[26] The multifactorial insults to the developing lung include intrauterine and postnatal infections, inflammation in the immature lung, effects of resuscitation techniques, patent ductus arteriosus, as well as ventilator- and oxygen-induced injury. Inadequate nutrition may also impair alveolar development and surfactant production and inhibit lung growth and repair.[22] The uneven damage to the airways and lungs results in marked V/Q mismatch. Bronchomalacia increases airway resistance because of inflammation and partial collapse of small and large airways during expiration. Lung compliance is also reduced secondary to edema and fibrosis.[28–30] As the disease progresses, atelectasis with areas of hyperinflation are seen on chest radiograph (**Fig. 6**).

Management includes judicious use of oxygen to maintain Sao_2 value between 90% and 94%, use of noninvasive ventilation to minimize further pressure-induced lung

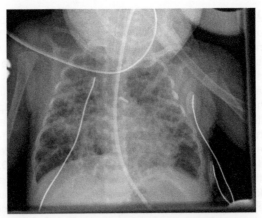

Fig. 6. Radiograph of chest showing bronchopulmonary dysplasia with hyperexpanded lung fields with cystic areas showing air trapping. Note clip showing ligation of patent ductus arteriosus.

damage, and fluid restriction.[26–29] Some patients may transiently respond to diuretics, bronchodilators, and inhaled steroids, hence their prolonged use is not recommended.[28,31] Adequate nutrition with micronutrients and macronutrients is essential to optimize lung and somatic growth and should be monitored closely.[22] Patients with severe BPD are at risk of developing pulmonary hypertension diagnosed by echocardiogram in consultation with cardiologist. These patients are at risk of sudden death because of pulmonary hypertension or bronchospasm. Use of iNO to prevent BPD has not been validated across clinical trials. Oral slidenifil has been used in some studies to treat pulmonary hypertension; its response is variable perhaps because of inconsistent absorption.[28] Before discharge from the NICU, careful planning should be done.[24] Home environment should be checked because there is an increased chance of rehospitalization (up to 50%) in them. If the infant is discharged on oxygen and receives medications or feeding via gastrostomy tube, parents should room-in and learn how to administer medications and feeds under nursing supervision. Use of home oxygen and ventilator should be coordinated by specially trained staff and home health services conversant with care of infants with BPD.[24] All immunizations should be up to date before discharge. The respiratory syncytial virus (RSV) prophylaxis is recommended within 6 months of the RSV season for all infants younger than 2 years. Influenza vaccine is administered to all care providers, siblings, and infants with BPD older than 6 months. Parents should be counseled to avoid second-hand smoke, to keep people with cold away from the infant, and to not take these infants to day care facility. Growth and nutrition should be monitored. Some infants have gastroesophageal reflux requiring therapy. Respiratory symptoms may persist beyond infancy into childhood. Patients with BPD may have delayed development, learning disorders, and neurologic problems.[28–30] Hence it is important for the pediatrician to work with subspecialist and community support agencies to help the family. Although most patients with BPD do well, patients with severe disease develop worsening respiratory failure, pulmonary hypertension, and cor pulmonale requiring repeated hospitalization in the intensive care unit, which may prolong suffering and death. Hence, end-of-life care should be discussed with parents including withdrawing assisted ventilation.

Interstitial Lung Disease

On rare occasions, neonates and infants have other chronic respiratory disorders. This category encompasses a group of diseases called childhood interstitial lung diseases (chILDs) or diffuse lung disease (DLD).[32] The American Thoracic Society has published an official clinical practice guideline for classification, evaluation, and management of childhood interstitial lung disease in infancy.[33] Causes include surfactant function abnormalities, persistent tachypnea of infancy or neuroendocrine cell hyperplasia of infancy, alveolar capillary dysplasia associated with misalignment of pulmonary veins, and pulmonary interstitial glycogenosis (**Box 4, Fig. 7**).

All neonates and infants (<2 years of age) with DLD should have common diseases excluded, which include GERD, cystic fibrosis, congenital or acquired immune deficiency, congenital heart disease, BPD, pulmonary infection, H-type TEF, primary ciliary dyskinesia presenting with newborn respiratory distress, and recurrent aspiration. After they have been eliminated, a neonate or infant with DLD is regarded as having chILD syndrome if at least 3 of the following are present: (1) respiratory symptoms (cough, rapid and difficult breathing, or exercise intolerance), (2) respiratory signs (tachypnea, rales, retractions, digital clubbing, failure to thrive, or respiratory failure), (3) hypoxemia, and (4) diffuse abnormalities on a chest radiograph or CT. Newborns who present with chILD syndrome and severe disease, or family history of adult or

> **Box 4**
> **Disorders causing severe neonatal childhood interstitial lung disease syndrome**
>
> - Acinar dysplasia
> - Pulmonary hypoplasia/alveolar simplification
> - Alveolar capillary dysplasia with misalignment of the pulmonary veins (*FOXF1* mutations)
> - PIG
> - Surfactant protein B deficiency (homozygous *SFTPB* mutations) *ABCA3* gene mutations
> - TTF-1 *(NKX2.1)* mutations
> - Pulmonary hemorrhage syndromes
> - Pulmonary lymphangiectasia
>
> *Abbreviations:* PIG, pulmonary interstitial glycogenosis; TTF, thyroid transcription factor.
>   *Data from* Kurland G, Deterding RR, Hagood JS, et al. An official American Thoracic Society clinical practice guideline: classification, evaluation, and management of childhood interstitial lung disease in infancy. Am J Respir Crit Care Med 2013;188:376–94.

chILD, should be tested for genetic diseases, such as mutation in genes *SFTPB, SFTBC, and ABACA3,* which encode proteins *SP-B, SP-C,* and *ABCA3.* Newborns presenting with chILD syndrome, congenital hypothyroidism, and hypotonia should be tested for *NKX2.*1 (ie, thyroid transcription factor).

Congenital Lung Diseases

Various congenital malformations of the lung such as congenital diaphragmatic hernia (**Fig. 8**), TEF (**Fig. 9**), sequestration of lung, congenital cystic adenomatous

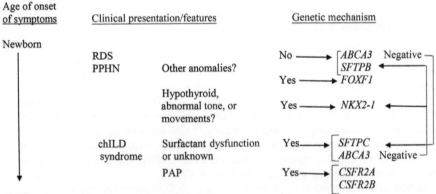

Fig. 7. Genetic approach to chILD diagnosis. Possible genetic mechanisms are listed on the right, ordered depending on age of the patient at presentation (top to bottom), as well as selected phenotypic characteristics. Arrows point to initial gene or genes to be analyzed; if results of initial studies were negative, arrows on right indicate additional genetic studies to be considered. PAP, pulmonary alveolar proteinosis; PPHN, persistent pulmonary hypertension of the newborn. (*From* Kurland G, Deterding RR, Hagood JS, et al. An official American Thoracic Society clinical practice guideline: classification, evaluation, and management of childhood interstitial lung disease in infancy. Am J Respir Crit Care Med 2013;188:376–94; with permission.)

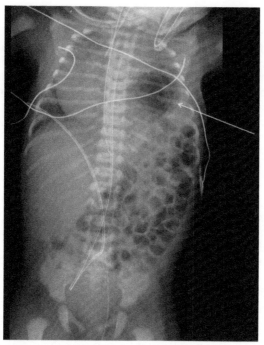

Fig. 8. Radiograph of chest showing congenital diaphragmatic hernia (Bochdalek). Note stomach bubble in the left side of chest (*arrow*) and cardiothymic silhouette displaced into the right side of chest.

malformation of lung, congenital lobar emphysema, lymphangiectesis, or mass in the chest may present with respiratory distress either in the newborn period or during infancy.[5–8,34–36] If these are diagnosed antenatally, the patient should be transferred to a perinatal center for further management. A pediatric surgeon should be consulted.

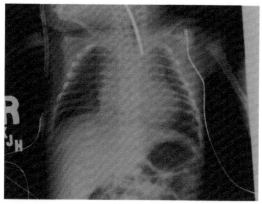

Fig. 9. Tracheoesophageal fistula. Note upper blind pouch (radio opaque tube) with fistula (air in stomach and intestines).

SUMMARY

Respiratory distress presents with varying degrees of tachypnea, grunting, chest retractions, nasal flaring, and/or cyanosis. After initial stabilization, followed by history taking and physical examination, chest radiograph, as well as blood gases, a diagnosis should be made in most instances,[1,9] which includes TTN, RDS, MAS, pneumonia, CLD of prematurity, interstitial lung disease, or upper airway disorders. Cyanotic heart disease should be suspected if Sao_2 value is less than 90% after 15 minutes of age.[5] In critically ill infants or when the diagnosis in unclear, a neonatologist, cardiologist, pulmonologist, or ENT surgeon must be promptly consulted.

REFERENCES

1. Edwards MO, Kotecha SJ, Kotecha S. Respiratory distress of the term newborn infant. Paediatr Respir Rev 2013;14:29–37.
2. te Pas AB, Davis PG, Hooper SB, et al. From liquid to air: breathing after birth. J Pediatr 2008;152(5):607–11.
3. Sweet DG, Carnielli V, Greisen G, et al. European consensus guidelines on the management of neonatal respiratory distress syndrome in preterm infants-2010 update. Neonatology 2010;97:402–17.
4. Dargaville PA, Copnell B, for Australian and New Zealand Neonatal Network. The epidemiology of meconium aspiration syndrome: incidence, risk factors, therapies and outcomes. Pediatrics 2006;117(5):1712–72.
5. Johnson LC, Lieberman E, O'Leary E, et al. Prenatal and newborn screening for critical congenital heart disease: findings from a nursery. Pediatrics 2014;134: 916–22.
6. Lee HJ, Song MJ, Cho JY, et al. Echogenic fetal lung masses: comparison of prenatal sonographic and postnatal CT findings. J Clin Ultrasound 2003;31(8): 419–24.
7. Duncombe GJ, Dickinson JE, Kikiros CS. Prenatal diagnosis and management of congenital cystic adenomatoid malformation of the lung. Am J Obstet Gynecol 2002;187(4):950–4.
8. Ankerman T, Oppermann HC, Engler S, et al. Congenital masses of the lung, cystic adenomatoid malformation versus congenital lobar emphysema. J Ultrasound Med 2004;23:1379–84.
9. Martin RJ, Fanaroff AA, Walsh MC. The respiratory system in Fanaroff and Martin's neonatal-perinatal medicine. In: Diseases of the fetus and infants. 10th edition. Elsevier, Mosby; 2014. p. 1075–206.
10. Bland RD. Lung fluid balance during development. Neoreviews 2005;6(6): e255–65.
11. Special report-neonatal resuscitation: 2010 American Heart Association Guidelines for Cardiopulmonary Resuscitation and Emergency Cardiovascular Care. Circulation 2010;122:S909–19.
12. Mathew OP. Apnea of prematurity: pathogenesis and management strategies. J Perinatol 2011;31(5):302–10.
13. te Pas AB, Wong C, Kamlin CO, et al. Breathing patterns in preterm and term infants immediately after birth. Pediatr Res 2009;65(3):352–6.
14. Peter CS, Sprodowski N, Bohnhorst B, et al. Gastroesophageal reflux and apnea of prematurity: no temporal relationship. Pediatrics 2002;109(1):8–11.
15. Yurdakök M. Transient tachypnea of the newborn: what is new? J Matern Fetal Neonatal Med 2010;23(Suppl 3):24–6.

16. Clark RH. The epidemiology of respiratory failure in neonates born at an estimated gestational: age of 34 weeks or more. J Perinatol 2005;25:251–7.
17. Morris SJ. Radiology of the chest in neonates. Curr Paediatr 2003;13:460–8.
18. Pramanik AK. Respiratory Distress Syndrome. 2012. Available at: http://emedicine.medscape.com/article/976034-overview. Accessed October 2014.
19. Roberts D. Antenatal corticosteroids in late preterm infants. BMJ 2011;342:d1614.
20. SUPPORT Study Group of the Eunice Kennedy Schiver NICHD Neonatal Research Network, Finer NN, Carlo WA, et al. Early CPAP versus surfactant in extremely preterm infants. N Engl J Med 2010;362:1970–9.
21. Engle WA. American Academy of Pediatrics Committee on Fetus and Newborn. Surfactant-replacement therapy for respiratory distress in the preterm and term neonate. Pediatrics 2008;121:419–32.
22. Ehrenkrantz RA, Dusick AM, Vohr BR, et al. Growth in the neonatal intensive care unit influences neurodevelopmental and growth outcomes of extremely low birth weight infants. Pediatrics 2006;117:1253–61.
23. American Academy of Pediatrics Committee on Fetus and Newborn. Apnea, sudden infant death syndrome, and home monitoring. Pediatrics 2011;111(4 Pt 1): 914–7.
24. American Academy of Pediatrics Committee on Fetus and Newborn. Hospital discharge of the high-risk neonate. Pediatrics 2008;122(5):1119–26.
25. Goldsmith JP. Continuous positive airway pressure and conventional mechanical ventilation in the treatment of meconium aspiration syndrome. J Perinatol 2008; 28(Suppl 3):S49–55.
26. Jobe AH, Bancalari E. Bronchopulmonary dysplasia. Am J Respir Crit Care Med 2001;163(7):1723–9.
27. Ehrenkranz RA, Walsh MC, Vohr BR, et al. Validation of the National Institutes of Health consensus definition of bronchopulmonary dysplasia. Pediatrics 2005; 116(6):1353–60.
28. Baraldi E, Fillipone M. Chronic lung disease after premature birth. N Engl J Med 2007;357:1946–55.
29. Allen J, Zwerdling R, Ehrenkranz R, et al. Statement on the care of the child with chronic lung disease of infancy and childhood. Am J Respir Crit Care Med 2003; 168(3):356–96.
30. Vollsæter M, Roksund OD, Bide GE, et al. Lung function after preterm birth: development from mid-childhood to adulthood. Thorax 2013;68(8):767–76.
31. Slaughter JL, Stenger MR, Reagan PB. Variation in the use of diuretic therapy for infants with bronchopulmonary dysplasia. Pediatrics 2013;131:716–23.
32. Deterding RR. Infants and young children with children's interstitial lung disease. Pediatr Allergy Immunol Pulmonol 2010;23(1):25–31.
33. Kurland G, Deterding RR, Hagood JS, et al. An official American Thoracic Society clinical practice guideline: classification, evaluation, and management of childhood interstitial lung disease in infancy. Am J Respir Crit Care Med 2013;188: 376–94.
34. Truitt AK, Carr SR, Cassese J, et al. Perinatal management of congenital cystic lung lesions in the age of minimally invasive surgery. J Pediatr Surg 2006; 41(5):893–6.
35. Stanton M, Davenport M. Management of congenital lung lesions. Early Hum Dev 2006;82(5):289–95.
36. Ozcelik U, Göçmen A, Kiper N, et al. Congenital lobar emphysema: evaluation and long-term follow-up of thirty cases at a single center. Pediatr Pulmonol 2003;35(5):384–91.

Cardiac Evaluation of the Newborn

Donald J. Fillipps, MD[a], Richard L. Bucciarelli, MD[b,c],*

KEYWORDS

- Term newborn cardiovascular examination
- Term newborn with congenital heart disease (CHD)
- Common types of neonatal congenital heart disease • Pulse oximetry screening
- Critical congenital heart disease (CCHD)

KEY POINTS

- Although congenital heart defects can be diagnosed using fetal cardiac ultrasonography, some defects can be challenging to identify.
- Even with a careful complete physical examination, some infants seem normal and are discharged home undiagnosed.
- The persistence of fetal channels can mask the presence of critical congenital heart disease, and the rather short postpartum hospital stay contributes to the diagnostic challenges.
- It is essential for the examiner to use all physical examination skills, including inspection, palpation, and auscultation, and to perform more than one physical assessment before discharge or shortly thereafter.
- The recent introduction of Pulse Oximetry Screening has been an extremely helpful adjuvant in assisting with the diagnosis of CCHD.

CARDIAC EVALUATION OF THE NEWBORN

The approach to the cardiac evaluation of a newborn can be challenging. As a result, many pediatricians report that they often feel uncomfortable when it comes to differentiating the normal from the abnormal state with regard to a newborn's

Declaration of conflict of interest: Both R.L. Bucciarelli, MD and D.J. Fillipps, MD attest that they have no conflicts of interest to declare in relation to the materials and information provided in this article.
[a] Division of General Pediatrics, College of Medicine, University of Florida, 1701 Southwest 16th Avenue, Building A, Gainesville, FL 32608, USA; [b] Division of Neonatology, College of Medicine, University of Florida, 2400 Archer Road, Gainesville, FL 32610, USA; [c] Division of Pediatric Cardiology, College of Medicine, University of Florida, 2400 Archer Road, Gainesville, FL 32610, USA
* Corresponding author. Division of Neonatology, College of Medicine, University of Florida, 2400 Archer Road, Gainesville, FL 32610.
E-mail address: buccirl@ufl.edu

cardiovascular examination. It is the authors' goal for this article to provide the reader with the background knowledge that will make the cardiac evaluation of newborns less intimidating and assist the general pediatrician in understanding, detecting, and treating a newborn with congenital heart disease (CHD).

CHD is the most common congenital disorder in newborns, occurring in approximately 8 out of 1000 live births, and is responsible for almost 30% of infant deaths related to birth defects. Of those children with CHD, about 1 in 4 (25%) babies born with a heart defect will have critical CHD (CCHD), defined as needing intervention within the first year of life.[1-3]

Although CHD can be diagnosed using fetal cardiac ultrasonography, some defects can be challenging to identify. Similarly, even with a careful complete physical examination, some infants seem normal and are discharged home undiagnosed. The persistence of fetal channels can mask the presence of CCHD, and the rather short postpartum hospital stay contributes to the diagnostic challenges. Thus it is essential for the examiner to use all physical examination skills, including inspection, palpation, and auscultation, and to perform more than one physical assessment before discharge or shortly thereafter. The recent introduction of pulse oximetry screening (POS) has been an extremely helpful adjuvant in assisting with the diagnosis of CCHD before signs of decompensation occur.[4]

Initial Evaluation

The first step in the assessment of the newborn infant's cardiovascular system is a careful review for conditions that are associated with an increased risk of CHD (**Table 1**). The presence of any of these factors should raise the index of suspicion, but a complete physical examination should be performed regardless.[5-7]

Inspection and Palpation of the Skin and Mucous Membranes

The color of the skin and briskness of capillary refill can be indicators of the adequacy of oxygenation and cardiac output. The mucous membranes of a normal newborn should be pink. This is usually checked by looking at the tongue and lips. When light

Table 1	
Common conditions associated with CHD	
Maternal	**Perinatal**
Diabetes	TORCH infection
Obesity	Premature delivery <37 wk
Hypertension	Genetic/chromosomal disorders
Systemic lupus erythematosus	VACTERL
Epilepsy	Omphalocele
Influenza or flulike symptoms	Congenital diaphragmatic hernia
First-trimester smoking	
Maternal thyroid conditions	
Maternal CHD	
Maternal alcohol/medication use	
Multifetal pregnancy	

Abbreviations: TORCH, toxoplasmosis, other agents, rubella, cytomegalovirus, herpes simplex; VACTERL, vertebral, anal, cardiac, tracheal, esophageal, renal, and limb.
    Data from Refs.[1-3,5]

pressure is applied to the skin or nail beds, normal color should return within 3 to 4 seconds after the pressure is released (capillary refill time).

Acrocyanosis is usually described as cyanosis of the distal portions of the extremities but can be seen around the mouth and in the nail beds. However, the mucous membranes generally remain pink. Acrocyanosis is common in newborns and is normal. It can be caused by vasomotor instability, vasoconstriction caused by cold, or polycythemia. The degree of acrocyanosis can be related to the level of hematocrit and is most obvious with a central hematocrit of 65% or greater.[7] Acrocyanosis is increased with crying and fades when sleeping. It is usually uniformly distributed in the arms and legs but may have an asymmetric pattern being more obvious in certain extremities. However, distinct differences in appearance between upper and lower parts of the body should raise concern and be investigated. Determination of a central hematocrit and peripheral hemoglobin saturation can be helpful. With acrocyanosis caused by polycythemia, the hematocrit will be elevated and hemoglobin saturation will be 90% to 95%. A normal hematocrit and/or abnormal hemoglobin saturation should prompt further investigation.

Central cyanosis is always abnormal. This condition may be caused by primary pulmonary disease or CCHD, which restricts pulmonary blood flow (PBF) (**Box 1**). Cyanosis caused by pulmonary disease is often responsive to the administration of oxygen. Central cyanosis caused by CCHD does not change significantly when patients are placed in an oxygen-enriched environment.

Mottling or pallor can be a sign of diminished cardiac output as blood is shunted away from the skin to support more central organs and tissues. The capillary refill time is prolonged, and a significant metabolic acidosis may be present. There are both common cardiac and noncardiac causes of compromised cardiac output, and they must be investigated (**Box 2**).

Assessment of Peripheral Pulses

Palpation of the brachial and femoral pulses is an essential element of the cardiovascular examination of the newborn. On first palpation, the examiner should assess the pulse rate (normal between 100 and 160 beats per minute) and rhythm (consistent rhythm without irregular beats). Although it is acceptable to palpate the pulses in each extremity separately, it is a good practice to also palpate one femoral pulse simultaneously with each of the brachial pulses. This practice gives one the opportunity to not only assess the pulse amplitude but also the timing of the pulses in the arms and the legs. Delays in the timing of the pulses between the upper and lower extremities is suggestive of abnormality in the aortic arch.[8]

Box 1
Congenital heart lesions producing a decrease in PBF

PS with intact ventricular septum

PA with intact ventricular septum

Tetralogy of Fallot (PS/PA with VSD)

Tricuspid atresia

Hypoplastic right heart syndrome

Epstein anomaly of the tricuspid valve

Abbreviations: PA, pulmonary atresia; PS, pulmonary valve stenosis; VSD, ventricular septal defect.

Box 2
Common causes of compromised cardiac output

Sepsis

Hypoplastic left heart syndrome

Myocardial dysfunction with tricuspid regurgitation caused by asphyxia

Great vein of Galen aneurysm

Sustained supraventricular tachycardia

Inborn errors of metabolism

After noting the rate and timing of the pulses, their amplitude and character should be noted. Amplitude of the peripheral pulses is frequently graded as 0 to 4+, with 0 being not palpable and 4+ being bounding.

Assessment of the Breathing Pattern

The normal respiratory pattern of a term neonate is regular and effortless. The breath sounds are usually very quiet and distant and may frequently be detected only with close observation and auscultation. Babies generally show an abdominal breathing pattern because of their weak chest wall muscles and diaphragm-directed breathing. A common additional pattern known as *periodic breathing* may also be noted. Periodic breathing is a normal variation of breathing found in premature and full-term infants. The examiner will notice pauses in breathing for less than 10 seconds, followed by a series of rapid, shallow breaths. Breathing then returns to normal without any stimulation or intervention.[8]

Changes in respiratory rate and effort are frequently the result of changes in lung compliance, a reflection of the stiffness of the lung and its ability to change volume in relation to a change in pressure.[9] Various types of CCHD can have a profound effect on pulmonary compliance, leading to predictable signs on physical examination.

When PBF is reduced, there is less blood in the lungs and compliance increases. Breathing becomes easier. Diminished PBF also produces hypoxemia, which stimulates the respiratory center in the brain stem and results in hyperpnea, effortless tachypnea with increased tidal volume. The baby seems cyanotic but has no significant respiratory distress. Because of the hyperpnea, $PaCO_2$ is often low. Effortless tachypnea in a cyanotic baby is the hallmark of CCHD caused by right heart obstructive lesions.[6,8]

CCHD that increases PBF increases the amount of blood in the lungs, leading to pulmonary edema and congestive heart failure (CHF). Pulmonary compliance is reduced; work of breathing is increased leading to tachypnea, grunting, alar flaring, and intercostal retractions. Because cardiac output is frequently diminished, the skin is mottled with increased capillary refill time. Often a mixed metabolic and respiratory acidosis is present. The possibility of CCHD should be considered in any term infant presenting with significant respiratory distress but whose history and initial evaluation does not support primary pulmonary disease.[10]

Inspection, Palpation, and Auscultation of the Heart

Similar to the examination of the lungs, the normal cardiac activity in the term neonate is barely visible with inspection and the precordium is usually quiet to palpation. A slight parasternal lift can usually be seen and palpated along the left sternal boarder, secondary to the normal right ventricular dominance seen in term newborns.

Auscultation of the heart should be performed using a high-quality stethoscope with a small bell and diaphragm. The examination is best performed by starting at the base of the heart (second left and right intercostal spaces), moving down the sternal boarder to the apex. Both the bell and diaphragm should be used while the examiner concentrates on heart rate, rhythm, cardiac sounds, and any murmurs heard.[8]

The normal heart rate of a term neonate is usually between 100 and 160 beats per minute. However, heart rates may exceed 180 when the baby is crying and can go as low as 70 when in a deep sleep. The rhythm should be regular without extra or skipped beats. The examiner may notice a predictable change in rate associated with respirations, the sinus arrhythmia, which is entirely benign.[6]

Normal heart sounds are generated by closure of the tricuspid and mitral valves (S_1) and by closure of the pulmonary and aortic valves (S_2). As PBF increases after birth, the pulmonary valve closes later causing audible splitting of S_2. A split S_2 indicates the presence of 2 normally positioned great vessels, suggests that the pulmonary vascular resistance is low, and indicates the presence of 2 normal ventricles separated by a ventricular septum. Thus the presence of splitting strongly suggests normal cardiac anatomy; however, its absence does not imply the presence of CHD. Occasionally extra heart sounds (S_3, S_4, or a summation S_3/S_4) can be heard. Although these sounds can be heard in some normal situations, their presences should prompt further evaluation.

Cardiac Murmurs

Murmurs are caused by turbulent blood flow, either by increased flow through normal vessels and valves or normal flow through abnormal valves, vessels, or septal defects. Murmurs are graded 1 to 6 and described as to whether they occur in systole or diastole. Attention should be also given to the quality of the murmurs (harsh, smooth, or vibratory) and whether or not they are only heard in a small area or radiate more widely throughout the chest. There are numerous common innocent murmurs that can be detected in newborns. The pulmonary flow murmur is probably one of the most common. It is heard best in the upper left sternal border (ULSB) and transmits well to both sides of the chest, axilla, and the back. It is usually soft and generally not louder than grade 2/6 intensity. Another innocent murmur is the transient systolic patent ductus arteriosus (PDA) murmur, which is audible at the ULSB and in the left infraclavicular area during the first days of life. It is thought to be caused by a closing ductus arteriosus and usually disappears shortly after the first day. Frequently a transient grade 1-2/6 murmur of tricuspid regurgitation can be heard in the fourth intercostal space to the right of the sternum. Transient tricuspid regurgitation is most commonly heard in stressed newborns with mild to moderate pulmonary hypertension and generally resolves before discharge as pulmonary vascular resistance falls.[11,12] Finally a soft, vibratory, low-frequency murmur is often best heard at the left lower sternal boarder, which may persist for some time. This murmur is also benign and often referred to as merely a *functional murmur*.

Pathologic murmurs heard in the neonatal period are often of grade 3 to 6 intensity. They are usually harsh in quality, occur in systole, and can be heard all over the chest and into the back. These murmurs are frequently associated with CCHD.[5,10]

Examination of the Abdomen

When assessing for CCHD, it is also important to inspect and palpate the abdomen. A neonate with cyanosis most likely will have a normal abdominal examination. However, infants with overcirculation of the lungs and respiratory distress may develop abdominal distention caused by aerophagia, which can further compromise respiratory mechanics. These infants would benefit from gastric decompression. Infants with CHF may have liver enlargement and, if a metabolic acidosis is present, may develop an ileus with diminished or absent bowel sounds on auscultation.

Blood Pressure

Determination of blood pressure in both arms and at least one leg is important in the evaluation of an infant suspected of having CCHD. The pattern of variation in pressure between the extremities can suggest the presence of significant CCHD (**Table 2**).[13]

COMMON CONGENITAL HEART DEFECTS

In this section, the authors discuss only the most common congenital heart defects. It is not important that the examiner arrive at the correct anatomic diagnosis in their assessment of a newborn with suspected CCHD. Rather, it is important to recognize the general presenting signs of CCHD and how to stabilize the infant until further evaluation can be accomplished.

Uncomplicated Congenital Heart Defects

Simple atrial septal defects (ASD), ventricular septal defects (VSD), endocardial cushion defects, and a patent ductus arteriosus (PDA) do not significantly affect the cardiopulmonary physiology of the newborn and, although possible, are not usually associated with symptoms in the first few days after birth. The blood crossing these defects is usually small in volume and nonturbulent, producing little to no murmur. With simple ASDs, even very large ones, the amount of blood that goes from the left atrium to the right atrium is very limited until several months after birth, when the right ventricular muscle becomes thinner, more compliant, and can accommodate additional blood. With VSDs, flow depends on the reduction in pulmonary vascular resistance, which occurs over the first 3 to 6 weeks after delivery.[13,14] This evolution in the pulmonary vascular bed occurs more rapidly in premature infants, leading to earlier identification and an increased likelihood of symptoms.[15] One exception to this rule is a very small muscular VSD that may be heard within the first days of life because flow through the defect is turbulent.[13,16] Although the murmur may be a grade 2-3/6, it is very short in duration, smooth in character, and mid to high frequency. These infants should be asymptomatic.

Lesions Causing Decreased Pulmonary Blood Flow

The lesions discussed in this section and presented in **Box 1** all have a significant degree of obstruction of blood flow into and/or out of the right ventricle.

Pulmonary valve stenosis and pulmonary valve atresia with an intact ventricular septum

In pulmonary valve stenosis (PS), the pulmonary valve is thickened and only allows a jet of blood to pass into the lungs. Because this jet is turbulent, it creates a loud,

Table 2			
Pulse and blood pressure patterns with left-sided obstructive lesions			
Site of Obstruction	**Right Arm**	**Left Arm**	**Legs**
AA/AS	Diminished	Diminished	Diminished
Long segment COA	Normal	Diminished	Diminished
Isolated COA	Normal	Normal	Diminished

Abbreviations: AA, aortic valve atresia; AS, aortic valve stenosis; COA, coarctation of aorta.

harsh systolic murmur at the base of the heart in the second intercostal space along the left and right sternal boarder. The murmur is also well heard along the back. Because the valve does not close properly, S_2 is single and diminished. With severe pulmonary stenosis, there is often massive tricuspid regurgitation, producing a grade 3 to 6 (murmur plus a thrill) at the third to fourth intercostal space along the right sternal margin. If there is no opening to the valve at all (pulmonary atresia [PA]), the obstruction is complete. The pulmonary valve and the main pulmonary arteries are underdeveloped. The baby is deeply cyanotic, but no murmur is heard over the precordium. There may be a faint (grade 2-3), smooth systolic murmur of a PDA heard along the ULSB and under the left clavicle. In this instance, the infant's entire PBF depends on the ductus. Because the tricuspid valve is competent, the pressure in the right ventricle is greater than systemic levels. Blood flow into the ventricle is minimal and leaves the chamber through the myocardium sinusoids, which drain into the coronary system. As a result, the right ventricle is small, underdeveloped, and nonfunctional. This combination of lesions is also known as the hypoplastic right heart syndrome (**Fig. 1**). However, when PS or PA exists in association with tricuspid valve incompetence, the pressure in the right ventricle is very low, allowing blood to enter during ventricular diastole and then flow retrograde into the right atrium during ventricular systole. This antegrade/retrograde flow creates enough volume variation to allow near-normal development of the right ventricle. Babies with PS/PA may

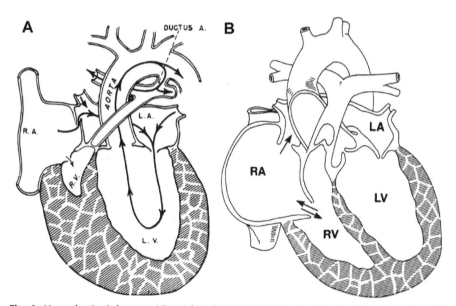

Fig. 1. Hypoplastic right ventricle with pulmonary atresia. An infant with severe PS or PA and a competent tricuspid valve (*A*) may have a severely underdeveloped and nonfunctional right ventricle. The infant is deeply cyanotic with little to no audible murmur. However, if the tricuspid valve is better developed and incompetent (*B*), there is both antegrade and retrograde flow into and out of the right ventricle, which remodels the ventricular wall, resulting in a much larger, functional chamber. In this situation there will be a loud murmur (grade iv/vi) along the right lower sternal boarder. A palpable thrill may also be present. Ductus A, Ductus Arteriosus; LA, left atrium; LV, left ventricle; RA, right atrium; RV, right ventricle. (*Adapted from* Krovetz LJ, Gessner IH, Schiebler GL. Handbook of pediatric cardiology. 2nd edition. Baltimore: University Park Press; 1979. p. 301; with permission.)

develop a large right atrium and are at risk for developing supraventricular tachycardia (SVT), which is briefly discussed later.

Pulmonary valve stenosis/pulmonary valve atresia with a ventricular septal defect
This combination of lesions is one of the most common types of CHD and is also known as tetralogy of Fallot (TOF). The 4 elements of TOF are PS or PA, VSD, overriding aorta, and right ventricular hypertrophy (RVH) (**Fig. 2**). RVH is not obvious because right ventricular dominance is common in the term neonate. The presenting signs depend on the degree of pulmonary obstruction. Severe obstruction produces deep cyanosis, whereas minor degrees of stenosis may affect color only slightly, hence the term *Pink Tetralogy*. In addition to PS, there is usually narrowing below the pulmonary valve, which is called muscular infundibular stenosis. S_2 is single because of PS and subvalvular stenosis. The VSD is always large with little restriction of flow such that blood flows easily from the right ventricle to the left ventricle with little turbulence, generating no murmur and allowing normal ventricular development. The aorta straddles the ventricular septum (overrides) and receives blood from both ventricles. The murmur heard in an infant with TOF is similar to the murmur of the PS. If tetralogy exists with pulmonary atresia, there may be no murmur at all or only the faint murmur of a PDA, which supplies all of the PBF.

Dextro-transposition of the great vessels
D-transposition of the great vessels (TGV) is one of the more common defects. In this case, the main pulmonary artery arises from the left ventricle and the aorta from the

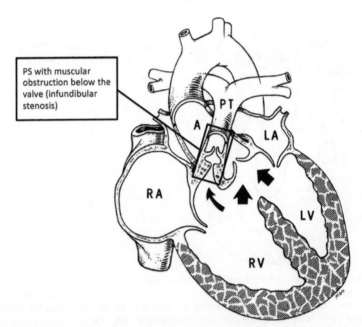

Fig. 2. Cyanotic TOF. Note the presence of PS with additional muscular narrowing in the infundibular region. The aorta is overriding the ventricular septum and receives blood from both the right and left ventricle. A, aorta; LA, left atrium; LV, left ventricle; PT, pulmonary trunk; PS, pulmonary valve stenosis; RA, right atrium; RV, right ventricle. (*Adapted from* Krovetz LJ, Gessner IH, Schiebler GL. Handbook of pediatric cardiology. 2nd edition. Baltimore: University Park Press; 1979. p. 288; with permission.)

right ventricle. The volume of PBF is normal; but because the origin of the great vessels is switched, oxygenated blood merely recirculates to the lungs and deoxygenated blood recirculates to the body. Mixing of the circulations only occurs across the atrial septum and the PDA. There are usually no murmurs because there is no turbulent flow. S_2 is single because the pulmonary artery is malpositioned and hidden by the aorta. Most frequently TGV occurs with an intact ventricular septum, presenting with deep cyanosis. However, it can also be associated with a VSD or a VSD and PS. It then takes on the characteristics of the other lesions described throughout this section.

Lesions Causing Increased Pulmonary Blood Flow

Lesions that cause increased PBF almost always involve obstruction to flow on the left side of the heart (**Box 3**). These lesions can quickly produce severe CHF because they often involve pressure overload of the left ventricle associated with the obstruction and volume overload of the right ventricle caused by an associated ASD and VSD. It is important to consider the possibility of left heart obstruction in any term neonate who has a period of well-being and then develops respiratory distress, a mottled appearance of the skin, with hypotension and shock. Unlike defects associated with right-sided lesions, left-sided lesions create turbulent flow and demonstrate increased heart activity with loud systolic murmurs. Careful attention to the pattern of blood pressure and pulse can give the examiner insight into the location of the lesion (see **Table 2**).

Aortic valve stenosis

Patients with mild, uncomplicated aortic valve stenosis (AS) usually do not have difficulty as newborns. However, more significant degrees of stenosis, so-called critical AS, cause symptoms at an early age. They present with a loud harsh systolic murmur at the base of the heart to the right of the sternum, radiating well into the carotids. Blood pressure and pulses are normal with mild disease but are uniformly diminished in all extremities with critical AS. S_2 is single because of delayed aortic valve closure. Extra sounds (ejection clicks and S_3–S_4) may be heard. CHF can develop quickly in infants with critical AS.

Coarctation of the aorta and coarctation of the aorta with a ventricular septal defect

A discrete, isolated coarctation of the aorta does not usually cause symptoms in the first few days of life. It is often detected on follow-up examination when upper

---

Box 3
Congenital heart lesions producing an increase in PBF

Atrial septal defect

Ventricular septal defect

Endocardial cushion defect

Aortic valve stenosis

Aortic valve atresia

Hypoplastic left heart syndrome

Discrete coarctation of the aorta

Long segment coarctation of the aorta with VSD

Total anomalous pulmonary venous return

Single ventricle, double inlet left ventricle, and double outlet right ventricle

extremity hypertension is noted in both arms and diminished blood pressure and pulses are present in the legs. The coarctation itself does not produce any audible murmurs; however, an abnormal aortic valve is often associated with coarctation and could be the cause of an AS murmur.

However, a coarctation of the aorta associated with a VSD frequently produces symptoms within the first few days after birth. The coarctation produces pressure overload of the left ventricle, and blood flowing through the VSD causes volume overload of the right ventricle leading to early CHF. Coarctation with a VSD often has a long segment narrowing of the aorta, which classically occurs after the origin of the left common carotid artery and before the origin of left subclavian artery. This area can be so hypoplastic that it is completely obstructed, creating an interruption of the aortic arch. There is a marked increase in precordial activity. Loud murmurs and signs of CHF with significant respiratory distress are obvious. There is usually a profound metabolic acidosis. Significant hypocalcemia can be present because the area of the aortic arch hypoplasia is also associated with the embryologic origin of the parathyroid glands, which are important in calcium homeostasis (Di George syndrome).

The pulse pattern in long segment coarctation may be helpful. The right arm blood pressure and pulse will be normal to elevated, whereas the left arm and lower extremity pulses and blood pressures are diminished or absent (see **Table 2**).

Hypoplastic left heart syndrome

The counterpart to the hypoplastic right heart syndrome is the hypoplastic left heart syndrome (**Fig. 3**). It may involve severe mitral stenosis or atresia, hypoplastic or absent left ventricle, severe AS or atresia, hypoplastic aortic arch, and long segment coarctation of the aorta. The entire systemic blood flow is supplied through a PDA. When the PDA is functioning, symptoms may be minimal. But when the PDA constricts, CHF with shock and metabolic acidosis occurs suddenly. Intervention must be quick and decisive.

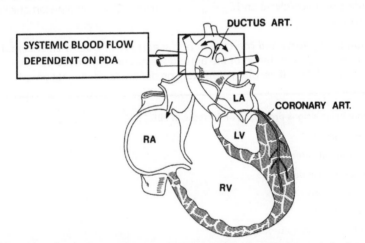

Fig. 3. Hypoplastic left heart syndrome. Note the atretic aortic valve and the hypoplastic, nonfunctional left ventricle. Ductal closure results in severe limitation of systemic blood flow, leading to profound shock. Coronary Art, coronary artery; Ductus Art, Ductus arteriosus; LA, left atrium; LV, left ventricle; PDA, patent ductus arteriosus; RA, right atrium; RV, right ventricle. (*Adapted from* Krovetz LJ, Gessner IH, Schiebler GL. Handbook of pediatric cardiology. 2nd edition. Baltimore: University Park Press; 1979. p. 346; with permission.)

Total anomalous pulmonary venous return

With total anomalous pulmonary venous return, the pulmonary veins do not attach to the left atrium directly. Rather they take one of 3 persistent fetal pathways to return to the right atrium. Once in the right atrium, oxygenated blood then crosses the foramen ovale into the left atrium and then out the left ventricle to the body. When the persistent fetal channels are nonrestrictive, signs may be minimal and presentation can be delayed for days to weeks. However, when there is obstruction within these fetal pathways or within the pulmonary venous system, pulmonary venous hypertension and CHF develops rapidly.

SPECIAL CONSIDERATIONS
Conditions Causing Central Cyanosis Without Congenital Heart Disease

Several common conditions can mimic CHD by causing central cyanosis and should be considered in the evaluation of the cyanotic newborn (**Box 4**). Infants with neurologic depression can be cyanotic because of central nervous system–induced hypoventilation. In addition to hypoxemia and cyanosis, the $PaCO_2$ is frequently elevated. Patients with rare hemoglobinopathies are cyanotic because the abnormal hemoglobin cannot load oxygen.[7] Because $PaCO_2$ is a measure of oxygen dissolved in plasma, it is normal. However, hemoglobin saturation, a measure of the oxygen contained within the red cell, is extremely low. Inborn errors of metabolism can also cause cyanosis, acidemia, or CHF.[17]

Arteriovenous Malformation of the Great Vein of Galen

The vein of Galen is located under the cerebral hemispheres and drains the anterior and central regions of the brain into the sinuses of the posterior cerebral fossa. A vein of Galen aneurysmal malformation (AVM) is formed early in gestation, and the amount of blood crossing the AVM can become massive.[18,19] The vein dilates and obstructs the third ventricle, causing significant hydrocephalus. Because CHF secondary to the AVM occurs in utero, babies with this AVM can present as nonimmune hydrops fetalis with cardiomegaly, pleural effusions, and ascites at delivery. Auscultation for a bruit over the anterior fontanel and over the temporal bones in term infants with CHF within the first hours after delivery can help make the diagnosis.

Box 4
Conditions mimicking CHD

Sepsis

Asphyxia neonatorum

CNS depression/apnea/seizures

Primary pulmonary disease

Pulmonary hypertension

Hypoglycemia

Methemoglobinemia

Nonimmune hydrops fetalis

Inborn errors of metabolism

Abbreviation: CNS, central nervous system.

DYSRHYTHMIAS

Sinus tachycardia and sinus bradycardia are common in term neonates and are benign. All ventricular complexes are preceded by a normal P wave originating at the sinus node and are positive in the electrocardiogram in lead I. Sinus tachycardia can have rates close to 200 beats per minute during crying. Sinus bradycardia can have rates as low as 70 beats per minute during sleep. Although these rates are concerning to the observer, they are benign as long as they change with activity and the pulse oximetry during the variations is normal. Sometimes with deep sleep and bradycardia, the P wave on an electrocardiogram (ECG) or cardiac monitor will have a different appearance or may be absent. This is an escape rhythm, usually junctional or low atrial in origin, and is usually a normal variant. In cases of concern, consultation with a specialist could be considered.

Premature Beats

The most common cause of an irregular rhythm in a term neonate is the presence of premature atrial contractions (PAC). Most often they are benign and will resolve in a matter of days.[20] The ECG shows an early beat preceded by a normal or inverted P wave and a pause following the premature beat. If the interval between the sinus beat and PAC shortens, the premature electrical activity from the atrium finds the ventricles in their relative refractory period and the beat is conducted with aberration, making the beat look like a premature ventricular contraction (PVC) but the complex is preceded by a P wave. If the interval shortens even further, the ventricular response may be dropped entirely, leaving a long pause (**Fig. 4**). The variation in QRS morphology may lead one to think that there is a combination

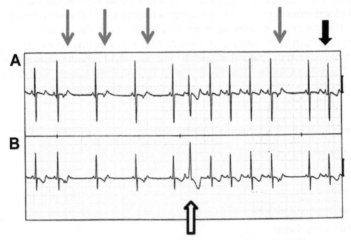

Fig. 4. PACs with varying coupling intervals. The tracings (*A, B*) are simultaneous. Note PACs (*gray arrows*) followed by a long pause. The PAC occurs during the refractory period of the ventricles and is not conducted. If the PAC occurs a bit later, it finds the ventricles in their relative refractory period and the PAC is conducted with aberration, looking like a PVC in strip (*B*) (*black and white arrow*), but the beat is clearly preceded by a P wave. When the PAC occurs even later, it is conducted normally (*solid black arrow*). (*Adapted from* Scagilotti D, Deal BJ. Benign cardiac arrhythmias in the newborn. In: Emmanouilides GC, Riemenschneider, TA, Allen HD, et al, editors. Moss and Adams heart disease in infants, children, and adolescents. 5th edition. Williams and Wilkins; 1995. p. 629; with permission.)

of PACs and PVCs, but that is not the case.[21] All are isolated PACs and are entirely benign.

PVCs are less common unless the patient is on cardiac drugs, postoperative from cardiac surgery, or has significant hyperkalemia. Isolated PVCs are usually also benign and will resolve within a few days. However, obtaining serum electrolytes and an echocardiogram could be considered to rule out pathologic causes.

Congenital Third-Degree Heart Block

With congenital third-degree heart block, the atria beat at their inherent rate, 110 to 150 beats per minute, and the ventricles beat at their rate of 60 to 70 beats per minute with no relationship between the two (**Fig. 5**).[21] Congenital third-degree heart block is frequently seen in babies born to women with systemic lupus erythematosus; if not already known, the diagnosis should be suspected when the dysrhythmia is discovered. Because this condition can be present for quite some time in utero, the infant's cardiovascular system can compensate for the low rate by increasing stroke volume to maintain cardiac output. It is uncommon for a neonate to be symptomatic and need pacing, but consultation with a specialist is advised.

Supraventricular Tachycardia

SVT is not uncommon in the neonate and must be distinguished from sinus tachycardia (**Fig. 6**).[21] Most times it occurs in the absence of structural heart disease but can be associated with lesions that produce a large right atrium, such as PS/PA with massive tricuspid regurgitation. SVT in utero is also a common cause of nonimmune hydrops fetalis, caused by CHF, which may resolve when the SVT breaks.

SVT is also frequent in instances of the various pre-excitation syndromes (ie, Wolf-Parkinson-White). Heart rates are in the range of 210 to 220 beats per minute and do not change with activity of the infant. SVT in the presence of a normal heart can be tolerated for several hours; unless the baby is symptomatic, with signs of CHF and metabolic acidosis, there is usually sufficient time to diagnose and treat the infant safely. Although maneuvers that produce vagal stimulation, ice to the forehead, and

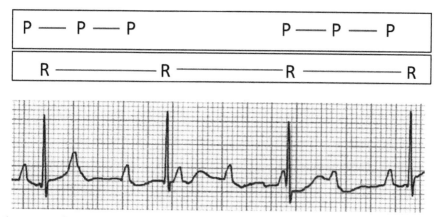

Fig. 5. Complete heart block (third-degree heart block). Atrial rate is 145 beats per minute (P-P interval 0.42 seconds) and regular. Ventricular rate is 60 beats per minute (R-R interval 1.0 second) and regular. P waves and QRS complexes are independent of each other. (*From* Artman M, Mahony L, Teitel DF. Neonatal cardiology. New York: McGraw-Hill; 2002. p. 165; with permission.)

A

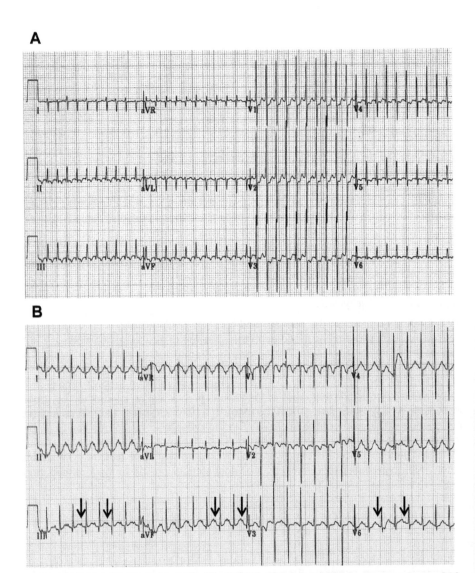

B

Fig. 6. SVT (*A*) and sinus tachycardia (*B*). SVT (*A*) with rate of 315 beats per minute. QRS complexes are normal, but no P waves are seen. With sinus tachycardia (*B*) rate is 230 beats per minute. P waves (*arrows*) are visible preceding a normal QRS. Running the paper at 2× speed helps to uncover and identify the P waves. (*From* Artman M, Mahony L, Teitel DF. Neonatal cardiology. New York: McGraw-Hill; 2002. p. 166, 171; with permission.)

painful stimuli can break the SVT, their benefit is questionable because SVT frequently recurs until maintenance medication is administered. When used in excess, these interventions have their own inherent risks. Consultation with a specialist is usually indicated.

PULSE OXIMETRY SCREENING

Universal newborn screening is the process by which newborns are tested shortly after birth for conditions that can cause severe illness, disability, or death. Through early identification and treatment, newborn screening provides an opportunity to reduce morbidity and mortality. Babies with CCHD are at significant risk of disability or even death if their condition is not timely diagnosed and treated. With the vast improvements in fetal cardiac ultrasonography and the addition of POS, great strides are being made in our diagnostic abilities for detecting CCHD. However, even when prenatal ultrasounds are performed by those with specific training in CHD, fewer than 50% of cases of proven CHD are identified. Further, it has been estimated that up to 30% of infants with unrecognized CCHD may be discharged each year from newborn nurseries in the United States.[22,23] The Centers for Disease Control and Prevention (CDC) estimates that each year about 1200 more newborns with CCHD could be identified at birth hospitals using POS.[23]

Universal POS was added to the federally recommended uniform screening panel through endorsement by the Secretary of Health and Human Services (HHS) in September 2011.[24,25] In December 2011, the American Academy of Pediatrics (AAP) published their endorsement of the HHS recommendations for POS for CCHD in the January issue of the journal *Pediatrics*.[26] POS for CCHD has now become a national standard of care and is part of most but not all state newborn screening panels. Data regarding US state participation in POS for CCHD can be found online on the AAP Web site.[27] The method of using POS for CCHD as a compliment to existing practices of care has been shown to be cost-effective and associated with improved detection and outcomes for babies. Estimated costs run from about $5 to $14 per newborn screened.[4,27–31]

In a 2012 meta-analysis of 13 studies with data for 229,421 newborn infants, the overall sensitivity of pulse oximetry for detection of CCHD was 76.5% (95% confidence interval [CI] 67.7–83.5) and specificity was 99.9% (95% CI 99.7–99.9).[32]

A recommended standard protocol for POS of well newborns and best-practice advice regarding implementation are now readily available to newborn health care providers. Utilization of the AAP-endorsed CCHD POS algorithm is recommended (**Fig. 7**).[26]

Newborn POS is most successful in identifying 7 primary and 5 secondary cardiac lesions (**Table 3**).[26,30] Obtaining both preductal and postductal pulse oximetry measurements is essential because defects with right-to-left shunting of desaturated blood through the ductus arteriosus will not be detected with only preductal readings. It is recommended that the probes be placed on both the right hand and one foot. Screening at least 24 hours after delivery substantially reduces the false-positive rate (0.05% after 24 hours vs 0.5% before 24 hours).[32]

Table 3 Screening targets for pulse oximetry	
Primary Screening Targets	**Secondary Screening Targets**
Hypoplastic left heart syndrome	Coarctation of the aorta
Pulmonary atresia	Interrupted aortic arch
Tetralogy of Fallot	Ebstein anomaly of the tricuspid valve
Total anomalous pulmonary venous return	Double outlet right ventricle
Transposition of the great vessels	Single ventricle
Tricuspid atresia	
Persistent truncus arteriosus	

It is important to remember that the current POS protocol will not detect all forms of CHD whether they are critical lesions or not.
Data from Refs.[26,29,30]

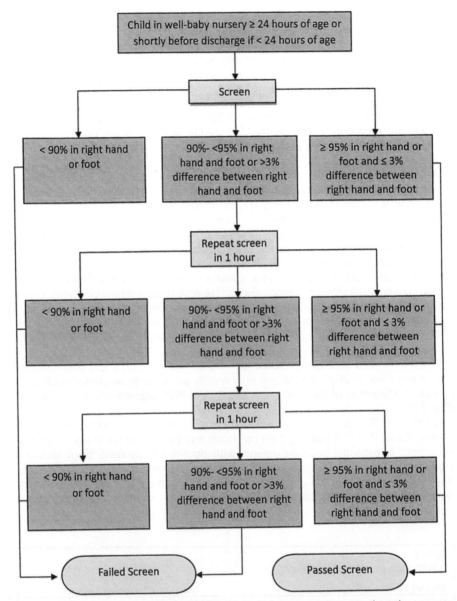

Fig. 7. Algorithm for POS. Effect of altitude: It is important to note that the oxygen saturation thresholds for a positive screening result may vary at high altitude. Appropriate studies need to be performed at higher altitudes to establish reliable thresholds. (*Adapted from* Kemper AR, Mahle WT, Martin GR, et al. Strategies for implementing screening for critical congenital heart disease. Pediatrics 2011;128(5):e1267; with permission.)

Pulse Oximetry Clinical Assessment

Babies with saturation less than 90% in the right hand or foot should be *immediately referred for clinical assessment* (see **Fig. 7**). Babies with 3 failed readings (pulse oximetry <95% in the right hand and foot OR >3% difference between the right hand and foot) should receive

- Clinical assessment (infectious and pulmonary pathology should be excluded)
- Echocardiogram
- Referral to pediatric cardiology, immediately if symptomatic, expeditiously if asymptomatic

1. Passed Screens
   A screen is considered passed if:
   - The oxygen saturation is 95% or greater in the right hand and foot with less than 4% difference between the two readings; screening would then be complete.
2. Failed Screens
   A screen is considered failed if:
   - Any oxygen saturation measure is less than 90% (in the initial screen or in repeat screens).
   - Oxygen saturation is less than 95% in the right hand and foot following 3 measurements, each separated by 1 hour.
   - A greater than 3% absolute difference exists in oxygen saturation between the right hand and foot on 3 measurements, each separated by 1 hour.

Any infant who fails the screen should have a diagnostic echocardiogram performed and be referred to a pediatric cardiologist for further management.

It is important to remember that it is possible for a baby to have a normal POS and still have a congenital heart defect.

EVALUATION AND STABILIZATION WHEN CRITICAL CONGENITAL HEART DISEASE IS SUSPECTED

After careful review of the history and physical examination, the physician must decide about the need for further intervention. If the term neonate seems well and has passed POS but has a benign dysrhythmia or has a grade i to ii mid- to high-frequency murmur that is localized, a follow-up examination in 24 hours should be sufficient to decide on the need for further referral. However, if the baby does not pass POS, obtaining both an echocardiogram and consulting with a pediatric cardiologist would be prudent.

When the infant seems ill, general interventions should be initiated. Obtain a serum glucose to screen for hypoglycemia. Check 4 extremity blood pressures. Screening for sepsis and the initiation of antibiotics should also be considered. A chest radiograph can be obtained and may show cardiomegaly or abnormal pulmonary vascularity. However, in many instances, the chest radiography will be normal even in the presence of a CCHD lesion. The real value of the chest film is not to support or dismiss the diagnosis of CHD but rather to identify other causes of distress in the newborn, such as a pneumothorax or primary pulmonary disease. Unless a dysrhythmia is present, an ECG is usually not helpful.

If the infant is extremely ill, early control of the airway and placement of umbilical artery and venous catheters would be strongly advised. When the index of suspicion of CCHD is high, consideration should be given to initiating an infusion of prostaglandin E_2 (PGE$_2$).

PGE$_2$ stabilizes a PDA and will usually reopen a constricted or closed ductus, providing a reliable means of PBF in patients with CCHD and improvement in

CHF. PGE_2 is infused at 0.02 to 0.1 μg/kg/min.[33] The infusion is usually begun at 0.05 μg/kg/min and can be titrated depending on the changes in oxygenation, increase in blood pressure, and decrease in acidosis. Ideally PGE_2 is infused into a reliable peripheral intravenous line; however, administration through an umbilical venous catheter or an umbilical artery catheter will suffice at least temporarily. Apnea can occur when initiating therapy, especially at higher doses. Therefore, it is important to be ready to establish a stable airway when initiating therapy.

Taking these measures should aid in stabilizing the newborn allowing for subsequent transport to an appropriate critical care unit while awaiting further interventions.

REFERENCES

1. Tennant PW, Pearce MS, Bythell M, et al. 20-year survival of children born with congenital anomalies: a population-based study. Lancet 2010;375(9715):649.
2. Reller MD, Strickland MJ, Riehle-Colarusso T, et al. Prevalence of congenital heart defects in metropolitan Atlanta, 1998–2005. J Pediatr 2008;153(6):807.
3. Botto LD, Correa A, Erickson JD. Racial and temporal variations in the prevalence of heart defects. Pediatrics 2001;107(3):e32.
4. Mahle WT, Martin GR, Beekman RH 3rd, et al. Endorsement of Health and Human Services recommendation for pulse oximetry screening for critical congenital heart disease. Pediatrics 2012;129:190.
5. Flanagan MR, Yeager SB, Weindling SN. Cardiac disease. In: MacDonald MG, Muller MD, Seshia MM, editors. Avery's neonatology: pathophysiology and management of the newborn. 6th edition. Philadelphia: Lippincott Williams and Wilkins; 2005. p. 636–767.
6. Vargo L. Cardiovascular assessment. In: Tappero EP, Honeyfield ME, editors. Physical assessment of the newborn: a comprehensive approach to the art of physical examination. 4th edition. Petaluma: NICU INK Book Publishers; 2009. p. 87–103.
7. Blanchette V, Dror Y, Chan A. Hematology. In: MacDonald MG, Muller MD, Seshia MM, editors. Avery's neonatology: pathophysiology and management of the newborn. 6th edition. Philadelphia: Lippincott Williams and Wilkins; 2005. p. 1189–90.
8. Allen HD, Phillip JR, Chan DR. History and physical examination. In: Allen HD, Gutgesell HP, Clark EB, editors. Moss and Adams' heart disease in infants, children, and adolescents: including the fetus and young adult. 6th edition. Philadelphia: Lippincott, Williams & Wilkins; 2007. p. 58–65.
9. Koff PB, Eitzman DV, Neu JF. Neonatal and pediatric respiratory care. St. Louis: Mosby; 1993. p. 42–3.
10. Fletcher MA. Physical diagnosis in neonatology. Philadelphia: Lippincott-Raven; 1998. p. 343, 363.
11. Bucciarelli RL, Nelson RM, Egan EA, et al. Transient tricuspid insufficiency in the newborn: a form of myocardial dysfunction of stressed newborns. Pediatrics 1977;59:330–7.
12. Rao SP. Other tricuspid valve anomalies. In: Long WA, editor. Fetal & neonatal cardiology. St. Louis: W.B. Saunders; 1990. p. 548–9.
13. Moller JH. Physical examination. In: Moller JH, Neal WA, editors. Fetal, neonatal, and cardiac disease. Norwalk (CT): Appleton & Lange; 1990. p. 167–78.
14. Nath H, Soto B. Angiography. In: Long WA, editor. Fetal & neonatal cardiology. St. Louis: W.B. Saunders; 1990. p. 368–70.

15. Rudolph AM. Congenital diseases of the heart. Chicago: Year Book Medical Publishers; 1974. p. 46.
16. Krovetz LJ, Gessner IH, Schiebler GL. Handbook of pediatric cardiology. 2nd edition. Baltimore: University Park Press; 1979. p. 267–349.
17. Cox GF. Diagnostic approaches to pediatric cardiomyopathy of metabolic genetic etiologies and their relations to therapy. Prog Pediatr Cardiol 2007;24(1):15–25.
18. Teitel D, Heymann MA, Liebman JT. The heart. In: Klaus MH, Fanaroff AA, editors. Care of the high risk neonate. 3rd edition. St. Louis: W.B. Saunders; 1986. p. 298–9.
19. Madsen JR, Frim DM, Hansen AR. Neurosurgery of the newborn. In: MacDonald MG, Mullett MD, Seshia MM, editors. Avery's neonatology: pathophysiology and management of the newborn. 6th edition. Philadelphia: Lippincott Williams and Wilkins; 2005. p. 1425.
20. Scagilotti D, Deal BJ. Benign cardiac arrhythmias in the newborn. In: Emmanouilides GC, Riemenschneider TA, Allen HD, et al, editors. Moss and Adams heart disease in infants, children, and adolescents. 5th edition. Baltimore: Williams and Wilkins; 1995. p. 629.
21. Artman M, Mahony L, Teitel DF. Neonatal cardiology. New York: McGraw-Hill; 2002. p. 165–71.
22. Peterson C, Ailes E, Riehle-Colarusso T, et al. Late detection of critical congenital heart disease among US infants: estimation of the potential impact of proposed universal screening using pulse oximetry. JAMA Pediatr 2014;168(4):361–70. http://dx.doi.org/10.1001/jamapediatrics.2013.4779.
23. Peterson C, Grosse SD, Oster ME, et al. Cost-effectiveness of routine screening for critical congenital heart disease in US newborns. Pediatrics 2013;132:e595–603.
24. Ewer AK. Review of pulse oximetry screening for critical congenital heart defects in newborn infants. Curr Opin Cardiol 2013;28(2):92–6.
25. Centers for Disease Control and Prevention. Rapid implementation of pulse oximetry newborn screening to detect critical congenital heart defects: New Jersey, 2011. MMWR Morb Mortal Wkly Rep 2013;62(15):292–4.
26. Kemper AR, Mahle WT, Martin GR, et al. Strategies for implementing screening for critical congenital heart disease. Pediatrics 2011;128(5):e1259–67.
27. Pulse oximetry screening for CCHD. Available at: http://www.aap.org/search/pulseoxscreening. Accessed September 21, 2014.
28. Oster ME, Lee KA, Honein MA, et al. Temporal trends in survival among infants with critical congenital heart defects. Pediatrics 2013;131(5):e1502–8. http://dx.doi.org/10.1542/peds.2012-3435.
29. Mahle WT, Newburger JW, Matherne GP, et al. Role of pulse oximetry in examining newborns for congenital heart disease: a scientific statement from the AHA and AAP. Pediatrics 2009;124:823–36.
30. De-Wahl Granelli A, Wennergren M, Sandberg K, et al. Impact of pulse-oximetry screening on the detection of duct-dependent congenital heart disease: a Swedish prospective screening study in 39,821 newborns. BMJ 2009;338:a3037.
31. Peterson C, Gross SD, Glidewell J, et al. A public health economic assessment of hospitals' cost to screen newborns for critical congenital heart disease. Public Health Rep 2014;129(1):86–93.
32. Thangaratinam S, Brown K, Zamora J, et al. Pulse oximetry screening for critical congenital heart defects in asymptomatic newborn babies: a systematic review and meta-analysis. Lancet 2012;379(9835):2459–64.
33. Allen HD, Gutgesell HP, Clark EB, editors. Moss and Adams heart disease in infants, children, and adolescents. 6th edition. New York: Lipincott Williams & Wilkens; 2001. p. 1462.

A Practical Guide to the Diagnosis, Treatment, and Prevention of Neonatal Infections

CrossMark

Roberto Parulan Santos, MD, MSCS[a],*, Debra Tristram, MD[b]

KEYWORDS

- Neonatal infections • Newborn sepsis • Early-onset sepsis • Late-onset sepsis
- Respiratory viral infections in infants • Antibacterial therapy • Antiviral therapy
- Neonatal antimicrobial stewardship

KEY POINTS

- Neonatal infections continue to cause morbidity and mortality in infants. Group B streptococcus and *Escherichia coli* are the most common agents of early-onset sepsis, whereas coagulase-negative *Staphylococcus* is the predominant cause of late-onset sepsis.
- Other important agents include *Listeria monocytogenes*, syphilis, *Staphylococcus aureus*, herpes simplex virus, cytomegalovirus, and *Candida* spp.
- There is increasing recognition of respiratory viral infections contributing to ruling out sepsis in very young infants whose presentations are similar to bacterial infections.
- Initial work up for neonatal infection consists of complete blood count and blood culture, with the option of performing cerebrospinal fluid analyses and culture if clinically indicated. Serial determinations of biomarkers (C-reactive protein, procalcitonin, or neutrophil CD64) may be used adjunctively in the diagnosis and management of neonatal infection.
- Ampicillin and gentamicin remains the cornerstone of initial antimicrobial regimen for neonatal infections. Third-generation cephalosporins should be used judiciously.
- The use of antiviral (acyclovir, ganciclovir, valganciclovir, and oseltamivir) and antifungal agents (fluconazole, amphotericin B, and voriconazole) may reduce mortality and morbidity due to specific viral and fungal disease.
- Different strategies, such as group B streptococcal prophylaxis, hand hygiene, immunization and immunoprophylaxis, antimicrobial stewardship, probiotics, and prebiotics, and care bundles may be used in preventing infections in neonates.

Disclosures: None.

[a] Pediatric Infectious Diseases, Bernard & Millie Duker Children's Hospital, Albany Medical Center, 47 New Scotland Avenue (MC88), Albany, NY 12208, USA; [b] Pediatric Infectious Disease, Department of Pediatrics, Albany Medical Center, 47 New Scotland Avenue (MC88), Albany, NY 12208, USA
* Corresponding author.
E-mail address: SantosR@mail.amc.edu

Pediatr Clin N Am 62 (2015) 491–508
http://dx.doi.org/10.1016/j.pcl.2014.11.010
0031-3955/15/$ – see front matter © 2015 Elsevier Inc. All rights reserved.

INTRODUCTION

Neonatal infections continue to cause morbidity and mortality in infants. Among approximately 400,000 infants followed nationally, the incidence rates of early-onset sepsis (EOS) infection within 3 days of life were 0.98 cases per 1000 live births.[1] More than two-thirds of the frequently isolated organisms were associated with group B streptococcus (GBS) (43%) and *Escherichia coli* (29%). Although 20% of the term infants were treated in the newborn nursery, 77% of the infected infants required intensive care management. Of those who survived beyond 3 days of life, about 21% had an episode of late-onset sepsis (LOS) infection after 3 days of life. The overall mortality rate of infected infants was 16%.

Newborn infants are at increased risk for infections because they have relative immunodeficiency. This may be due to decreased passage of maternal antibodies in preterm infants and to immaturity of the immune system in general.[2,3] The innate immune functions in infants are impaired with decreased production of inflammatory markers (interleukin 6 and tumor necrosis factor)[4] and with decreased dendritic and neutrophil functions.[5] The adaptive immune system is less than optimal with decreased cytotoxic functions,[2] decreased cell mediated immunity,[6] and delayed or lack of isotype switching.[2,3] Complement is important in opsonization and bacterial killing. In term infants, complement levels are approximately half compared with adults.[2] Taken together, these predispose infants to severe, prolonged, or recurrent infections associated with bacterial, viral, or fungal infections.

Suspected sepsis, presumed infection, and ruling out sepsis remain the most common diagnoses in the nursery intensive care unit (NICU). The American Academy of Pediatrics (AAP) Committee on Fetus and Newborn[7] has published a clinical report extensively discussing clinically relevant challenges: identifying newborns with signs of sepsis with high likelihood of EOS requiring antimicrobial regimen and identifying healthy-appearing newborns with high likelihood of EOS requiring antimicrobial regimen. The committee concluded that, although these guidelines are evidence-based, they may be modified by the clinical judgment of the provider. The primary reason is that the clinical presentation of neonatal infection may be subtle and nonspecific, and may overlap with noninfectious causes.[7,8] Many clinicians empirically start broad spectrum antimicrobial regimen for infants considered at risk for sepsis but antibiotics are occasionally continued despite a negative blood culture. This practice may be detrimental to the infant[8] because it increases the risk of invasive fungal infections,[9] necrotizing enterocolitis (NEC), or death,[10,11] which increases the pressure for selecting multidrug-resistant organisms[12] and even the risk of LOS.[11]

The purpose of this article is to provide evidence-based practical approaches to the diagnosis, management, and prevention of neonatal infections.

MICROBIOLOGIC AGENTS

The timing of transmission is one of the factors contributing to the cause of neonatal infections. Different pathogens may be acquired during pregnancy (prenatal), during delivery (perinatal), or after delivery (postnatal). **Table 1** shows the different periods of transmission of various neonatal pathogens.

The introduction of new molecular-based assays, such as quantitative real-time polymerase chain reaction (PCR),[13] has paved the way for increasing recognition of respiratory viral infections contributing to ruling out sepsis in late-onset infections.[14] **Table 1** includes respiratory viral infections (coronavirus, enterovirus, human metapneumovirus, influenza, parainfluenza virus, respiratory syncytial virus [RSV], and rhinovirus) as possible causes of postnatal infections in infants.[14–16]

Table 1
Periods of transmission in neonatal infections

Pathogens	During Pregnancy	During Delivery	After Delivery
Bacteria			
Chlamydia trachomatis	—	+[a]	—
GBS	++[b]	++	++
Enterococcus spp	—	+	+
Enterobacteriaceae	—	++	++
Listeria monocytogenes	+	+	+
Neisseria gonorrhea	—	+	—
Staphylococcus spp	—	—	++
Treponema pallidum	+	—	—
Ureaplasma urealyticum	—	+	—
Viruses			
Coronavirus	—	—	+
Cytomegalovirus	+	+	+
Enterovirus	+	+	+
Hepatitis B virus	+	+	—
Herpes simplex virus	+	—	—
Human immunodeficiency virus	+	+	+
Human metapneumovirus	—	—	+
Influenza	—	—	+
Parainfluenza virus	—	—	+
Parvovirus B19	+	—	—
Respiratory syncytial virus	—	—	+
Rhinovirus	—	—	+
Rubella virus	+	—	—
Varicella-zoster virus	+	+	+
Fungi			
Candida spp	—	+	+
Aspergillus spp	—	—	+
Protozoa			
Toxoplasma gondii	+	—	—

[a] common.
[b] most common.
Data from Refs.[1,8,14–18]

CLINICAL PRESENTATIONS
Early-Onset Infections

EOS is arbitrarily defined as infection within the first 3 days of life. The most common organisms associated with EOS include GBS and *E coli*.[1,19] In general, the risk of bacterial infection in a healthy-appearing newborn remains relatively low.[20] The most common clinical findings include hypoglycemia (<40 mg/dL, 22%) and hypothermia (<36.5°C, 20%), followed by hyperglycemia (>140 mg/dL, 19%) and apnea (18%).[19]

Edwards and Baker[21] summarized that newborn infants with sepsis manifest similar clinical signs as those with meningitis, including hyperthermia; hypothermia;

respiratory distress; anorexia or vomiting; jaundice; and lethargy. Hypotension may be more frequently found in infants with sepsis, whereas irritability, convulsions, and bulging or full fontanel is found in those with meningitis. However, they cautioned that absence of any of the aforementioned signs do not exclude central nervous system involvement. Furthermore, it was suggested to evaluate infants for various foci of infections such as acute otitis media, conjunctivitis, osteomyelitis, pyogenic arthritis, and skin soft-tissue infections.

Late-Onset Infections

LOS is arbitrarily defined as infection after 3 days of life. The most common organisms isolated with LOS include coagulase-negative staphylococci in more than a third of the cases, which may or may not be associated with a medical device.[19] Yeast or *Candida* spp infection is another important pathogen.[19] Also, there is increasing recognition of viral respiratory infections as a possible cause in LOS.[14] The most common clinical findings include hypothermia (41%), hyperglycemia (38%), apnea (38%), and bradycardia (30%).[19]

There are several factors that may increase the risk for LOS. There are significantly more infants with LOS who have an indwelling central vascular catheter at the time of infection than those infants with EOS (78% vs 10%, $P<.0001$).[19] Additionally, there are more infants with LOS who had a surgical procedure before infection (8% vs 1%, $P<.0001$).

DIAGNOSTIC EVALUATIONS

The clinical presentations of infections may overlap with noninfectious causes in newborns. It has been previously demonstrated that relying on symptoms alone may not be sufficient in diagnosing neonatal infections.[22] Bacteremia has been reported in infants without clinical signs of sepsis.[23] There are several diagnostic tests and principles that may guide clinicians in evaluating infants with infections.

Algorithm-Based Guideline

The AAP Committee on Fetus and Newborn have published a clinical report on the evaluation of asymptomatic infants (<37 and ≥37 week gestation) with risk factors for sepsis.[7] Evaluation of asymptomatic preterm infants (<37-week) with risk factors for sepsis is shown in **Fig. 1**.[7] Similar algorithms for the evaluation of asymptomatic term infants (≥37 week gestation) are available from the AAP Committee on Fetus and Newborn. (http://www.ncbi.nlm.nih.gov/pubmed/22547779).[7]

Additional principles in the evaluation of infants with risk factors for sepsis[7] follow:

- Major risk factors for neonatal sepsis include chorioamnionitis, prolonged rupture of membrane 18 or more hours, and colonization of GBS with inadequate intrapartum antimicrobial prophylaxis (IAP).
- Chorioamnionitis usually presents as maternal fever greater than 38°C (100.4°F) and its diagnosis should be discussed with the obstetric providers. Maternal fever may be the only abnormal finding in chorioamnionitis.
- Adequate IAP means maternal treatment with penicillin, ampicillin, or cefazolin at or earlier than 4 hours before delivery.
- At least 1 mL of blood may be sufficient for a single blood culture from a peripheral vein. Blood culture from umbilical artery catheter or umbilical vein may be a reliable alternative following aseptic techniques
- Screening blood cultures have not been proven of value and are not recommended.

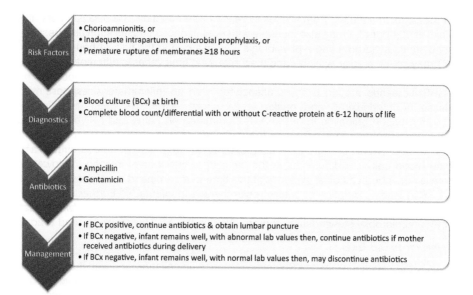

Fig. 1. Evaluation of asymptomatic preterm infants (<37-week gestation) with risk factors for sepsis. (*Adapted from* Polin RA, Committee on Fetus and Newborn. Management of neonates with suspected or proven early-onset bacterial sepsis. Pediatrics 2012;129(5): 1006–15.)

- Complete blood count with differential has poor positive predictive value and it is suggested waiting 6 to 12 hours after birth to avoid falsely normal values at birth.
- Platelet counts remain low days to weeks after sepsis; thus this cannot be used in following response to treatment.
- The sensitivity of C-reactive protein (CRP) improves if done 6 to 12 hours after birth. Bacterial sepsis is unlikely if CRP remains normal.
- Lumbar puncture may be indicated in infants whom sepsis is highly suspected, those infants with bacteremia, and in infants who fail to respond to antimicrobial therapy.
- Urinary tract infection in newborns is associated with episodes of bacteremia; thus urine culture should not be part of routine sepsis workup.
- Microbiologic evaluation using gastric aspirates, tracheal aspirates, or superficial body sites cultures are of limited value and are not routinely recommended for sepsis.

Biomarkers

Several acute-phase reactants or biomarkers (neutrophil CD64 [nCD64], procalcitonin [PCT], or CRP) may be used adjunctively in the evaluation and management of neonatal infection. The diagnostic usefulness of the various surrogate markers depends on the phases of neonatal sepsis: early phase or 2 to 12 hours (nCD64), mid phase or 12–24 hours (PCT), and late phase or greater than 24 hours (CRP).[24]

nCD64 is a high-affinity Fc receptor that increases with exposure to bacterial or fungal agents.[2,24] The usefulness of nCD64 is related to its high negative predictive value as well as decreasing concentration on serial determinations on infants undergoing antimicrobial treatment of bacteremia.[24] However, there is a scarcity of medical evidence to recommend nCD64 for routine evaluation of neonatal infection and this may not be readily available.

Procalcitonin released from tissues increases with infection at around 2 hours and peaks at 12 hours.[7] It may also increase with noninfectious causes such as in respiratory distress syndrome and a physiologic increase during the first 24 hours of birth.[7] PCT may not be readily available and the turnaround time varies in different institutions from 20 minutes to 5 hours.[24]

CRP increases around 6 hours associated with an inflammatory response with release of interleukin-6 and peaks at 24 hours.[7] CRP has been used in the algorithm-based guideline from the AAP Committee on Fetus and Newborn for the evaluation of asymptomatic term and preterm infants with a risk factor for sepsis.[7] It is best used as part of a group of diagnostic tests[2] together with blood culture and white blood cell with differential in the evaluation of neonatal infection.[7] However, there is not enough medical evidence at this time to recommend serial determinations of CRP in guiding duration of antimicrobial therapy in infants.[7,24] Further studies are needed to evaluate the usefulness of sequential determination of CRP and biomarkers for an antimicrobial stewardship program (ASP) in the NICU setting.

Molecular-Based Tests

In 2013, the Infectious Disease Society of America, in collaboration with the American Society for Microbiology, affirmed the importance of close collaboration and positive working relationships between clinicians and microbiologists[25] to better serve patients. The most up-to-date edition of the *Red Book* provides contact information for expert advice and national collaborative study groups that give guidance on diagnostic assays regarding specific agents causing mother-to-child transmission. It is important to know the various microbiologic resources available locally, which include but are not limited to PCR and matrix-assisted laser desorption ionization-time of flight mass spectrometry (MALDI-TOF).

Rapid antigen tests for respiratory viruses may lack sensitivity,[25] which is important in the NICU setting in controlling local outbreaks. There are several nucleic acid amplification test platforms currently available that differ in the number of analytes detected.[25] It is important to obtain adequate specimens and to use suitable viral transport media following manufacturer instructions.

MALDI-TOF is a valuable alternative to the conventional microbiologic assays; however, it may not be a readily available resource for diagnostic testing in most institutions. However, if it is available, it has several practical applications that may benefit clinical management even in the NICU settings:

- Earlier and accurate diagnosis of neonatal sepsis due to various bacteria[26]
- Rapid identification of highly virulent GBS that causes meningitis and LOS in infants[27]
- Identification of maternal-to-child transmissions (chorioamnionitis and neonatal infections) of opportunistic pathogen[28]
- Accurate identification of bloodstream infection associated with fungal infections in the NICU[29]
- Identification and monitoring the spread of nosocomial outbreak (eg, methicillin-resistant *Staphylococcus aureus* [MRSA][30] and *Candida parapsilosis*[31] in the NICU).

THERAPEUTIC MANAGEMENT

When appropriate specimens for diagnostic evaluations are collected in clinically stable patients, then empirical antimicrobial therapy should be initiated for neonatal sepsis. It is recommended to discuss complicated cases, such as multidrug resistant organisms and infants not improving while on therapy or those requiring unconventional dosing regimens and antimicrobial agents, with pediatric infectious disease specialists.

Antibiotic Treatment

Ampicillin and gentamicin remains the cornerstone of initial antimicrobial regimen for early-onset neonatal infections. The combination of such broad-spectrum antibiotic regimens cover the most common cause (GBS and *E coli* in more than 70%)[1] of EOS and has synergistic activity (against GBS and *Listeria monocytogenes*).[7,32] The dosing regimen for ampicillin may change over time based on the chronologic age of the infant and body weight.[32] For example, an 8-day-old infant weighing greater than 2000 g may need dosing adjustment of ampicillin from 150 mg/kg/d intravenous (IV) divided every 8 hours to 200 mg/kg/d IV divided every 6 hours.

Once-daily dosing of gentamicin (4 mg/kg IV qd)[32] has been used in the term newborn for more than a decade. The pharmacodynamic characteristics of aminoglycosides that allow the use of once-daily dosing include concentration-dependent killing (peak concentration to minimal inhibitory concentration [peak/MIC] ratio),[33,34] postantibiotic effect with leukocyte enhancement,[35,36] and prevention of adaptive resistance.[37]

Third-generation cephalosporins should be used judiciously. There is significant association between the use of third-generation cephalosporins and invasive candidiasis in preterm infants.[9] Cefotaxime has excellent penetration to the cerebrospinal fluid and its therapeutic use should be limited to Gram-negative meningitis.[7] Routine use of cefotaxime for EOS may lead to rapid development of drug-resistant organisms.[38] Ceftriaxone is contraindicated in neonates for 2 reasons: (1) it is highly protein bound and may displace bilirubin progressing to hyperbilirubinemia[7] and (2) concurrent administration with calcium-containing solutions may produce insoluble precipitates (ceftriaxone-calcium salts) leading to cardiorespiratory complications.[39]

The AAP periodically updates the dosing regimens and recommended therapy for selected neonatal infections through *Nelson's Pediatric Antimicrobial Therapy*.[32] It provides various antimicrobial regimens (antibiotic, antiviral, and antifungal agents) based on body weight of infants and their chronologic age or gestational and postnatal age. Between new editions, a monthly update of short and interesting reports related to pediatric antimicrobial therapy is posted at www.aap.org/en-us/aap-store/Nelsons/Pages/Whats-New.aspx. Suggested durations of antibiotic therapy for EOS adapted from *2014 Nelson's Pediatric Antimicrobial Therapy*[32] and the AAP Committee on Fetus and Newborn[7] are shown in **Table 2**.

Antiviral Therapy

There are several antiviral agents that can be used for the treatment of neonatal viral infections. Acyclovir (60 mg/kg/d IV divided every 8 hours) is the treatment of choice for term infants with herpes simplex virus (HSV) and varicella-zoster infections.[32] There are several topical agents (0.15% ganciclovir ophthalmic gel, 0.1% iododeoxyuridine, or 1% trifluridine) that may be added to systemic antiviral regimen if there is eye involvement.[32] After parenteral therapy with acyclovir, it is recommended to give HSV suppressive regimen (300 mg/m^2/dose po tid), which improves neurodevelopmental outcomes of infants with central nervous system involvement.[40] There is currently no dosing regimen for valacyclovir in infants younger than 3 months of age.[32] The AAP Committee on Infectious Diseases and the Committee on Fetus and Newborn recently published an algorithm-based guideline on the evaluation and treatment of asymptomatic infants born to mothers with active herpes lesions[41] (http://www.ncbi.nlm.nih.gov/pubmed/23359576).

Table 2
Duration of antibiotic therapy for early-onset sepsis

Conditions	Duration & Comments
Newborns with early onset pulmonary infiltrates (within 3 d of life)	4 d, may be sufficient based on limited data with no additional risk factors, including • No chorioamnionitis • No bacteremia • Does not require O_2 >8 h • Asymptomatic at 48 h of treatment
Mild or presumed sepsis	5 or 7 d, no prospective controlled studies; remains controversial
Bacteremia without a focus	10 d
Uncomplicated GBS meningitis and other gram-positive bacteria	14–21 d
Gram-negative meningitis	21 d or 14 d after a negative cerebrospinal fluid culture, whichever is longer

Data from Polin RA, Committee on Fetus and Newborn. Management of neonates with suspected or proven early-onset bacterial sepsis. Pediatrics 2012;129(5):1006–15; and American Academy of Pediatrics. Antimicrobial therapy for newborns. In: Bradley JS, editor. 2014 Nelson's pediatric antimicrobial therapy. Elk Grove Village (IL): American Academy of Pediatrics; 2014. p. 17–36.

Oral valganciclovir (16 mg/kg/dose po bid) is the drug of choice for infants with symptomatic congenital cytomegalovirus (CMV) disease with or without central nervous system involvement.[32,42] The treatment of congenital CMV should be initiated in the first month of life. Kimberlin and colleagues[42] concluded from the phase III randomized double-blind placebo-controlled multinational study that 6 months of valganciclovir regimen for symptomatic congenital CMV disease significantly improves hearing and neurodevelopmental outcomes. There is significant improvement in language and receptive communication at 2 years of age. There was less grade 3 to 4 neutropenia at 6 weeks oral valganciclovir (~19%) compared with 6 weeks of IV ganciclovir (63%) reported previously.

IV ganciclovir (6 mg/kg/dose bid) can be used initially for infants with symptomatic congenital CMV disease if oral valganciclovir is contraindicated due to extreme prematurity or NEC.[32] The same dosing regimen is the treatment of choice for perinatally or postnatally acquired CMV disease associated encephalitis, hepatitis, pneumonitis, or persistent thrombocytopenia.

Oral oseltamivir (3 mg/kg/dose bid) remains the treatment of choice for term infants with influenza infections.[32,43] Oral suspension formulation is available (6 mg/mL) and should be offered to young infants with suspected or confirmed influenza infection regardless of severity because they are at higher risk for complications.[43] Limited data are available for the weight-based dosing regimen for preterm infants using postmenstrual age (ie, gestational age plus chronologic age):

• Less than 38 weeks postmenstrual age, 1 mg/kg/dose po bid
• 38 to 40 weeks, 1.5 mg/kg/dose po bid
• Greater than 40 weeks, 3 mg/kg/dose po bid.

There is currently no dosing regimen for inhalational zanamivir for young infants.

Suggested durations of antiviral therapy, prophylaxis, and suppressive regimen for congenital and perinatal or postnatally acquired viral infections adapted from *2014 Nelson's Pediatric Antimicrobial Therapy*[32] and the AAP Committee on Infectious Diseases and the Committee on Fetus and Newborn[41] are shown in **Table 3**.

Table 3
Duration of antiviral therapy and suppressive regimen for congenital and perinatal or postnatally acquired viral infections

Conditions	Duration & Comments
HSV: central nervous system or disseminated disease	Acyclovir IV for 21 d, continue treatment until repeat cerebrospinal fluid HSV PCR negative
HSV: skin, eye, or mouth disease	Acyclovir IV for 14 d
HSV suppressive regimen after IV therapy	Acyclovir po for 6 mo, monitor for neutropenia
Congenital CMV disease	Valganciclovir po for 6 mo
Perinatally or postnatally acquired CMV disease associated encephalitis, hepatitis, pneumonitis, or persistent thrombocytopenia	Ganciclovir IV for 14–21 d, monitor for relapse after treatment completion
Influenza A and B viruses therapy	Oseltamivir po for 5 d
Influenza A and B viruses prophylaxis	Generally not recommended because of limited safety and efficacy data, discuss with pediatric infectious disease specialist

Data from Refs.[32,40–43]

Antifungal Treatment and Prophylaxis

For candidiasis, IV amphotericin B deoxycholate (1 mg/kg/d) and IV fluconazole (loading dose 25 mg/d on day 1, then 12 mg/kg/d on day 2) may be used for susceptible isolates.[32] Lipid-based amphotericin (3–5 mg/kg/d) can be used if there is no renal involvement because of inadequate kidney penetration. For aspergillosis, voriconazole (loading dose 18 mg/kg/d divided every 12 hours on day 1, then 16 mg/kg/d on day 2) is the drug of choice. Local debridement may be needed for cutaneous aspergillosis. However, if there is clinical deterioration and if the infant is unstable for surgical intervention, consultation with pediatric infectious diseases specialists is recommended.[18] **Fig. 2** shows an extensive cutaneous aspergillosis on a preterm infant who was a poor surgical risk successfully treated with combination antifungal agents.

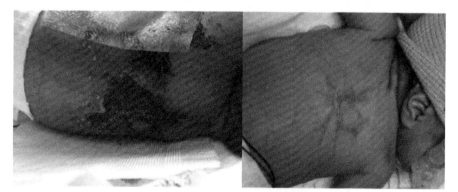

Fig. 2. 4 × 6 cm necrotic black eschar on the back of a preterm infant due to *Aspergillus fumigatus* and the residual scarring after several weeks of combination antifungal agents. (*From* Santos RP, Sanchez PJ, Mejias A, et al. Successful medical treatment of cutaneous aspergillosis in a premature infant using liposomal amphotericin B, voriconazole and micafungin. Pediatr Infect Dis J 2007;26(4):364–6; with permission.)

Fluconazole prophylaxis (6 mg/kg/d twice a week) may be indicated in high-risk infants with birth weight of less than 1000 g from institutions with high incidence of candidiasis (ie, above 10%).[32] Fluconazole prophylaxis (25 mg/kg once weekly) may be offered to young infants younger than 4 months old on extracorporeal membrane oxygenation.

Suggested durations of antifungal treatment of candidiasis and aspergillosis adapted from *2014 Nelson's Pediatric Antimicrobial Therapy*[32] are shown in **Table 4**.

SURGICAL TREATMENT OPTIONS

Surgical interventions may be indicated for the source control of neonatal infections. In a single-center 20-year retrospective study, NEC-associated blood stream infection (BSI) occurred within 3 days of NEC diagnosis and was noted in approximately 43% (69 out of 158 infants with one episode of BSI). Infants with NEC-associated BSI had higher odds (adjusted odds ratio 3.51; 95% CI 1.98–6.24) of having surgical interventions compared with those without BSI.[44] It is of utmost importance to correspond with pediatric surgery regarding source control of infection if clinically indicated because NEC-associated BSI had higher odds of death (adjusted odds ratio 2.88; 95% CI 1.39–5.97).[44]

The following includes disease-specific conditions that may require surgical interventions for adequate source control of infections if the infant is clinically stable. Pediatric providers are encouraged to discuss with their surgical colleagues the following surgical treatment options[32]:

- Early debridement of cutaneous lesions with disseminated aspergillosis
- Surgical drainage of peritonitis with bowel rupture
- Wound cleaning and debridement rapidly spreading cellulitis (*S aureus*), necrotizing fasciitis (group A or B streptococci), tetanus neonatorum
- Surgical drainage of pus in osteomyelitis and suppurative arthritis
- Thoracostomy drainage of empyema
- Surgical drainage of breast abscess may be needed to minimize damage to breast tissue.

Surgical interventions for primary diseases in infants may also increase the risk for neonatal infections. Higher rates of surgical site infection defined as superficial, deep, and organ infections within 30 days of surgical procedures were noted among infants following closure of gastroschisis.[45] It is important to closely monitor infants with surgical site infection because they require significantly longer hospital stay.[45]

Table 4 Duration of antifungal treatment regimen for candidiasis and aspergillosis	
Conditions	**Duration & Comments**
Candidiasis	Usually 3 wk, depending on disease; persistent disease requires: • Removal of infected catheters • Dissemination studies (eg, lumbar puncture if stable, cardiac echo, eye examination, ultrasound of abdomen) • Antifungal susceptibility assay
Aspergillosis	Depends on disease and local debridement

Data from American Academy of Pediatrics. Antimicrobial therapy for newborns. In: Bradley JS, editor. 2014 Nelson's pediatric antimicrobial therapy. Elk Grove Village (IL): American Academy of Pediatrics; 2014. p. 17–36.

PREVENTIVE STRATEGIES

There are various measures that can be used, depending on the availability of local resources, to prevent neonatal infections. These include but are not limited to GBS prophylaxis, hand hygiene, immunization and immunoprophylaxis, ASP, probiotics and prebiotics, and care bundles.

Group B Streptococcal Prophylaxis

IAP is the only preventive strategy that substantially reduces the incidence of early-onset GBS.[7,46] The following are indications for IAP:

- Previous infant with invasive GBS disease
- GBS bacteriuria during the current pregnancy
- Positive GBS vaginal-rectal screening (at 35–37 week gestation) except for cesarean delivery without labor or ruptured membrane
- Unknown maternal GBS status with delivery at less than 37 weeks, rupture of membrane at or before 18 hours, or fever equal to or greater than 100.4°F ($\geq$38°C).

Adequate IAP means receiving penicillin, ampicillin, or cefazolin for at least 4 hours before delivery. Cefazolin may be used if with nonserious β-lactam allergy. If there is history of serious β-lactam allergy (anaphylaxis, angioedema, respiratory insufficiency, or urticarial rash) and if GBS isolate is susceptible, clindamycin may be used. Otherwise, vancomycin is an alternative. Because of high resistance rates, erythromycin is not recommended.

The Center for Disease Control and Prevention has an extensive online resource on GBS for clinicians, including the algorithm-based guidance on secondary prevention of EOS in newborns.[47] The Web page also provides an application, Prevent Group B Strep, which includes guidance on various patient scenarios in collaboration with different medical societies, such as the AAP and the American College of Obstetricians and Gynecologists (http://www.cdc.gov/groupBstrep/guidelines/index.html).

Hand Hygiene

There is no doubt that hand hygiene remains the cornerstone in decreasing health care–associated infections in different hospital settings, including the NICU. In fact, there are various educational programs, multidisciplinary quality-improvement teams, and guidelines on the proven effectiveness of hand hygiene in decreasing infection; however, this is significantly affected by compliance.[48,49] The Center for Disease Control and Prevention has a Web site (http://www.cdc.gov/handhygiene/) containing resources for hand hygiene in health care settings including an application, iScrub, for monitoring hand hygiene compliance using an iPhone or iPod Touch.[50] Thus, hand hygiene guidelines are effective in reducing infections only if we use it.

Soap and water is recommended for decontaminating visibly soiled hands by rubbing hands together vigorously for 15 seconds.[48,49] Alcohol-based gel or foam or an antiseptic soap may be used for routine hand hygiene if not grossly contaminated.[48,49] Hand hygiene compliance is improved if with available alcohol-based products at the infant's bedside.[48] Antimicrobial-impregnated towelettes or wipes are considered alternatives but not substitutes for washing with soap and water or alcohol-based gel or foam.[49]

Immunization and Immunoprophylaxis

The development of a safe and effective vaccine is arguably one of the greatest medical interventions in the last century.[51] Hepatitis B vaccine is the only agent in the

United States recommended to be administered at birth. The various brands available in the United States have an efficacy of 90% to 95% in preventing hepatitis B virus infection and disease.[52] Additional information regarding recommended dosages of hepatitis B vaccines are available in the most recent edition of the *Red Book*[52] and in the annual publication from the Advisory Committee on Immunization Practices.[53] The first dose in the primary series of the subsequent vaccines (diphtheria and tetanus toxoids and acellular pertussis vaccine [DTaP], *Haemophilus influenza* type B, inactivated polio, pneumococcal, or rotavirus vaccine) can be administered at a minimum age of 6 weeks.[53]

Care givers at home should be advised on the importance of immunizing family members to protect infants who are too young to be vaccinated. This is called cocooning[54] and prevents vaccine-preventable diseases, such as pertussis and influenza, in young infants. Educational materials on cocooning for parents and clinicians are available at the AAP Web site http://www2.aap.org/immunization/families/cocooning.html.

In October 2012, the use of tetanus toxoid, reduced diphtheria toxoid, and acellular pertussis vaccine (Tdap) during every pregnancy was recommended because of increasing cases of pertussis in young infants in the recent years.[55] The mother's protective antibodies against pertussis are short-lived and a dose of Tdap in a previous pregnancy may not be protective to the infants of subsequent pregnancies.[56]

Young preterm infants (<1 year of age born at <29 weeks and 0-day gestation) should receive palivizumab during the RSV season for immunoprophylaxis.[57] Five monthly doses of palivizumab at 15 mg/kg given intramuscularly will provide adequate protection for 6 months. Other indications during the RSV season include preterm infants (<1 year of age born at <32 weeks and 0-day gestation) with chronic lung disease of prematurity who required greater than 21% oxygen for at least the first 28 days of life and young infants (<1 year of age) with certain hemodynamically significant heart disease.[57] Clinicians should consult the most current guidelines or policy statement from the AAP regarding palivizumab prophylaxis among young children at increased risk for hospitalization for RSV infection.

Antimicrobial Stewardships

Injudicious use of antibiotics can alter the neonates' microflora that increases exposure and pressure that leads to antimicrobial resistance. The NICU milieu and interventions are permissive for the development of antibiotic-resistant organisms.[48,58] The AAP Committee on Fetus and Newborn[48] have listed ASP strategies that may be useful in the NICU setting based on the guideline from the Infectious Diseases Society of America and the Society for Healthcare Epidemiology of America (**Box 1**).[59]

Probiotics and Prebiotics

There is some medical evidence supporting the use of probiotics in the prevention of NEC in preterm infants. Probiotic is an oral supplement containing sufficient amount of viable microorganisms that alters the host microflora with potential for health benefits.[60] A meta-analysis based on 9 randomized control trials involving approximately 1400 infants born before or at 37 weeks gestation and/or weighing less than or equal to 2500 g at birth showed that enteral use of probiotic significantly decreased the incidence of severe NEC and mortality.[61] There were no severe adverse events or systemic infections directly related to the probiotics used were reported.

The AAP Committee on Nutrition,[60] however, cannot recommend the use of all probiotics in young infants until further studies are done to resolve problematic issues. They noted the large heterogeneity of the studies included in the review, the different

---

Box 1
Antimicrobial stewardship strategies in the nursery intensive care unit

- Audit antimicrobial use and provide feedback to providers
- Formulary restriction and preauthorization requirements for selected antibiotics
- Education of care providers regarding antibiotic use or misuse and the development of resistance
- Development of clinical guidelines for selected medical conditions
- Antimicrobial order forms
- Specific plans for streamlining (broad-to-narrow spectrum antibiotic agents) and de-escalation (elimination of redundant or unnecessary) antibiotic agents
- Optimize dosing regimen based on individual patient characteristics such as weight, renal status, or drug-drug interactions
- Change from parenteral to oral antibiotic agents when appropriate and feasible

Data from Polin RA, Denson S, Brady MT, Committee on Fetus and Newborn, Committee on Infectious Diseases. Strategies for prevention of health care-associated infections in the NICU. Pediatrics 2012;129(4):e1085–93; and Dellit TH, Owens RC, McGowan JE Jr, et al. Infectious Diseases Society of America and the Society for Healthcare Epidemiology of America guidelines for developing an institutional program to enhance antimicrobial stewardship. Clin Infect Dis 2007;44(2):159–77.

---

mixture of probiotics used, and that the combinations of probiotics used in the studies are not available in the United States. Further, there remains some gap in knowledge on which probiotic bacteria species to use, the microbial dose, as well as the duration of administration.

In 2014, an updated review of the aforementioned meta-analysis of randomized controlled trials continues to support a change in practice of supplementing preterm infants with probiotics. The review provided similar results involving more than 5000 infants in whom probiotics significantly reduced severe NEC and mortality.[62] However, the previously mentioned gap in knowledge remains, as well as the need for comparative studies.

There is scarcity of medical evidence to recommend the addition of prebiotics such as oligosaccharides in infant formula. Prebiotics are nondigestible food ingredients that occur naturally or as dietary supplements that enhance growth of probiotic bacteria such as *Bifidobacterium* spp.[60] Several studies had reported that the addition of prebiotics in infant formula significantly increased the bifidobacteria counts in their stool without adverse effects noted. However, clinical efficacy as well as cost-benefit analyses regarding the addition of oligosaccharides to infant formulas is lacking.[60]

For infants, human milk remains the best source of naturally occurring prebiotics and probiotics, and immunoprotective compounds known to decrease the incidence of respiratory and gastrointestinal infections.[48,60]

Nursery Intensive Care Unit Care Bundles

There are invasive procedures that may increase the infant's risk of health care–associated infections in the NICU setting. These infections include central line–associated BSIs (CLABSIs), pneumonia, skin, and soft tissue infections; and, occasionally, vaccine-preventable diseases and outbreak of respiratory viral infections. Care bundles are sets of interventions aimed at reducing health care–associated infections in the NICU.[48]

The most common cause of CLABSI[48] and LOS[8] are coagulase-negative staphylo-cocci. Several randomized clinical trials on the use of low-dose vancomycin in paren-teral solutions in preterm infants did not show significant decrease in the length of stay and mortality.[48] There is an antibiotic-lock therapy done in neonates that significantly decrease CLABSI however it was not powered to answer whether vancomycin resis-tance occurred. Both are currently not recommended because of the lack of long-term efficacy evidence as well as concern for development of drug-resistant organisms.

Infection control intended to decrease CLABSI in the NICU should include measures to decrease extraluminal and intravascular catheter–related infections. Various tech-niques and guidelines in the prevention of CLABSI in infants adapted from the AAP Committee on Fetus and Newborn are shown in **Box 2**.[48]

There are specific practices that may be adapted in the local setting for preventing vaccine-preventable diseases and outbreaks of respiratory viral infections. These include but are not limited to vaccination of health care providers against influenza and pertussis (Tdap), visitation guidelines to screen ill or symptomatic visitors, and cohorting in cases of clustering of infections or in outbreak situations.[48] Cohorting may only be possible if early screening procedures, such as the use of PCR-based as-says, are in place if available in cases of clustering of respiratory viral infections.[14–16] Further, appropriate isolation (eg, contact precautions for MRSA, droplet precautions for influenza, and airborne precautions for measles) should be observed if the infant is

---

Box 2
Techniques and guidelines in the prevention of central line–associated bloodstream infections in the nursery intensive care unit

Techniques in the prevention of extraluminal catheter contamination

- Hand hygiene
- Aseptic catheter insertion and the use of maximal sterile barrier for catheter insertion and care
- Use of topical antiseptic
- Use of sterile dressing

Guidelines in the prevention of intravascular catheter infection

- Remove and do not replace umbilical artery catheters if signs of CLABSI, thrombosis, or vascular insufficiency in the lower extremities are present.
- Remove and do not replace umbilical venous catheters if signs of CLABSI or thrombosis are present.
- Clean the umbilical insertion site using an antiseptic such as povidone-iodine before catheter insertion.
- Avoid using topical antibiotic ointment or creams on insertion sites to prevent fungal infections and antimicrobial resistance.
- Use low doses of heparin (0.25–1.0 U/mL) to the fluid infused through umbilical arterial catheter.
- Remove umbilical catheters as soon as no longer needed or if signs of vascular insufficiency to the lower extremities (for umbilical artery access) are present; they may be replaced if malfunctioning. Umbilical artery catheters should not be left in place for more than 5 days. Umbilical venous catheters may be used up to 14 days if managed aseptically.

Data from Polin RA, Denson S, Brady MT, Committee on Fetus and Newborn, Committee on Infectious Diseases. Strategies for prevention of health care-associated infections in the NICU. Pediatrics 2012;129(4):e1085–93.

colonized or infected with a pathogen requiring additional protection beyond standard precautions.[63]

SUMMARY

Neonatal infections continue to cause morbidity and mortality in infants. GBS and *E coli* are the most common agents of EOS, whereas coagulase-negative *Staphylococcus* is the predominant cause for LOS. There is increasing recognition of respiratory viral infections contributing to ruling out sepsis in very young infants whose presentations are similar to bacterial infections. Blood culture at birth and white blood cell with or without CRP has been used in the algorithm-based guideline for the evaluation of asymptomatic term and preterm infants with risk factors for sepsis. Ampicillin and gentamicin remains the cornerstone of initial antimicrobial regimen for neonatal infections. Third-generation cephalosporins should be used judiciously. The use of antiviral (acyclovir, ganciclovir, valganciclovir, and oseltamivir) and antifungal (fluconazole, amphotericin B, and voriconazole) treatment and prophylactic regimens may reduce mortality and morbidity to specific viral and fungal disease in infants. There are various strategies, such as GBS prophylaxis, hand hygiene, immunization, and immunoprophylaxis, ASP, probiotics, and prebiotics, and NICU care bundles, which may be used in preventing infections in infants.

REFERENCES

1. Stoll BJ, Hansen NI, Sanchez PJ, et al. Early onset neonatal sepsis: the burden of group B Streptococcal and *E. coli* disease continues. Pediatrics 2011;127(5): 817–26.
2. Camacho-Gonzalez A, Spearman PW, Stoll BJ. Neonatal infectious diseases: evaluation of neonatal sepsis. Pediatr Clin North Am 2013;60(2):367–89.
3. Schelonka RL, Maheshwari A. The many faces of B cells: from generation of antibodies to immune regulation. NeoReviews 2013;14:e438–47.
4. Kollmann TR, Crabtree J, Rein-Weston A, et al. Neonatal innate TLR-mediated responses are distinct from those of adults. J Immunol 2009;183(11):7150–60.
5. Levy O. Innate immunity of the newborn: basic mechanisms and clinical correlates. Nat Rev Immunol 2007;7(5):379–90.
6. Randolph D. The neonatal adaptive immune system. NeoReviews 2005;6: e454–62.
7. Polin RA, Committee on Fetus and Newborn. Management of neonates with suspected or proven early-onset bacterial sepsis. Pediatrics 2012;129(5):1006–15.
8. Tripathi N, Cotten CM, Smith PB. Antibiotic use and misuse in the neonatal intensive care unit. Clin Perinatol 2012;39(1):61–8.
9. Cotten CM, McDonald S, Stoll B, et al. The association of third-generation cephalosporin use and invasive candidiasis in extremely low birth-weight infants. Pediatrics 2006;118(2):717–22.
10. Cotten CM, Taylor S, Stoll B, et al. Prolonged duration of initial empirical antibiotic treatment is associated with increased rates of necrotizing enterocolitis and death for extremely low birth weight infants. Pediatrics 2009;123(1):58–66.
11. Kuppala VS, Meinzen-Derr J, Morrow AL, et al. Prolonged initial empirical antibiotic treatment is associated with adverse outcomes in premature infants. J Pediatr 2011;159(5):720–5.
12. Cordero L, Ayers LW. Duration of empiric antibiotics for suspected early-onset sepsis in extremely low birth weight infants. Infect Control Hosp Epidemiol 2003;24(9):662–6.

13. Rhedin S, Lindstrand A, Rotzen-Ostlund M, et al. Clinical utility of PCR for common viruses in acute respiratory illness. Pediatrics 2014;133(3):e538–45.
14. Ronchi A, Michelow IC, Chapin KC, et al. Viral respiratory tract infections in the neonatal intensive care unit: the VIRIoN-I study. J Pediatr 2014;165(4):690–6.
15. Bennett NJ, Tabarani CM, Bartholoma NM, et al. Unrecognized viral respiratory tract infections in premature infants during their birth hospitalization: a prospective surveillance study in two neonatal intensive care units. J Pediatr 2012;161(5): 814–8.
16. Steiner M, Strassl R, Straub J, et al. Nosocomial rhinovirus infection in preterm infants. Pediatr Infect Dis J 2012;31(12):1302–4.
17. Smith PB, Benjamin DK. Clinical approach to the infected neonate. In: Long SS, Pickering LK, Prober CG, editors. Principles and practice of pediatric infectious diseases. 4th edition. Philadelphia: Elsevier Saunders; 2012. p. 536–8.
18. Santos RP, Sanchez PJ, Mejias A, et al. Successful medical treatment of cutaneous aspergillosis in a premature infant using liposomal amphotericin B, voriconazole and micafungin. Pediatr Infect Dis J 2007;26(4):364–6.
19. Bizzarro MJ, Raskind C, Baltimore RS, et al. Seventy-five years of neonatal sepsis at Yale: 1928-2003. Pediatrics 2005;116(3):595–602.
20. Escobar GJ, Li DK, Armstrong MA, et al. Neonatal sepsis workups in infants >/=2000 grams at birth: a population-based study. Pediatrics 2000;106(2 Pt 1):256–63.
21. Edwards MS, Baker CJ. Bacterial infections in neonate. In: Long SS, Pickering L, Prober CG, editors. Principles and practice of pediatric infectious diseases. 4th edition. Philadelphia: Elsevier Saunders; 2012. p. 538–43.
22. Piantino JH, Schreiber MD, Alexander K, et al. Culture negative sepsis and systemic inflammatory response syndrome in neonates. NeoReviews 2013;14: e294–305.
23. Ottolini MC, Lundgren K, Mirkinson LJ, et al. Utility of complete blood count and blood culture screening to diagnose neonatal sepsis in the asymptomatic at risk newborn. Pediatr Infect Dis J 2003;22(5):430–4.
24. Effective biomarkers for diagnosis of neonatal sepsis. J Ped Infect Dis 2014;3(3): 234–45.
25. Baron EJ, Miller JM, Weinstein MP, et al. A guide to utilization of the microbiology laboratory for diagnosis of infectious diseases: 2013 recommendations by the Infectious Diseases Society of America (IDSA) and the American Society for Microbiology (ASM)(a). Clin Infect Dis 2013;57(4):e22–121.
26. Mussap M. Laboratory medicine in neonatal sepsis and inflammation. J Matern Fetal Neonatal Med 2012;25(Suppl 4):32–4.
27. Lartigue MF, Kostrzewa M, Salloum M, et al. Rapid detection of "highly virulent" Group B Streptococcus ST-17 and emerging ST-1 clones by MALDI-TOF mass spectrometry. J Microbiol Methods 2011;86(2):262–5.
28. Mekouar H, Voortman G, Bernard P, et al. Capnocytophaga species and perinatal infections: case report and review of the literature. Acta Clin Belg 2012;67(1): 42–5.
29. Iatta R, Cafarchia C, Cuna T, et al. Bloodstream infections by Malassezia and Candida species in critical care patients. Med Mycol 2014;52(3):264–9.
30. Schlebusch S, Price GR, Hinds S, et al. First outbreak of PVL-positive nonmultiresistant MRSA in a neonatal ICU in Australia: comparison of MALDI-TOF and SNP-plus-binary gene typing. Eur J Clin Microbiol Infect Dis 2010;29(10):1311–4.
31. Pulcrano G, Roscetto E, Iula VD, et al. MALDI-TOF mass spectrometry and microsatellite markers to evaluate Candida parapsilosis transmission in neonatal intensive care units. Eur J Clin Microbiol Infect Dis 2012;31(11):2919–28.

32. American Academy of Pediatrics. Antimicrobial therapy for newborns. In: Bradley JS, editor. 2014 Nelson's pediatric antimicrobial therapy. Elk Grove Village (IL): American Academy of Pediatrics; 2014. p. 17–36.
33. de Hoog M, Mouton JW, van den Anker JN. The use of aminoglycosides in newborn infants. In: Choonara I, Nun AJ, Kearns G, editors. Introduction to paediatric and perinatal drug therapy. Notthingham (England): Nottingham University Press; 2003. p. 117–40.
34. Begg EJ, Barclay ML, Kirkpatrick CJ. The therapeutic monitoring of antimicrobial agents. Br J Clin Pharmacol 1999;47(1):23–30.
35. Novelli A, Mazzei T, Fallani S, et al. In vitro postantibiotic effect and postantibiotic leukocyte enhancement of tobramycin. J Chemother 1995;7(4):355–62.
36. Craig WA. Once-daily versus multiple-daily dosing of aminoglycosides. J Chemother 1995;7(Suppl 2):47–52.
37. Rotschafer JC, Zabinski RA, Walker KJ. Pharmacodynamic factors of antibiotic efficacy. Pharmacotherapy 1992;12(6 Pt 2):64S–70S.
38. Bryan CS, John JF Jr, Pai MS, et al. Gentamicin vs cefotaxime for therapy of neonatal sepsis. Relationship to drug resistance. Am J Dis Child 1985;139(11): 1086–9.
39. Bradley JS, Wassel RT, Lee L, et al. Intravenous ceftriaxone and calcium in the neonate: assessing the risk for cardiopulmonary adverse events. Pediatrics 2009;123(4):e609–13.
40. Kimberlin DW, Whitley RJ, Wan W, et al. Oral acyclovir suppression and neurodevelopment after neonatal herpes. N Engl J Med 2011;365(14):1284–92.
41. Kimberlin DW, Baley J, Committee on Infectious Diseases, et al. Guidance on management of asymptomatic neonates born to women with active genital herpes lesions. Pediatrics 2013;131(2):e635–46.
42. Kimberlin DW, Jester P, Sanchez PJ, et al. Six months versus six weeks of oral valganciclovir for infants with symptomatic congenital cytomegalovirus (CMV) disease with and without central nervous system (CNS) involvement: Results of a Phase III, randomized, double-blind, placebo-controlled, multinational study. 2013 ID Week. Infectious Disease Society of America. San Francisco (CA), October 5, 2013. Available at: https://idsa.confex.com/idsa/2013/webprogram/Paper43178.html. Accessed October 7, 2014.
43. Committee On Infectious Diseases. Recommendations for prevention and control of influenza in children, 2014-2015. Pediatrics 2014;134(5):e1503–19.
44. Bizzarro MJ, Ehrenkranz RA, Gallagher PG. Concurrent bloodstream infections in infants with necrotizing enterocolitis. J Pediatr 2014;164(1):61–6.
45. Segal I, Kang C, Albersheim SG, et al. Surgical site infections in infants admitted to the neonatal intensive care unit. J Pediatr Surg 2014;49(3):381–4.
46. Verani JR, McGee L, Schrag SJ, et al. Prevention of perinatal group B streptococcal disease—revised guidelines from CDC, 2010. MMWR Recomm Rep 2010;59(RR-10):1–36.
47. Prevention CfDCa. Group B Strep (GBS). 2014. Available at: http://www.cdc.gov/groupBstrep/guidelines/index.html. Accessed October 8, 2014.
48. Polin RA, Denson S, Brady MT, et al. Strategies for prevention of health care-associated infections in the NICU. Pediatrics 2012;129(4):e1085–93.
49. Boyce JM, Pittet D, Healthcare Infection Control Practices Advisory Committee, et al. Guideline for hand hygiene in health-care settings: recommendations of the Healthcare Infection Control Practices Advisory Committee and the HICPAC/SHEA/APIC/IDSA Hand Hygiene Task Force. Infect Control Hosp Epidemiol 2002;23(12 Suppl):S3–40.

50. CDC. Hand Hygiene in Healthcare Settings. 2014. Available at: http://www.cdc. gov/handhygiene/. Accessed September 30, 2014.
51. Healy CM, Pickering LK. How to communicate with vaccine-hesitant parents. Pediatrics 2011;127(Suppl 1):S127–33.
52. American Academy of Pediatrics. Hepatitis B. In: Pickering LK, editor. Red Book. Elk Grove Village (IL): American Academy of Pediatrics; 2012. p. 369–90.
53. Committee on Infectious Diseases, American Academy of Pediatrics. Recommended childhood and adolescent immunization schedule—United States, 2014. Pediatrics 2014;133(2):357–63.
54. Lessin HR, Edwards KM, Committee On Practice And Ambulatory Medicine, et al. Immunizing parents and other close family contacts in the pediatric office setting. Pediatrics 2012;129(1):e247–53.
55. Sawyer M, Liang JL, Messonnier N, et al. Updated recommendations for use of tetanus toxoid, reduced diphtheria toxoid, and acellular pertussis vaccine (Tdap) in pregnant women—Advisory Committee on Immunization Practices (ACIP), 2012. MMWR Recomm Rep 2013;62(7):131–5.
56. Healy CM, Rench MA, Baker CJ. Importance of timing of maternal combined tetanus, diphtheria, and acellular pertussis (Tdap) immunization and protection of young infants. Clin Infect Dis 2013;56(4):539–44.
57. American Academy of Pediatrics Committee on Infectious Diseases, American Academy of Pediatrics Bronchiolitis Guidelines Committee. Updated guidance for palivizumab prophylaxis among infants and young children at increased risk of hospitalization for respiratory syncytial virus infection. Pediatrics 2014; 134(2):415–20.
58. Basu S. Neonatal sepsis: the gut connection. Eur J Clin Microbiol Infect Dis 2014. [Epub ahead of print].
59. Dellit TH, Owens RC, McGowan JE Jr, et al. Infectious Diseases Society of America and the Society for Healthcare Epidemiology of America guidelines for developing an institutional program to enhance antimicrobial stewardship. Clin Infect Dis 2007;44(2):159–77.
60. Thomas DW, Greer FR, American Academy of Pediatrics Committee on Nutrition, et al. Probiotics and prebiotics in pediatrics. Pediatrics 2010;126(6):1217–31.
61. Alfaleh K, Anabrees J, Bassler D, et al. Probiotics for prevention of necrotizing enterocolitis in preterm infants. Cochrane Database Syst Rev 2011;(3):CD005496.
62. AlFaleh K, Anabrees J. Probiotics for prevention of necrotizing enterocolitis in preterm infants. Cochrane Database Syst Rev 2014;(4):CD005496.
63. American Academy of Pediatrics. Transmission-based precautions. In: Pickering LK, Baker CJ, Kimberlin DW, et al, editors. Red ook: 2012 report of the committee on infectious diseases. 29th edition. Elk Grove Village (IL): American Academy of Pediatrics; 2012. p. 164–7.

Common Hematologic Problems in the Newborn Nursery

Jon F. Watchko, MD

KEYWORDS

- Hyperbilirubinemia • Hemolysis • Anemia • Polycythemia • Thrombocytopenia
- Rh disease • G6PD deficiency

KEY POINTS

- Early clinical jaundice or rapidly developing hyperbilirubinemia are often signs of hemolysis, the differential diagnosis of which commonly includes immune-mediated disorders, red-cell enzyme deficiencies, and red-cell membrane defects.
- Knowledge of the maternal blood type and antibody screen is critical in identifying non-ABO alloantibodies in the maternal serum that may pose a risk for severe hemolytic disease in the newborn.
- Moderate to severe thrombocytopenia in an otherwise well-appearing newborn strongly suggests immune-mediated (alloimmune or autoimmune) thrombocytopenia.

INTRODUCTION

Hematologic problems often arise in the newborn nursery, particularly those related to the red blood cell (RBC), the primary focus of this review. Their timely identification is important to ensure appropriate care of the neonate. Common RBC disorders include hemolytic disease of the newborn, anemia, and polycythemia. Another clinically relevant hematologic issue in neonates to be covered herein is thrombocytopenia. Disorders of white blood cells will not be reviewed.

RED BLOOD CELL

Clinical signs of an RBC disorder in the immediate newborn period are jaundice (hemolysis), pallor (anemia), and plethora (polycythemia). Of these RBC disorders, hemolysis is the most frequently encountered and often heralded by early-onset jaundice

Disclosure Statement: Dr J.F. Watchko reports providing expert testimony in legal cases related to neonatal jaundice. No other potential conflict of interest was reported.
Division of Newborn Medicine, Department of Pediatrics, Magee-Womens Hospital, 300 Halket Street and Children's Hospital of Pittsburgh, University of Pittsburgh School of Medicine, 4401 Penn Avenue, Pittsburgh, PA 15213, USA
E-mail address: jwatchko@mail.magee.edu

Pediatr Clin N Am 62 (2015) 509–524
http://dx.doi.org/10.1016/j.pcl.2014.11.011
0031-3955/15/$ – see front matter © 2015 Elsevier Inc. All rights reserved.
pediatric.theclinics.com

($\leq$24 hours of age).[1] In the current era of birth hospitalization, bilirubin screening using total serum bilirubin (TSB) or transcutaneous bilirubin (TcB) measurements,[2,3] an elevated hour specific bilirubin greater than 75% on the Bhutani nomogram also is a marker for hemolysis.[4] Although there are many diagnostic considerations in the interpretation of RBC disturbances in the neonatal period,[5] a systematic approach based on mechanism(s) of disease highlighted herein make this process more straightforward.

HEMOLYTIC DISEASE OF THE NEWBORN

Catabolism of RBC-derived heme produces bilirubin that results in jaundice, the most prevalent clinical condition requiring evaluation and management in neonates.[6–8] Although hepatic and gastrointestinal immaturities that limit bilirubin clearance contribute to neonatal jaundice, it is increasingly clear that accelerated RBC turnover (hemolysis) plays a pivotal role in the risk for subsequent severe hyperbilirubinemia.[4,8–11] Moreover, hemolysis potentiates the risk of bilirubin neurotoxicity[9–12] and treatment interventions are therefore recommended at lower TSB levels when hemolysis is present.[13,14] Pediatricians must therefore have a strong working knowledge of hemolytic disorders to properly care for the jaundiced neonate. These conditions are outlined in **Box 1** and include immune-mediated disorders, red-cell enzyme defects, red-cell membrane abnormalities, and, for completeness but exceedingly rare in neonates, hemoglobinopathies.[7–9]

Immune-Mediated Hemolytic Disorders

Immune-mediated disorders are the most common cause of hemolysis in neonates and should be suspected when there is (1) a heterospecific mother-infant pair in which

---

Box 1
Hemolytic conditions in the neonate

1. Immune-mediated (positive direct Coombs test)
    a. Rhesus blood group: Anti-D, -c, -C, -e, -E, C^W, and several others
    b. Non-Rhesus blood groups: Kell, Duffy, Kidd, Xg, Lewis, MNS, and others
    c. ABO blood group: Anti-A, -B
2. Red blood cell (RBC) enzyme defects
    a. Glucose-6-phosphate dehydrogenase (G6PD) deficiency
    b. Pyruvate kinase deficiency
    c. Others
3. RBC membrane defects
    a. Hereditary spherocytosis
    b. Elliptocytosis
    c. Stomatocytosis
    d. Pyknocytosis
    e. Others
4. Hemoglobinopathies
    a. alpha-thalassemia
    b. gamma-thalassemia

the infant expresses a red-cell antigen(s) foreign to the mother, (2) the presence of a maternal antibody directed to the infant RBC antigen, (3) and a positive direct Coombs test in the neonate indicating maternal antibody bound to the infant RBC. An initial priority in evaluating every newborn is therefore knowledge of the maternal blood type and the maternal antibody screen. The latter deserves specific comment and emphasis.

The maternal antibody screen is a routine test performed at maternal registration on pregnancy diagnosis. The goal of screening is to identify non-ABO alloantibodies in the maternal serum that may pose a risk for hemolytic disease in the newborn. A standard screening panel for alloantibodies is shown in **Table 1**. In addition, women who are Rh-D negative and have a negative antibody screen at registration will have a repeat screen at 24 to 28 weeks' gestation before Rhogam (RhD-Ig) administration, and another screen at delivery along with a type and Coombs on the infant to determine the need for postpartum Rhogam. Interpreting the results of the maternal antibody screen by pediatricians is critical in identifying mothers who carry a non-ABO alloantibody, several of which can cause moderate to severe hemolytic disease of the newborn as detailed in **Table 2**.[15,16]

Indeed, in addition to the classic Rhesus hemolytic disease of the newborn secondary to Rh-D isoimmunization, alloantibodies directed to non-D Rhesus antigens and a broad range of non-Rhesus blood group antigens are seen. Increasingly, the latter 2 categories comprise a clinically relevant proportion of hemolytic disease of the newborn. Identical maternal and infant blood grouping with respect to the ABO system and Rh-D status ("Rh positive" or "Rh negative") does not preclude the presence of a clinically significant maternal alloantibody. Only a review of the maternal antibody screen and the direct Coombs test on the infant will uncover such cases.[15–17] Indeed, a type and direct Coombs test are indicated at delivery (cord or infant blood) on all infants born to women with potentially significant alloantibodies.[17]

Table 3 outlines several clinical scenarios in which the maternal antibody screen is positive, accompanied by the likely clinical explanation for the positive screen. It should be readily apparent that the clinical details outlined in each case must be sought out and appreciated by caretakers to identify infants at risk for non-ABO immune-mediated hemolytic disease. The only scenario shown that does not indicate maternal sensitization is that secondary to Rhogam administration. The latter positive anti-D maternal antibody screen finding must be distinguished from the rare occurrence of late Rh-D sensitization by confirming that the mother was anti-D antibody

Table 1
Standard maternal antibody screening

Alloantibody	Blood Group
D, C, c, E, e, f, C^W, V	Rhesus
K, k, Kp^a, Js^a	Kell
Fy^a, Fy^b	Duffy
Jk^a, Jk^b	Kidd
Xga	Xg
Le^a, Le^b	Lewis
S, s, M, N	MNS
P1	P
Lu^b	Lutheran

Table 2
Non-ABO alloantibodies reported to cause moderate to severe hemolytic disease of the newborn

Within Rh system	Anti-D, -c, -C, -C^W, -C^x, -e, -E, -E^W, -ce, -Ce^s, -Rh29, -Rh32, -Rh42, -f, -G, -Go^a, -Be^a, -Evans, -Rh17, -Hr$_o$, -Hr, -Tar, -Sec, -JAL, -STEM
Outside Rh system	Anti-LW, -K, -k, -Kp^a, -Kp^b, -Jk^a, -Js^a, -Js^b, -Ku, -K11, -K22, -Fy^a, -M, -N, -S, -s, -U, -PP$_1$^{pk}, -Di^b, -Far, -MUT, -En^3, -Hut, -Hil, -Vel, -MAM, -JONES, -HJK, -REIT

Data from Liley HG. Immune hemolytic disease. In: Nathan DG, Orkin SH, Look AT, et al, editors. Nathan and Oski's hematology of infancy and childhood. 6th edition. Philadelphia: WB Saunders; 2003. p. 56–85; and Eder AF. Update on HDFN: new information on long-standing controversies. Immunohematology 2006;22:188–95.

negative before Rhogam administration, and that she did indeed receive the Rhogam. At times, the infant also will have a positive direct Coombs test secondary to maternal Rhogam administration.[18–20] This finding is generally not thought to indicate a hemolytic risk,[18–20] albeit one recent case report suggests in rare circumstances it may.[21] The latter has yet to be confirmed.[22]

It is also important to note that infants who are Rh-D positive and delivered to women who are Rh-D negative during the first isoimmunized pregnancy (conversion from negative to positive maternal antibody titer in that pregnancy) are at an approximately 20% risk of developing hemolytic disease of the newborn requiring treatment, including the possibility of an exchange transfusion.[23] This risk likely holds true for all non-ABO alloantibodies. An infant born of a pregnancy during which maternal antibody conversion occurs will by definition carry the foreign antigen and may have a positive direct Coombs test. Such infants are at risk of hemolytic disease of the newborn, should be monitored closely for the development of severe hyperbilirubinemia with serial TSB measurements, and should not be discharged early from the birth hospital.

ABO HEMOLYTIC DISEASE

Hemolytic disease related to ABO incompatibility is generally limited to mothers who are blood group O and infants of blood group A or B.[1,7–9,24] Although this association exists in approximately 15% of pregnancies, only a subset of such infants will develop significant hyperbilirubinemia.[1,7–9,24] Defining which infants will be affected is difficult to predict using standard laboratory screening tests.[1,7–9,24] Ozolek and colleagues[24] observed that of infants who are type A or B born to mothers who are blood group O, approximately one-third had a positive direct Coombs test, and of those with a positive direct Coombs test, approximately 15% had peak serum bilirubin levels greater than 12.8 mg/dL. Others have reported a higher percentage (approximately 50%) of hyperbilirubinemia (defined by an hour specific TSB >95% on the Bhutani nomogram) in infants who are type A or B who demonstrate a positive direct Coombs test born to mothers who are type O.[9,25] Regardless, only a subset evidence symptomatic hemolytic disease.[1,7–9,24,25]

Infants born of ABO-incompatible mother-infant pairs who have a negative direct Coombs test as a group appear to be at no greater risk for developing hyperbilirubinemia than their ABO-compatible counterparts[24] and the development of significant hyperbilirubinemia in such neonates should prompt an evaluation for a cause other than isoimmunization.[26] Similarly, infants who are group A or B born to mothers who

Table 3
Interpreting maternal antibody status in Rh-D negative women at delivery

Maternal Antibody Status at Beginning of Pregnancy	Maternal Antibody Status at 24–28 wk Before Rhogam	Was Rhogam Administered?	Maternal Antibody Status at Delivery	Maternal Antibody	Diagnosis	Infant at Risk for Hemolytic Disease of the Newborn
Negative	Negative	Yes	Positive	Anti-D	Passive anti-D; Rhogam effect	Unlikely[a]
Negative	Negative	No	Positive	Anti-D	Late sensitization to Rh-D	Yes
Negative	Positive	No	Positive	Anti-D	Early sensitization to Rh-D	Yes
Positive	Positive	No	Positive	Anti-D	Sensitized pregnancy to Rh-D	Yes
Negative	Negative	Yes	Positive	Non-D antibody	Late sensitization to non-D antigen	Yes

[a] At times, the infant will also have a positive direct Coombs test secondary to maternal Rhogam administration.[18–20] This finding is generally not thought to indicate a hemolytic risk,[18–20] albeit one recent case report suggests in rare circumstances it may.[21] The latter has yet to be confirmed.[22]

are, respectively, incompatible group B or A, are not likely to manifest symptomatic ABO hemolytic disease and fewer than 1% will have a positive direct Coombs test.[24]

Despite the difficulty in predicting its development, symptomatic ABO hemolytic disease does occur.[1,7–9] Hyperbilirubinemia seen with symptomatic ABO hemolytic disease is often detected within the first 12 to 24 hours of life[9,25] along with jaundice ("icterus neonatorum praecox")[27] and accompanied by microspherocytosis on peripheral blood smear and an increased reticulocyte count.[1,7–9,28] Indeed, of infants who were ABO-incompatible direct Coombs positive who developed a TSB greater than 95% on the Bhutani nomogram, 67% did so within the first 24 hours of life and only 1 of 85 such infants developed hyperbilirubinemia after 48 hours.[25] Hyperbilirubinemia in symptomatic ABO hemolytic disease is more often than not controlled with intensive phototherapy alone. Only a few affected infants will develop hyperbilirubinemia to levels requiring exchange transfusion, albeit this must be monitored for.

Some ABO heterospecific mother-infant pairs hold potential for more severe hemolytic disease than others. O-B heterospecificity is associated with greater hyperbilirubinemia risk than O-A,[9,25] in particular in mothers and neonates of African origin.[1,29–31] Although there is some conflicting literature regarding the latter,[1] our recent institutional experience and other reports[31,32] support the assertion that O-B heterospecificity poses some risk in African American individuals. The last 6 double-volume exchange transfusions we performed for symptomatic ABO hemolytic disease have all been in the context of O-B incompatibility and an African American mother. In each case there were markedly elevated maternal immunoglobulin G (IgG) anti-B titers in the range of 1:1024 to 1:2048, as contrasted with the more typical 1:8 to 1:32 titers in mothers who are type O. None of the affected neonates had coexistent glucose-6-phosphate dehydrogenase (G6PD) deficiency. High-titer anti-B IgG also has been reported in the rare case of ABO hemolytic disease in mothers who are group A.[33]

During robust hemolysis of any cause, the TSB may continue to rise despite intensive phototherapy. Indeed, if not previously considered, failure of phototherapy to produce a prompt decline in TSB should raise the possibility of an underlying hemolytic condition.[34] It follows that in hyperbilirubinemic newborns with symptomatic ABO hemolytic disease, TSB should be monitored during phototherapy to ensure the TSB does not rise to levels that merit exchange transfusion.

Routine screening of all ABO-incompatible cord blood has been recommended in the past and remains common practice in many nurseries. The literature, however, suggests that such screening is not warranted given the cost and low yield,[24,35,36] consistent with the tenor of recommendations of the American Association of Blood Banks,[17] the American Academy of Pediatrics,[13] and the implementation of universal newborn bilirubin screening during the birth hospitalization.[14] A blood type and direct Coombs test is indicated, however, in the evaluation of any newborn with early jaundice (<24 hours of age) and/or clinically significant hyperbilirubinemia, including those treated with phototherapy.

Red Blood Cell Enzymopathies

G6PD[9,37–40] and pyruvate kinase (PK)[41] deficiency are the 2 most common red-cell enzyme disorders associated with marked neonatal hyperbilirubinemia. Of these, G6PD deficiency is the more frequently encountered and it remains an important cause of kernicterus worldwide, including the United States, Canada, and the United Kingdom,[9,37–40,42,43] the prevalence in Western countries a reflection in part of immigration patterns and intermarriage. The risk of kernicterus in G6PD deficiency also relates to the potential for unexpected rapidly developing extreme hyperbilirubinemia in this disorder associated with acute severe hemolysis after exposure to oxidative stress.[9,40,42–44] Reported hemolytic triggers in neonates include among others naphthalene (moth balls), methylene blue, antimalarials, sulfonamides, maternal ingestion of fava beans (favism by proxy), and infection.[9,37–40,44] This mode of G6PD-deficiency–associated hazardous hyperbilirubinemia can result in kernicterus that may not always be preventable.[9,40,44]

More than 20% of neonates in the United States pilot kernicterus registry, a database of voluntarily submitted information on 125 infants who developed kernicterus between 1992 and 2004, had G6PD deficiency, as contrasted to an estimated 4% to 7% background population prevalence.[43] African American neonates comprised the most (73%),[43] reflecting the high prevalence of this condition (12.2% for boys; 4.1% for girls)[45,46] and risk for hazardous hyperbilirubinemia (TSB $\geq$30 mg/dL) in newborns of black race.[47] The latter belies the fact that black race is associated with a lower risk of TSB in the ranges of 13 to 15 mg/dL, 16 to 19 mg/dL, and $\geq$20 mg/dL.[44] This apparent discrepancy is best explained by G6PD deficiency itself and its potential to predispose to acute hemolysis, resultant rapid rise in TSB, and hazardous hyperbilirubinemia.[9,37–40,44]

G6PD deficiency is an X-linked enzymopathy affecting hemizygous males, homozygous females, and a subset of heterozygous females (via X chromosome inactivation). Hemolysis in G6PD deficient neonates, however, may be self-limited and overt anemia not necessarily noted, masked by other factors that modulate hemoglobin concentration in the immediate newborn period.[9,37–40] Severe jaundice rather than anemia may predominate in the clinical presentation.[48] In other neonates, the combination of G6PD deficiency with hepatic bilirubin conjugation defects of Gilbert syndrome significantly increases the risk of hyperbilirubinemia.[44,49] Pediatricians must have a high index of suspicion for G6PD deficiency in populations with increased risk (Mediterranean region, Africa, the Middle East, Asia), and in particular the African American neonate, with significant hyperbilirubinemia.[9,13,37–40,44]

PK deficiency typically presents with jaundice, anemia, and reticulocytosis.[41] Such jaundice may be severe, as reflected by one series in which a full third of affected infants required *exchange transfusion* to control hyperbilirubinemia[50] and kernicterus in PK deficiency, and is well described.[41,51] The diagnosis of PK deficiency is often difficult, as the enzymatic abnormality is frequently not simply a quantitative defect, but in many cases involves abnormal enzyme kinetics or an unstable enzyme that decreases in activity as the red cell ages.[41] It is inherited as an autosomal recessive disorder, but notably, most affected individuals are compound heterozygotes; that is, they express 2 different disease-causing alleles: 1 maternal and 1 paternal in origin.[41] The diagnosis of PK deficiency should be considered whenever persistent significant hyperbilirubinemia and a picture of nonspherocytic, Coombs-negative hemolytic anemia is observed, particularly in populations in which consanguinity is prevalent, including newborns of Amish descent[52] and in other remote communities where intermarriage is prevalent.[53,54]

RED BLOOD CELL MEMBRANE DEFECTS

Establishing a diagnosis of RBC membrane defects is classically based on the development of Coombs-negative hyperbilirubinemia, a positive family history, and abnormal RBC smear, albeit it is often difficult because newborns normally exhibit a marked variation in red-cell membrane size and shape.[7,55] Spherocytes, however, are not often seen on RBC smears of hematologically normal newborns and this morphologic abnormality, when prominent, may yield a diagnosis of hereditary spherocytosis (HS) in the immediate neonatal period.[7,28] Given that approximately 75% of families affected with hereditary spherocytosis manifest an autosomal dominant phenotype, a positive family history can often be elicited and provide further support for this diagnosis.[7] More recently, Christensen and Henry[56] highlighted the use of an elevated mean corpuscular hemoglobin concentration (MCHC) ($\geq$36.0 g/dL) and/or elevated ratio of MCHC to mean corpuscular volume, the latter they term the "neonatal HS index" (>0.36, likely >0.40)[28,57] as screening tools for HS. An index of greater than 0.36 had 97% sensitivity, greater than 99% specificity, and greater than 99% negative predictive value for identifying HS in neonates.[57] Christensen and colleagues[28] also provided a concise update of morphologic RBC features that may be helpful in diagnosing this and other underlying hemolytic conditions in newborns.

The diagnosis of HS can be confirmed using the incubated osmotic fragility test when coupled with fetal red-cell controls[7] or eosin-5-maleimide flow cytometry.[28] One must rule out symptomatic ABO hemolytic disease by performing a direct Coombs test, as infants so affected also may manifest prominent microspherocytosis.[26] Moreover, HS and symptomatic ABO hemolytic disease can occur in the same infant and result in severe hyperbilirubinemia and anemia.[58]

Of other red-cell membrane defects, only hereditary elliptocytosis, stomatocytosis, and infantile pyknocytosis have been reported to exhibit significant hemolysis in the newborn period.[7,59–61] Hereditary elliptocytosis and stomatocytosis are both rare.[7,59] Infantile pyknocytosis, a transient red-cell membrane abnormality manifesting itself during the first few months of life, is more common. The pyknocyte, an irregularly contracted red cell with multiple spines, can normally be observed in newborns, particularly premature infants, in whom up to approximately 5% of red cells may manifest this morphologic variant.[7,61] In newborns affected with infantile pyknocytosis, up to 50% of red cells exhibit the morphologic abnormality and this degree of pyknocytosis is associated with jaundice, anemia, and reticulocytosis.[7,61] Infantile pyknocytosis can cause hyperbilirubinemia that is severe enough to require control by exchange transfusion.[61] Red cells transfused into affected infants become pyknocytic and have a shortened life span, suggesting that an extracorpuscular factor mediates the morphologic alteration.[7,61] Whatever the mechanism underlying infantile pyknocytosis, the disorder tends to resolve after several months of life. Pyknocytosis also may occur in other conditions, including G6PD deficiency and hereditary elliptocytosis, and these must be excluded before a diagnosis of infantile pyknocytosis is made.[7]

HEMOGLOBINOPATHIES

Defects in hemoglobin structure or synthesis are rare disorders that infrequently manifest themselves in the neonatal period. Of these, the alpha-thalassemia syndromes are the most likely to be clinically apparent in newborns. Each human diploid cell contains 4 copies of the alpha-globin gene and, thus, 4 alpha-thalassemia syndromes have been described reflecting the presence of defects in 1, 2, 3, or 4 alpha-globin genes. Silent carriers have 1 abnormal alpha-globin chain and are asymptomatic. Alpha-thalassemia trait is associated with 2 alpha-thalassemia mutations and in neonates is not associated with hemolysis. Alpha-thalassemia trait, however, is common in black populations and can be detected by a low mean corpuscular volume of less than 95 μ^3 (healthy infants 100 to 120 μ^3).[62] Hemoglobin H disease results from the presence of 3 thalassemia mutations and can cause hemolysis and anemia in neonates.[63] Homozygous alpha-thalassemia (total absence of alpha-chain synthesis) results in profound hemolysis, anemia, hydrops fetalis, and almost always stillbirth or death in the immediate neonatal period.

The pure beta-thalassemias do not manifest themselves in the newborn period and the gamma-thalassemias are (1) incompatible with life (homozygous form), (2) associated with transient mild to moderate neonatal anemia if 1 or 2 genes are involved that resolves when beta-chain synthesis begins, or (3) in combination with impaired beta-chain synthesis, associated with severe hemolytic anemia and marked hyperbilirubinemia.[64]

DIAGNOSIS OF HEMOLYSIS

It is increasingly apparent that the diagnosis of hemolysis in neonates remains problematic and hemolytic conditions as a result are underrecognized. Several reports demonstrate that the etiology of extreme (>25 mg/dL) or hazardous (>30 mg/dL) hyperbilirubinemia is often unclear and not identified,[10,43,65] when almost assuredly a hemolytic process is an important contributor to its genesis in many if not most cases.[4,9,66] Indeed, Christensen and colleagues[66] recently reported that when an exhaustive search, including "next-generation" sequencing of a panel of hematologic and hepatic gene variants involved in neonatal hyperbilirubinemia was performed, a specific diagnosis was made in all infants with extreme hyperbilirubinemia (TSB >25 mg/dL) and without exception in this cohort was hemolytic in nature. Because the catabolism of heme derived from red-cell hemoglobin produces equimolar amounts of carbon monoxide (CO) and bilirubin, the point-of-care measurement of end-tidal CO corrected for ambient CO (ETCOc) may prove a useful adjunct in identifying infants with hemolysis at risk for subsequent severe hyperbilirubinemia and in further stratifying phototherapy and exchange transfusion treatment criteria.[67,68]

HEMOLYSIS AND NEUROTOXICITY RISK

Although bilirubin-induced brain injury is complex and multifactorial in nature,[69] the clinical impression that hemolysis potentiates bilirubin neurotoxicity in neonates is long-standing, dating back to the early work on Rh isoimmunization[70] and subsequent debates on the TSB treatment thresholds for exchange transfusion in hemolytic and nonhemolytic hyperbilirubinemia.[71,72] The neurotoxicity intensifying effect of hemolysis has recently been reaffirmed.[10–12] In one such study, Gamaleldin and coworkers[11] showed that the TSB threshold for identifying 90% of infants with bilirubin encephalopathy was 25.4 mg/dL (434 μmol/L) in infants with neurotoxicity risk factors (n = 138; primarily hemolytic disorders) as contrasted with 31.5 mg/dL (539 μmol/L) in those without (n = 111).[11] The presence of Rh hemolytic disease alone greatly increased the risk for bilirubin encephalopathy (odds ratio 48.6; 95% confidence interval 14–168).[11]

Other risk factors that might increase the risk of brain damage in an infant who has severe hyperbilirubinemia are shown in **Box 2**.[14] Treatment is recommended at a lower TSB when any of the neurotoxicity risk factors is present.[13,14]

Jaundice Evaluation and Management

The identification, evaluation, and management of neonatal jaundice are outlined in detail in the 2004 American Academy of Pediatrics hyperbilirubinemia practice guideline and is beyond the scope of the current review.[13] An update with clarifications published in 2009 highlighted the utility of universal bilirubin screening before birth hospitalization discharge and provided an algorithm for management and follow-up according to the predischarge bilirubin measurement(s), gestation, and risk factors for subsequent severe hyperbilirubinemia.[14]

Phototherapy and exchange transfusion remain the mainstays of treatment with intervention thresholds based on hour specific TSB measurement, gestation, and risk factors for neurotoxicity.[13,14] Phototherapy can be effectively administered in

---

Box 2
Risk factors for bilirubin neurotoxicity

Isoimmune hemolytic disease

G6PD deficiency

Asphyxia

Sepsis

Acidosis

Albumin less than 3.0 g/dL

Data from Maisels MJ, Bhutani VK, Bogen D, et al. Hyperbilirubinemia in the newborn infant > or =35 weeks' gestation: an update with clarifications. Pediatrics 2009;124:1193–8.

---

the newborn nursery, including during rooming-in, skin-to-skin contact, and breast-feeding.[73] Szucs and Rosenman[73] recently highlighted this family-centered method of phototherapy delivery in the mother's room, another example of which is shown in **Fig. 1**. Exchange transfusion, on the other hand, because of attendant risks and the need for intensive monitoring during the procedure, must be performed in the neonatal intensive care unit (NICU).[34,74]

ANEMIA

The causes of neonatal anemia (defined here as a hematocrit at birth <39)[75] are numerous and diagnostically categorized as those secondary to hemolysis, hemorrhage, and impaired RBC production. In the newborn nursery, hemolytic disorders

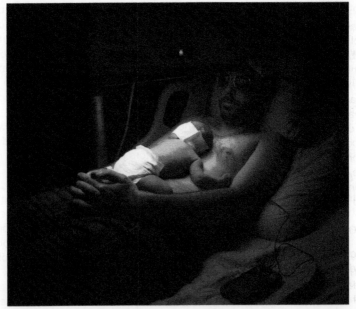

Fig. 1. Infant receiving family-centered care phototherapy delivery in mother's room and in skin-to-skin contact with father. Protective eye cover is worn by both the infant and parent.

are the most frequently encountered cause for anemia and any hemolytic condition can lead to anemia. In this regard, practitioners must monitor for progressive anemia in alloimmune-mediated disease and subsequent later need for packed RBC transfusion in the weeks after birth hospitalization discharge.[1]

Impaired RBC production is a rare cause of neonatal anemia, with the most frequent current etiology being fetal infection with parvovirus B-19; an important cause of fetal anemia and hydrops fetalis. If the degree of fetal anemia is modest and chronic in nature, such infants may appear otherwise well at birth. Pure RBC aplasia (Diamond-Blackfan anemia) is exceedingly uncommon.

Perinatal hemorrhage is the third diagnostic category and a commonly observed cause of neonatal anemia, particularly that secondary to fetomaternal hemorrhage and twin-twin transfusion syndrome. Like other etiologies, if the degree of anemia is modest and chronic in nature, such infants will not be compromised from a cardiorespiratory standpoint and will appear well without pallor . If fetal-neonatal blood loss is extensive and/or acute (regardless of cause), infants will be ill-appearing and managed in the NICU. The diagnosis of fetomaternal hemorrhage is made using Kleihauer-Betke testing on maternal blood. This test is based on the property of fetal hemoglobin (as opposed to adult hemoglobin) to resist elution from the RBC by strong acid to detect fetal RBCs in the maternal circulation. Twin-twin transfusion syndrome should be suspected in monochorionic twins and is often diagnosed in utero.

POLYCYTHEMIA

Polycythemia (venous hematocrit $\geq$65%) in seen in infants across a range of conditions associated with active erythropoiesis or passive transfusion.[76,77] They include, among others, placental insufficiency, the infant of a diabetic mother, recipient in twin-twin transfusion syndrome, and several aneuploidies, including trisomy 21.[76,77] The clinical concern related to polycythemia is the risk for microcirculatory complications of hyperviscosity. However, determining which polycythemic infants are hyperviscous and when to intervene is a challenge. Microviscometer measurements on blood are often not clinically available and the generalizability of normative data limited by several variables, including the site and time of sampling. Clinicians therefore screen for the presence of abnormal signs of hyperviscosity several of which are nonspecific and seen in other clinical contexts[76] and include lethargy, hypotonia, jitteriness, respiratory distress, hypoglycemia, and cyanosis. A hematocrit measurement should be part of the evaluation of infants with these signs to rule out the presence of polycythemia.

The management of the polycythemic neonate remains highly controversial because of the lack of evidence showing that aggressive treatment improves long-term outcome.[76,77] Most recent recommendations suggest limiting partial exchange transfusion to those polycythemic neonates with abnormal signs.[76,77] Partial volume exchange transfusion, if indicated, should be performed as early as possible and done so in the NICU with intensive monitoring. Polycythemia also is associated with increased risk for hyperbilirubinemia.

THROMBOCYTOPENIA

Thrombocytopenia (platelet count <150,000/μL) occurs in fewer than 1% of all newborns and is far more common in sick neonates in the NICU than the otherwise healthy-appearing term or late-preterm neonate in the newborn nursery. Analogous to anemia, the causes of thrombocytopenia can be grouped into (1) increased destruction, (2) loss (consumption), and (3) decreased production. For the otherwise healthy-appearing full-term neonate in the newborn nursery during the birth hospitalization, the most common etiology is immune-mediated destruction secondary to alloimmune and autoimmune-mediated mechanisms.[78,79] Indeed, the classic presentation of such disorders is a term neonate who appears well but manifests petechiae or bruising and has isolated thrombocytopenia.[78,79]

Neonatal alloimmune thrombocytopenia (NAIT) is often severe (median 19,000/ mm^3, range 1000–51,000 mm^3)[78] and affected newborns are frequently firstborns.[78] Fetomaternal incompatibility for human platelet antibodies 1a, 5b, and 15b account for 95% of NAIT with HPA-1a the most common.[78] Such infants are at risk for intracranial hemorrhage and should have neuroimaging to rule out this complication. Monitoring and treatment will require transfer to the NICU.

In contrast, autoimmune-mediated thrombocytopenia results from the passage of maternal antibodies directed to both maternal and infant platelet antigens and is associated with a history of or concurrent maternal thrombocytopenia and the diagnosis of a maternal autoimmune disorder, including among others maternal immune thrombocytopenic purpura, lupus, or other collagen vascular disorder.[79] In some cases, the maternal diagnosis is first made during the evaluation of her thrombocytopenic neonate.[79]

Other etiologies of thrombocytopenia encountered in the newborn nursery include congenital intrauterine infection and consumptive processes, such as vascular tumors in Kasabach-Merritt syndrome and renal vein thrombosis.[78,79] Inherited etiologies include those associated with aneuploidies (eg, trisomy 21), Fanconi anemia, thrombocytopenia absent radii syndrome, and congenital amegakaryocytic thrombocytopenia.[78,79] Thus, all thrombocytopenic infants in the healthy-infant nursery should have a careful examination for splenomegaly and lymphadenopathy (congenital infection), limb abnormalities, and cutaneous hemangiomas.[78] Infants with severe thrombocytopenia should be referred to the NICU for evaluation, monitoring, and management.

REFERENCES

1. Naiman JL. Erythroblastosis fetalis. In: Oski FA, Naiman JL, editors. Hematologic problems in the newborn. Philadelphia: W.B. Saunders; 1982. p. 283–346.
2. Kuzniewicz MW, Escobar GJ, Newman TB. Impact of universal bilirubin screening on severe hyperbilirubinemia and phototherapy use. Pediatrics 2009;124(4): 1031–9.
3. Darling EK, Ramsay T, Sprague AE, et al. Universal bilirubin screening and health care utilization. Pediatrics 2014;134(4):e1017–24.
4. Maisels MJ, Kring E. The contribution of hemolysis to early jaundice in normal newborns. Pediatrics 2006;118(1):276–9.
5. Brugnara C, Platt OS. The neonatal erythrocyte and its disorders. In: Nathan DG, Orkin SH, Look AT, et al, editors. Nathan and Oski's hematology of infancy and childhood. 6th edition. Philadelphia: W.B. Saunders; 2003. p. 19.
6. Keren R, Tremont K, Luan X, et al. Visual assessment of jaundice in term and late preterm infants. Arch Dis Child Fetal Neonatal Ed 2009;94:F317–22.
7. Watchko JF. Indirect hyperbilirubinemia in the neonate. In: Maisels MJ, Watchko JF, editors. Neonatal jaundice. Amsterdam: Harwood Academic Publishers; 2000. p. 51–66.
8. Maisels MJ. Jaundice. In: MacDonald MG, Seshia MM, Mullett MD, editors. Neonatology: pathophysiology and management of the newborn. 6th edition. Philadelphia: J.B. Lippincott; 2005. p. 768–846.
9. Kaplan M, Hammerman C. Hemolytic disorders and their management. In: Stevenson DK, Maisels MJ, Watchko JF, editors. Care of the jaundiced neonate. New York: McGraw-Hill; 2012. p. 145–73.

10. Kuzniewicz MW, Wickremasinghe AC, Wu YW, et al. Incidence, etiology, and outcomes of hazardous hyperbilirubinemia in newborns. Pediatrics 2014;134(3): 504–9.
11. Gamaleldin R, Iskander I, Seoud I, et al. Risk factors for neurotoxicity in newborns with severe neonatal hyperbilirubinemia. Pediatrics 2011;128:e925.
12. Iskander I, El Houchi S, El Shenawy A, et al. Validation of bilirubin/albumin ratio as a predictor of bilirubin-induced neurologic dysfunction (BIND). Pediatrics 2014;134(5):e1330–9.
13. Subcommittee on Hyperbilirubinemia, American Academy of Pediatrics. Clinical practice guideline: management of hyperbilirubinemia in the newborn infant 35 or more weeks of gestation. Pediatrics 2004;114:297–316.
14. Maisels MJ, Bhutani VK, Bogen D, et al. Hyperbilirubinemia in the newborn infant ≥ 35 weeks' gestation: an update with clarifications. Pediatrics 2009;124:1193–8.
15. Liley HG. Immune hemolytic disease. In: Nathan DG, Orkin SH, Look AT, et al, editors. Nathan and Oski's hematology of infancy and childhood. 6th edition. Philadelphia: WB Saunders; 2003. p. 56–85.
16. Eder AF. Update on HDFN: new information on long-standing controversies. Immunohematology 2006;22:188–95.
17. Judd WJ. Practice guidelines for prenatal and perinatal immunohematology, revisited. Transfusion 2001;41:1445–52.
18. Bowman JM, Chown B, Lewis M, et al. Rh isoimmunization during pregnancy: antenatal prophylaxis. Can Med Assoc J 1978;118:623–7.
19. Maayan-Metzger A, Schwartz T, Sulkes J, et al. Maternal anti-D prophylaxis during pregnancy does not cause neonatal haemolysis. Arch Dis Child Fetal Neonatal Ed 2001;84:F60–2.
20. Dillon A, Chaudhari T, Crispin P, et al. Has anti-D prophylaxis increased the rate of positive direct antiglobulin test results and can the direct antiglobulin test predict need for phototherapy in Rh/ABO incompatibility? J Paediatr Child Health 2011; 47:40–3.
21. Cohen DN, Johnson MS, Liang WH, et al. Clinically significant hemolytic disease of the newborn secondary to passive transfer of anti-D from maternal RhIG. Transfusion 2014;54(11):2863–6.
22. Watchko JF, Triulzi D. Need to clarify the cause of hemolysis in case report of newborn with clinically significant hemolytic disease and passive transfer of anti-D from maternal RhIG. Transfusion 2014;54(11):3017–8.
23. Goplerud CP, White CA, Bradbury JT, et al. The first Rh-isoimmunized pregnancy. Am J Obstet Gynecol 1973;115(5):632–8.
24. Ozolek JA, Watchko JF, Mimouni F. Prevalence and lack of clinical significance of blood group incompatibility in mothers with blood type A or B. J Pediatr 1994; 125:87–91.
25. Kaplan M, Hammerman C, Vreman HJ, et al. Hemolysis and hyperbilirubinemia in antiglobulin positive, direct ABO blood group heterospecific neonates. J Pediatr 2010;157:772–7.
26. Herschel M, Karrison T, Wen M, et al. Isoimmunization is unlikely to be the cause of hemolysis in ABO-incompatible but direct antiglobulin test-negative neonates. Pediatrics 2002;110:127–30.
27. Halbrecht I. Role of hemagglutinins anti-A and anti-B in pathogenesis of jaundice of the newborn (icterus neonatorum precox). Am J Dis Child 1944;68:248–9.
28. Christensen RD, Yaish HM, Lemons RS. Neonatal hemolytic jaundice: morphologic features of erythrocytes that will help you diagnose the underlying condition. Neonatology 2014;105:243–9.

29. Adewuyi JO, Gwanzura C, Mvere D. Characteristics of anti-A and anti-B in black Zimbabweans. Vox Sang 1994;67(3):307–9.
30. Adewuyi JO, Gwanzura C. Racial difference between white and black Zimbabweans in the haemolytic activity of A, B, O antibodies. Afr J Med Sci 2001; 30(1–2):71–4.
31. Murray NA, Roberts IAG. Haemolytic disease of the newborn. Arch Dis Child Fetal Neonatal Ed 2007;92(2):F83–8.
32. Ziprin JH, Payne E, Hamidi L, et al. ABO incompatibility due to immunoglobulin G anti-B antibodies presenting with severe fetal anemia. Transfus Med 2005;15: 57–60.
33. Wang M, Hays T, Silliman CC, et al. Hemolytic disease of the newborn caused by high titer anti-group B IgG from a group A mother. Pediatr Blood Cancer 2005;45: 861–2.
34. Maisels MJ, Stevenson DK, Watchko JF, et al. Phototherapy and other treatments. In: Stevenson DK, Maisels MJ, Watchko JF, editors. Care of the jaundiced neonate. New York: McGraw Hill; 2012. p. 195–227.
35. Shahid R, Graba S. Outcome and cost analysis of implementing selective Coombs testing in the newborn nursery. J Perinatol 2012;32:966–9.
36. Maisels MJ, Watchko JF. Routine blood typing and DAT in infants of group O mothers. J Perinatol 2013;33:579–80.
37. Beutler E. G6PD deficiency. Blood 1994;84:3613–36.
38. Luzzatto L. Glucose-6-phosphate dehydrogenase deficiency and hemolytic anemia. In: Nathan DG, Orkin SH, Look AT, et al, editors. Nathan and Oski's hematology of infancy and childhood. 6th edition. Philadelphia: WB Saunders; 2003. p. 721–42.
39. Valaes T. Neonatal jaundice in glucose-6-phosphate dehydrogenase deficiency. In: Maisels MJ, Watchko JF, editors. Neonatal jaundice. Amsterdam: Harwood Academic Publishers; 2000. p. 67–72.
40. Watchko JF, Kaplan M, Stark AR, et al. Should we screen newborns for glucose-6-phosphate dehydrogenase deficiency in the United States? J Perinatol 2013;33: 499–504.
41. Mentzer WC. Pyruvate kinase deficiency and disorders of glycolysis. In: Nathan DG, Orkin SH, Look AT, et al, editors. Nathan and Oski's hematology of infancy and childhood. 6th edition. Philadelphia: WB Saunders; 2003. p. 685–720.
42. Bhutani VK, Johnson LH, Maisels MJ, et al. Kernicterus: epidemiological strategies for its prevention through systems-based approaches. J Perinatol 2004; 24:650–62.
43. Johnson L, Bhutani VK, Karp K, et al. Clinical report from the pilot USA Kernicterus Registry (1992 to 2004). J Perinatol 2009;29(S1):S25–45.
44. Watchko JF. Hyperbilirubinemia in African American neonates: clinical issues and current challenges. Semin Fetal Neonatal Med 2010;15:176–82.
45. Nkhoma ET, Poole C, Vannappagari V, et al. The global prevalence of glucose-6-phosphate dehydrogenase deficiency: a systematic review and meta-analysis. Blood Cells Mol Dis 2009;42:267–78.
46. Chinevere TD, Murray CK, Grant E Jr, et al. Prevalence of glucose-6-phosphate dehydrogenase deficiency in US Army personnel. Mil Med 2006;171:905–7.
47. Wickremasinghe AC, Kuzniewicz MW, Newman TB. Black race is not protective against hazardous bilirubin levels. J Pediatr 2013;162:1068–9.
48. Kaplan M, Hammerman C, Vreman HJ, et al. Severe hemolysis with normal blood count in a glucose-6-phosphate dehydrogenase deficient neonate. J Perinatol 2008;28(4):306–9.

49. Kaplan M, Renbaum P, Levy-Lahad E, et al. Gilbert syndrome and glucose-6-phosphate dehydrogenase deficiency: a dose-dependent genetic interaction crucial to neonatal hyperbilirubinemia. Proc Natl Acad Sci U S A 1997;94: 12128–32.

50. Matthay KK, Mentzer WC. Erythrocyte enzymopathies in the newborn. Clin Haematol 1981;10:31–55.

51. Oski FA, Nathan DG, Sidel VW, et al. Extreme hemolysis and red-cell distortion in erythrocyte pyruvate kinase deficiency. I. Morphology, erythrokinetics and family enzyme studies. N Engl J Med 1964;270:1023–30.

52. Rider NL, Strauss KA, Brown K, et al. Erythrocyte pyruvate kinase deficiency in an old-order Amish cohort: longitudinal risk and disease management. Am J Hematol 2011;86(10):827–34.

53. Christensen RD, Eggert LD, Baer VL, et al. Pyruvate kinase deficiency as a cause of extreme hyperbilirubinemia in neonates from a polygamist community. J Perinatol 2010;30:233–6.

54. Christensen RD, Yaish HM, Johnson CB, et al. Six children with pyruvate kinase deficiency from one small town: molecular characterization of the *PK-LR* gene. J Pediatr 2011;159:695–7.

55. Stockman JA. Physical properties of the neonatal red blood cell. In: Stockman JA, Pochedly C, editors. Developmental and neonatal hematology. New York: Raven Press; 1988. p. 297–323.

56. Christensen RD, Henry E. Hereditary spherocytosis in neonates with hyperbilirubinemia. Pediatrics 2010;125(1):120–5.

57. Yaish HM, Henry E, Baer VL, et al. A simple method of screening newborn infants for hereditary spherocytosis. J Appl Hematol 2013;4:27–32.

58. Trucco JI, Brown AK. Neonatal manifestations of hereditary spherocytosis. Am J Dis Child 1967;113:263–70.

59. Oski FA. The erythrocyte and its disorders. In: Nathan DG, Oski FA, editors. Hematology of infancy and childhood. Philadelphia: W.B. Saunders; 1993. p. 18–43.

60. Caprari P, Maiorana A, Marzetti G, et al. Severe neonatal hemolytic jaundice associated with pyknocytosis and alterations of red cell skeletal proteins. Prenat Neonatal Med 1997;2:140–5.

61. Tuffy P, Brown AK, Zuelzer WW. Infantile pyknocytosis: common erythrocyte abnormality of the first trimester. Am J Dis Child 1959;98:227–41.

62. Schmaier A, Maurer HM, Johnston CL, et al. Alpha thalassemia screening in neonates by mean corpuscular volume and mean corpuscular hemoglobin concentration. J Pediatr 1973;83:794–7.

63. Pearson HA. Disorders of hemoglobin synthesis and metabolism. In: Oski FA, Naiman JL, editors. Hematologic problems in the newborn. Philadelphia: W.B. Saunders; 1982. p. 245–82.

64. Oort M, Heerspink W, Roos D, et al. Haemolytic disease of the newborn and chronic anemia induced by gamma-beta thalassemia in a Dutch family. Br J Haematol 1981;48:251–62.

65. Christensen RD, Lambert DK, Henry E, et al. Unexplained extreme hyperbilirubinemia among neonates in a multihospital healthcare system. Blood Cells Mol Dis 2013;50:105–9.

66. Christensen RD, Nussenzveig RH, Yaish HM, et al. Causes of hemolysis in neonates with extreme hyperbilirubinemia. J Perinatol 2014;34:616–9.

67. Tidmarsh GF, Wong RJ, Stevenson DK. End-tidal carbon monoxide and hemolysis. J Perinatol 2014;34:577–81.

68. Stevenson DK, Vreman HJ, Wong RJ. Bilirubin production and its measurement. In: Stevenson DK, Maisels MJ, Watchko JF, editors. Care of the jaundiced neonate. New York: McGraw-Hill; 2012. p. 29–39.
69. Watchko JF, Tiribelli C. Bilirubin-induced neurologic damage—mechanisms and management approaches. N Engl J Med 2013;369:2021–30.
70. Hsai DY, Allen FH, Gellis SS, et al. Studied of serum bilirubin in relation to kernicterus. N Engl J Med 1952;247:668–71.
71. Watchko JF, Oski FA. Bilirubin 20 mg/dL = vigintiphobia. Pediatrics 1983;71: 660–3.
72. Watchko JF. Vigintiphobia revisited. Pediatrics 2005;115:1747–53.
73. Szucs KA, Rosenman MB. Family-centered evidence-based phototherapy delivery. Pediatrics 2013;131:e1982.
74. Watchko JF. Exchange transfusion. In: Maisels MJ, Watchko JF, editors. Neonatal jaundice. Amsterdam: Harwood Academic Publishers; 2000. p. 169–76.
75. Brown MS. Physiologic anemia of infancy: normal red-cell values and physiology of neonatal erythropoiesis. In: Stockman JA, Pochedly C, editors. Developmental and neonatal hematology. New York: Raven Press; 1988. p. 249–74.
76. Mimouni FB, Merlob P, Dollber S, et al. Neonatal polycythaemia: critical review and a consensus statement of the Israeli Neonatology Association. Acta Paediatr 2011;100:1290–6.
77. Remon JI, Raghavan A, Maheshwari A. Polycythemia in the newborn. NeoReviews 2011;12:e20.
78. Blanchette VS. Neonatal alloimmune thrombocytopenia. In: Stockman JA, Pochedly C, editors. Developmental and neonatal hematology. New York: Raven Press; 1988. p. 145–68.
79. Fernandez KS, de Alarcon P. Neonatal thrombocytopenia. NeoReviews 2013;14: e74.

Neonatal Medications

Robert M. Ward, MD[a],*, Justin Stiers, MD[a], Karen Buchi, MD[b]

KEYWORDS

- Neonatal abstinence syndrome • Opioids • Circumcision • Analgesia
- Pharmacogenomics • Single nucleotide polymorphism

KEY POINTS

- Maternal substance use and abuse during pregnancy is dramatically increasing in North America.
- Despite increasing frequency of neonatal abstinence syndrome (NAS), high-quality evidence and treatment guidelines remain limited and there is wide interinstitution variability in treatment strategies.
- Newborns show physiologic responses to painful stimuli. Untreated or undertreated pain in the newborn period may have effects on future response to pain and anxiety.
- Current available evidence for nonpharmacologic and pharmacologic approaches to pain management for common medical procedures (including circumcision) are described.
- Single nucleotide polymorphisms contribute to diseases and differences in drug metabolism (pharmacogenomics/pharmacogenetics) and must be distinguished from developmental differences in the level of activity of drug-metabolizing enzymes.

MATERNAL DRUG ABUSE AND NEONATAL ABSTINENCE SYNDROME

The American Academy of Pediatrics (AAP) Committee on Drugs and the Committee on Fetus and Newborn recently updated their Clinical Report on Neonatal Withdrawal.[1,2] This was an extensive review of the topic. In it, they recommended that every nursery have a policy for assessing maternal substance abuse and have a standardized plan for the evaluation and management of infants at risk for or showing withdrawal. In this article, we work through an example of such a standardized plan.

Fig. 1 provides an algorithm that can be used by the nursery team to assess the newborn with in utero drug exposure and to make management decisions regarding neonatal abstinence syndrome (NAS). It represents a starting point for the organization of care and decision making regarding nursery management of in utero drug exposure.

Disclosure: The authors have no conflicts of interest related to the content of this article.
[a] Division of Neonatology, Department of Pediatrics, University of Utah, 295 Chipeta Way, Salt Lake City, UT 84108, USA; [b] Division of General Pediatrics, Department of Pediatrics, University of Utah, 295 Chipeta Way, Salt Lake City, UT 84108, USA
* Corresponding author.
E-mail address: robert.ward@hsc.utah.edu

Pediatr Clin N Am 62 (2015) 525–544
http://dx.doi.org/10.1016/j.pcl.2014.11.012
0031-3955/15/$ – see front matter © 2015 Elsevier Inc. All rights reserved.

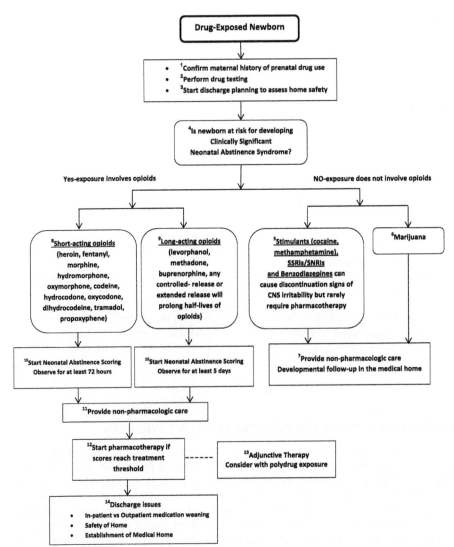

Fig. 1. Algorithm for assessment and treatment of neonatal abstinence syndrome (NAS). The numbers refer to sections in the text with discussions.

Assessment of the Drug-Exposed Newborn

1. Confirm the maternal history of prenatal drug use

It is important to know all of the drugs taken by the mother, because that will help to determine the risk to the newborn of developing withdrawal symptoms. It is also often the first opportunity for the pediatrician to meet the mother and start forming a positive relationship around the care of her infant.

2. Perform drug testing

Each nursery should have a uniform policy regarding which infants to test for drug exposure. Oral and Strang[3] surveyed drug screening practices in Iowa and compiled a list of maternal and neonatal characteristics that are used to determine which mother–infant dyads should undergo drug testing (**Table 1**). Other nurseries have a universal screening policy, for example, 7 hospitals in the greater Cincinnati area began universal drug testing on all expectant mothers in 2013.[4]

The most common type of drug testing is performed on urine and meconium, but umbilical cord analysis is gaining more acceptance. A drugs of abuse screen for urine reflects only recent exposure (within the last 72 hours). It is best to collect the first void after delivery, which is easily missed. Meconium analysis has become the "gold standard" for detection of in utero drug exposure because a positive test indicates exposure sometime after the 18th week of gestation. The first stool after birth is the best to use because it has been there the longest. Umbilical cord analysis also reflects exposure from 18 weeks gestation onward and has been shown to be similar to meconium in sensitivity.[5] It requires a cord segment, which can be collected at the time of delivery. This assay is commercially available and is gaining favor because the cord can be collected at delivery and there is no need to wait until passage of stool.

3. Start discharge planning and assess the safety of the home environment
The concern that a mother of a newborn has a substance use problem is a red flag that the home environment may not be safe. Many newborns exposed to drugs of abuse in utero are medically stable and may not require a lengthy in-hospital stay. It is imperative to involve the social work team as soon as possible to help assess the mother's ability to care for her newborn at home. Child protective services may need to be involved, depending on state law. It is equally important to identify the medical home, especially if discharge management involves medications and close follow-up.

4. Is the newborn at risk for developing clinically significant neonatal abstinence syndrome?
After assessing the type of in utero drug exposure, the pediatrician needs to assess whether this infant is at risk to develop clinically significant NAS. This step is important in medical decision making for the newborn.

Table 1	
Factors to be considered in perinatal illicit drug screening	
Maternal Risk Factors	**Infant Risk Factors**
Report of illicit drug use	Signs of withdrawal
Maternal or paternal incarceration	Unexplained low birth weight
Prostitution	Unexplained small head circumference
Domestic violence	Unexplained prematurity (<37 wk)
Multiparity (>3)	Congenital anomalies
Children removed from home owing to child abuse	
Poor prenatal care	
Tobacco/alcohol use during pregnancy	
Depression	
Unexplained acute hypertension	
Unexplained stroke, myocardial infarction	
Abruptio placenta	
Precipitous labor (<3 h)	
Sexually transmitted diseases (human immunodeficiency virus, hepatitis B, hepatitis C, and syphilis)	
Signs of withdrawal or drug influence, intravenous drug use	

Withdrawal, neurobehavioral dysregulation, and neonatal abstinence syndrome There remains a lack of consistency in the literature and in pediatric practice in the use of the term NAS. The term *neonatal abstinence syndrome* (NAS) has been principally used to describe neonatal symptoms occurring after in utero exposure to opioids.[5] This is because the majority of those newborns exposed to in utero opioids display a consistent neurobehavioral pattern, therefore qualifying as a syndrome. The pattern of neonatal neurobehaviors attributed to other substances such as cocaine or methamphetamine, as discussed herein, is not nearly as consistent and usually decreases progressively after birth. Non-narcotic drugs can cause neonatal psychomotor behavior that are consistent with withdrawal (often referred to as discontinuation signs), but rarely require pharmacotherapy when they are not used in conjunction with other drugs that affect the central nervous system. These include alcohol, barbiturates, caffeine, benzodiazepines, nicotine, selective serotonin reuptake inhibitors (SSRIs), serotonin–norepinephrine reuptake inhibitors (SNRIs) and other antidepressants.

5. Stimulants, selective serotonin reuptake inhibitors, serotonin–norepinephrine reuptake inhibitors, and benzodiazepines can cause discontinuation signs of neurologic irritability, but rarely require pharmacotherapy

- Methamphetamine
  - There are no identifiable patterns of neurobehavior that are consistent with a methamphetamine exposure "syndrome."[6]
  - The Infant Development, Environment, and Lifestyle (IDEAL) Study found that methamphetamine had a small but measurable impact on birth weight and gestational age, and that heavy methamphetamine use was related to lower arousal, more lethargy, and increased physiologic stress in the newborn. This is similar to the effects of cocaine and can be termed "neurobehavioral dysregulation."[6]
  - These subtle neurobehavioral findings are consistent with previous findings in cocaine- and nicotine-exposed children.
- Cocaine
  - There is no cocaine withdrawal syndrome because the neonatal presentation is not consistent. Both depressed and excitable profiles have been observed, which may be related to the dose and exposure.[7]
  - The Maternal Lifestyle Study (MLS) is a longitudinal cohort study focusing on cocaine-exposed children. It enrolled mother–infant dyads from 1993 to 1995 and has been providing longitudinal developmental follow-up ever since. The MLS found that cocaine-exposed infants showed more "soft signs" and behavioral effects in the newborn period.[7]
  - As with methamphetamine exposure, the most pressing management issues are those concerning the safety of the home environment
- Antidepressants: SSRIs and SNRIs
  - SSRIs and SNRIs are 2 of the most commonly prescribed classes of drugs in pregnancy, yet not much is known about their potential for adverse effects
  - They cross the placenta and accumulate in the fetus to varying degrees, depending on the specific drug and its pharmacologic properties.
  - It is uncommon to need pharmacotherapy to treat neonatal symptoms of withdrawal from SSRIs or SNRIs. It is important to be aware that clinical signs like irritability can develop over the first week of life. This is something to communicate with the parents and the medical home provider.[8,9]

Given that methamphetamine, cocaine, SSRIs, SNRIs, and benzodiazepines rarely require pharmacotherapy, the algorithm presented herein recommends observation, nonpharmacologic treatment and heightened awareness in the medical home of the infant's developmental risk.

6. Marijuana, a special case
There are changing attitudes regarding marijuana use in the United States. Twenty states have laws legalizing some form of marijuana use, and 2 states (Colorado and Washington) have legalized its recreational use. This means that the nursery provider will be encountering the marijuana-exposed neonate with increased frequency. The clinician should not anticipate that the marijuana-exposed newborn will develop clinically significant neonatal withdrawal signs requiring pharmacotherapy with exclusively gestational marijuana exposure.[10] The need to report to child protective services for marijuana positivity is state dependent.

7. Provide nonpharmacologic care and developmental follow-up in the medical home
Provision of nonpharmacologic care does not usually require use of a scoring tool. Some clinicians do decide to start using a scoring system (see step 10) to evaluate signs and symptoms of withdrawal in newborns exposed to these nonopioid drugs. This is an area that needs more research to assess the cost–benefit ratio of using a scoring system and requiring a predetermined length of stay.

All infants born to a mother who used drugs that affect the central nervous system should undergo periodic developmental assessment in the medical home. It is not only the direct exposure to these drugs that may place the infant at risk, but the myriad of other environmental factors that may accompany drug use that also may impact early development.

8. Short-acting opioids
If the newborn is exposed to opioids, then she is at risk for developing clinically significant NAS. The significant increases in NAS that we are all seeing in our nurseries is owing, for the most part, to the increase in prescription pain medication misuse and abuse across the country. Most of these are short-acting opioids. There is a difference in the risk to the infant in developing clinically significant NAS when exposed to short-acting opioids compared with those exposed to long-acting opioids, such as methadone and buprenorphine. Kellogg and colleagues[11] in 2011 reported a retrospective review from Mayo Clinic. Out of 26,314 deliveries from 1998 to 2009, they found 167 women who used prescription narcotics during pregnancy and NAS was seen in only 5.6% of the infants. The reasons for the mothers to be on these potent analgesics included headaches, chronic pain, genitourinary pathology (stones), and orthopedic issues. The AAP 2012 Clinical Report states that if it has been longer than 1 week since the mother last took the opioid, then the incidence of neonatal withdrawal is relatively low. This statement is based on an observation made by a pediatrician in a 1957 paper and referred to heroin exposure.[12] Despite the surge of short-acting pain medication use in pregnant women over the past decade, there has been no systematic analysis of the risk of NAS in relationship to the time of the last use of a narcotic analgesic before delivery.

9. Long-acting opioids
It is important to recognize when a newborn has been exposed to long-acting opioids in utero to evaluate the risk of developing NAS and determine the length of observation. Methadone is a long-acting opioid that remains the standard of care for narcotic addiction management in pregnancy in the United States. The elimination half-life in

neonates is longer than 24 hours; thus, the exposed newborn may not start manifesting signs of NAS for up to 3 days. Buprenorphine alone (Subutex) or in combination with naloxone (Suboxone) are also long-acting opioids whose use is increasing for opioid dependency in pregnancy. Newborns exposed to these long-acting opiates are very likely to develop clinically significant NAS.

10. Start neonatal abstinence scoring

The standard of care for the in-patient management of NAS begins with the use of an abstinence scoring tool to measure the severity of the withdrawal and help to guide treatment as it increases or decreases. The goal of NAS scoring tools is to quantify the severity of symptoms to determine the need for pharmacotherapeutic intervention. The scoring tools help to provide uniform assessments of newborns at risk for clinically significant NAS. Nurseries should establish a consistent method to train and periodically assess the use of the scoring system by the nursing staff to maximize interrater reliability for the score that physicians use to determine pharmacologic intervention. Several scoring systems are available; the most common are the modified Neonatal Abstinence Scoring System, The Lipsitz tool,[13] and the Neonatal Withdrawal Inventory.[14] Each of these tools uses a different "number" as the threshold for determining the need to initiate pharmacotherapy.

Length of observation The length of observation for the newborn at risk for developing clinically significant NAS should be standardized in nurseries.[15] Prenatal care providers need to be aware that NAS occurs in 55% to 94% of opioid exposed newborns[1] and that early discharge for the newborn may not be indicated medically. It is generally accepted that an infant born to a mother who took a low dose of a short-acting opioid during pregnancy may be safely discharged if asymptomatic after 3 days of observation.[1] Smirk and colleagues[16] at the University of Melbourne conducted a 10-year retrospective analysis of babies treated pharmacologically for NAS and found that 94% of the 142 infants exposed to long-acting opioids (methadone or buprenorphine) developed NAS symptomatology requiring treatment by day 5 of life.

11. Provide nonpharmacologic care

The goal of NAS treatment is to relieve symptoms that are interfering with physiologic stability, weight gain, the ability to be consoled, and sleep. There is also a paramount need to educate the mother (who in most cases will be involved with the ongoing care of her infant) about her newborn's neurobehavioral dysfunction and the best ways to interact with her newborn. **Box 1** lists common nonpharmacologic techniques. Velez and Jansson[17] wrote an in-depth article for physicians and nurses about the complexity and vulnerability of the opioid-dependent pregnant and post partum woman and her infant that offers practical advice to nursery staff to better understand these dyads.

Breastfeeding issues It is safe to breastfeed with methadone and other opioids if the mother is negative for the human immunodeficiency virus, and she is not using other substances of abuse, such as cocaine or methamphetamine. Methadone concentrations in breast milk are low and not related to maternal dose of the opioid.[18] A 2010 retrospective study looking for independent predictors of response to treatment for NAS found that infants born to mothers on methadone who were breastfed had a shorter median duration of pharmacotherapy for NAS and that the favorable response correlates with the volume of the breast milk ingested as a proportion of total intake.[19] Sudden cessation of breastfeeding by mothers treated with methadone has been

---

Box 1
Nonpharmacologic treatment

- Nursing support
  - Swaddling with soft blankets
  - Quiet, dark environment
  - Frequent small feedings of hypercaloric formula
  - Try a pacifier with simple syrup
  - Skin care
  - High degree of suspicion for other disease processes
  - Organize care to minimize handling
  - Swings; helpful for some
  - Determine level of stimulation infant can tolerate

Data from Velez M, Jansson LM. The opioid dependent mother and newborn dyad: non-pharmacologic care. J Addict Med 2008;2(3):113–20.

---

associated with recurrence of NAS.[19] The physician and mother should both be aware of this risk.

Rooming-in Some nurseries are allowing newborns with NAS to room in with their mothers. Hunseler and colleagues[20] in Germany found that infants with opioid-induced NAS required less pharmacotherapy for NAS and had shorter hospital stays when placed with their mothers in the postnatal unit compared with infants admitted to the neonatal unit.

12. Start pharmacotherapy if scores reach treatment threshold

There are numerous pharmacologic treatment strategies published. Reviews have, in general, concluded that there is a lack of strong evidence on the relative efficacy of the different drug regimens for the treatment of NAS.[1] Morphine remains the most widely used initial medication for treatment of NAS. Nurseries should establish dosing regimens for morphine based on their chosen scoring system to standardize the approach. Treatment algorithms available on-line specify initial dosing, escalation, and weaning parameters.[21,22] Treating NAS with methadone is also used in some nurseries. The Vermont Children's Hospital guidelines specify a dosing and weaning schedule.[21] No longer recommended for treatment of NAS are diazepam, paregoric, and diluted tincture of opium.

13. Adjunctive pharmacotherapy—consider with polydrug exposure

When morphine or methadone alone is not controlling symptoms to enable the newborn to sleep and eat adequately, adjunctive treatment may be considered. If the newborn has been exposed to multiple drug classes or has significant neurologic hyperirritability, oral phenobarbital can be considered. It is important to remember that phenobarbital does not control gastrointestinal symptoms. A neonatal loading dose of 16 mg/kg per day is recommended with a maintenance dose between 2 and 8 mg/kg per day, titrated to the symptoms.

Clonidine is also used for adjunctive and, at times, primary treatment for NAS.[23] It reduces the signs and symptoms of NAS while the newborn's neurons are reversing their tolerance to opioids. Because of its potential to cause hypotension, blood pressures and heart rates should be closely monitored before each dose for 24 hours after initiation or change in dosing.

14. Discharge issues: medication weaning, safety of the home environment, and establishing a medical home

The discharge of newborns treated for NAS depends on a number of factors. Although many treatment algorithms specify that the scores must be below the treatment threshold, it is more important to assess the goals of treatment and determine if the newborn is (1) gaining weight appropriately, (2) getting adequate sleep, and (3) has behavior that a nonprofessional caretaker can manage. Scoring helps to direct the uniform and consistent care given, but these characteristics, not a number on a scoring system, are what determines readiness for discharge.

As stated in step 3 of the algorithm, the safety of the home environment and assessment of support systems for the home care provider need to be determined. In addition, a medical home for the newborn needs to be established, with direct communication to the primary care provider about the out-patient management. One of the most important issues is the out-patient management of the drug(s) used to treat NAS. The decision to send the newborn home on NAS medications with a plan to wean the medication over time varies across the country. Medication options for home weaning include phenobarbital[24,25] and methadone.[26] There are no published studies on the outpatient weaning of clonidine. As with the in-patient management of NAS, the out-patient management has not been rigorously studied to assess the success of different weaning regimens.

The goal of out-patient pharmacologic management should be to wean the infant off the medications as efficiently as is safely possible while still maintaining adequate weight gain, sleep, and the ability to be consoled. This process can be challenging for both the medical home provider and the caregivers, especially when assessing infant behavior at 4 to 6 weeks of age. This is the age when all term newborns become fussier as a part of normal development. There is a risk that parents and medical care providers will perceive that any discomfort or annoying behavior in the infant needs to be treated with medications. This needs to be taken into consideration when assessing the infant exposed to opioids in utero and it should not be presumed that all irritability is owing to withdrawal. Nonpharmacologic intervention as described herein can be used. The medical home should also provide developmental surveillance of infants with NAS, as with other high-risk newborns.

Summary

The newborn exposed to a drug in utero is best managed with a standard team approach with flexibility to consider each infant individually and utilize outpatient management in the medical home.

PAIN

Pain Perception

All newborns have the ability to perceive pain during medical procedures after birth. However, the newborn's ability to perceive and remember painful experiences has not always been appreciated.[27,28] Before the 1980s, it was incorrectly believed that a newborn's nervous system was too underdeveloped and immature to perceive pain. Embryologic studies identified the presence of neuroanatomic, neurophysiologic, and neurochemical substrates for pain perception appearing as early as the 7th week of gestation and developing fully by 20 to 24 weeks' gestation.[29,30] These findings were further supported by clinical studies demonstrating improved outcomes of operative procedures when anesthesia was provided.[31] Not only do newborns experience pain, but more recent studies suggest that pain perception may actually be heightened in newborns compared with older children and adults.[32] There is growing evidence that untreated or undertreated pain in the newborn period has long-term negative consequences, including hypersensitivity to future pain as well as future emotional, behavioral, and learning disabilities.[32–35] These long-term consequences and altered pain sensitivity can be reduced or eliminated when adequate pain relief is provided.[36,37]

Inadequate Treatment of Pain in Newborns

Given what is now known about neonatal pain perception and the consequences of untreated pain, the AAP Committee on the Fetus and Newborn policy states, "Every health care facility caring for neonates should implement an effective pain-prevention program, which includes strategies for routinely assessing pain, minimizing the number of painful procedures performed, effectively using pharmacologic and nonpharmacologic therapies for the prevention of pain associated with routine minor procedures, and eliminating pain associated with surgery and other major procedures."[38] Multiple tools have been validated for the assessment of pain in newborns and many proven and safe therapies are available for treating pain in neonates.[38] Despite heightened awareness of neonatal pain and drastic improvements in the ability to recognize and treat pain in newborns, pain is underrecognized and undertreated for an alarming number of routine, minor and major, painful procedures.[39,40]

Nonpharmacologic Interventions for Pain

Developmentally appropriate swaddling, nonnutritive sucking, skin-to-skin contact, attention to behavioral cues, and breastfeeding have all been shown to reduce pain scores in neonates undergoing minor procedures.[38] The simple act of skin-to-skin contact can reduce crying and grimacing during minor procedures by as much as 82%.[41] The addition of breastfeeding with skin-to-skin contact nearly eliminates clinical symptoms of pain from a heel stick with reduction of crying by 91% and grimacing by 84% compared with swaddling alone.[42] Breastfeeding or breast milk feeding during painful procedures should be encouraged whenever feasible.[43,44]

Pharmacologic Interventions for Pain

Sucrose
Although breastfeeding provides superior analgesia compared with oral sucrose,[44–46] multiple studies have shown oral sucrose to be an effective analgesic for term and preterm neonates undergoing a minor procedure.[47–53] Although the optimal dose and formulation have not been defined, sucrose, glucose, and even artificial sweeteners at a variety of doses all have similar analgesic effects compared with placebo.[48,54–56] Guidelines were recently published with expert consensus for sucrose indications, dosage per painful procedure, age-related dosage over 24 hours, method of delivery, and contraindications.[57] Outside of the immediate newborn period, oral sucrose analgesia remains an effective pain management strategy for immunizations up to 6 months of age and venipuncture up to 3 months age.[47,52,56,58]

Further studies are needed to determine the mechanism of action, optimal dosing, and safety of repeated doses of oral sucrose (or glucose). Although the mechanism of action for "analgesic sweets" is unknown, it seems to be related to gustaoception, because intragastric sucrose administration does not have any effect on pain.[59] Studies in rodents suggest that sucrose analgesia is mediated through opioid and serotonin receptors.[60,61] However, opioid antagonists do not reduce the effect of glucose in term neonates, suggesting other neuronal pathways may be involved.[62] Neither the optimal dose nor safe cumulative exposure has been established for sucrose analgesia. Wide variability exists in sucrose dosing with studies utilizing a range of doses from 0.1 to 0.5 mL of 7.5% to 50% sucrose (or glucose) solutions.[53,63] In 1 study, the lower dose of 7.5% sucrose did not reduce the duration of crying and may be below the lowest effective dose.[64] Although single doses of glucose or sucrose are safe, well-tolerated, and recommended as an important component of routine newborn care, the safety of multiple doses, particularly in very preterm neonates, has been questioned.[65] Further study is needed on the long-term and developmental effects of repeated sucrose doses, as well as the safety and efficacy of using oral sucrose in very preterm, unstable, and/or ventilated infants.[53]

Topical anesthetics

Topical anesthetics, typically EMLA cream (a eutectic mixture of 2.5% lidocaine/2.5% prilocaine), are effective anesthetics for venipuncture, lumbar puncture, and starting an intravenous line.[66–70] EMLA cream has several limitations to its routine clinical use. EMLA must be applied at least 30 minutes (ideally 60–90 minutes) before a procedure,[71,72] has less pain attenuation compared with oral sucrose,[73] and is ineffective for heel sticks because the pain results primarily from squeezing the heel and not the heel lance itself.[74] EMLA cream also can result in skin irritation and blistering, particularly in preterm neonates.[52,72,75,76] Systemic absorption of EMLA increases methemoglobin levels, although rarely to a degree that is significant clinically.[71,72] Case reports of methhemoglobinemia have been reported in premature infants with prolonged exposure and should be considered when using EMLA in neonates.[77–79]

Circumcision

Currently approximately 60% of male infants in the United States undergo circumcision as newborns.[80] Although nonpharmacologic interventions (padded, developmentally appropriate swaddling/restraints and oral sucrose) improve patient comfort during circumcision,[81] they alone are insufficient as the sole method of treating pain associated with this surgical procedure.[82,83] Similarly, acetaminophen may be a useful adjunctive therapy, but is insufficient alone to treat the pain associated with circumcision.[84] Analgesic topical creams (EMLA and 4% lidocaine) are effective at reducing circumcision pain compared with placebo. Topical creams are less effective than dorsal penile nerve block (DPNB) or subcutaneous ring block[85] and may be less than ideal as the sole anesthetic for circumcision.

Dorsal penile nerve block and subcutaneous ring block

DPNB is performed by injecting 0.4 to 0.5 mL of 1% lidocaine without epinephrine on both sides ("10 o'clock and 2 o'clock" positions) of the base of the penis. This technique reduces behavioral and physiologic responses of pain, and has a low failure rate and few complications.[86] Peak serum lidocaine levels are well below toxic ranges[87] and we found no reported evidence of lidocaine toxicity (seizures or cardiovascular effects) from this technique.[80] The most common complication from DPNB is bruising and hematomas, reported to occur in 11% to 43% of cases using DPNB for circumcision.[86] In all cases, the bruising and hematomas were self-resolved.[75,86] Subcutaneous ring block is performed by injecting 0.8 mL of 1% lidocaine without epinephrine circumferentially in the subcutaneous tissue at the base or mid shaft of the penis.[80] This technique provides effective anesthesia for circumcision and may provide improved anesthesia compared with DPNB.[85,88] No complications of ring block have been reported; however, a failure rate of 5% has been reported.[80] Whether using DPNB or subcutaneous ring block, it is critical to use lidocaine without epinephrine and not to exceed the appropriate dose based on weight. Epinephrine can cause vasoconstriction, which may lead to distal ischemia and potentially necrosis of the penis.

Circumcision Technique

Circumcision is primarily performed utilizing one of the following 3 techniques: Gomco clamp, PlastiBell device, or Mogen clamp. Few studies have directly compared these techniques and there is no evidence that 1 technique results in less pain than the others. A moderate sized study of 350 neonates showed a slightly greater risk of infection and adhesions with Gomco clamp compared with the PlastiBell device[89]; however, this result has not been replicated in other studies and the AAP Task Force on Circumcision does not recommend 1 technique over another.[80] Regardless of the technique used, there is no evidence of persistent pain beyond the period of the procedure and, therefore, the routine use of analgesics after the local anesthetic dissipates is not necessary.[80]

Summary

Multiple nonpharmacologic and pharmacologic interventions are safe and efficacious for the reduction, and in some cases elimination, of pain in neonates, especially related to circumcision. All painful procedures, even "routine" minor interventions, should include a consideration, evaluation, and treatment of pain.

PHARMACOGENOMICS AND PHARMACOGENETICS
Inherited Variation in Pharmacology and the Human Genome Project

Inherited variations in the pharmacology of medications have been recognized for many decades and the history of their discovery was described recently by pioneers in this field.[90] In 1957, Motulsky recognized that "inheritance might explain why many individuals differ in drug efficacy and in experiencing adverse drug reactions." Two years later, Friedrich Vogel first coined the term "pharmacogenetics," defined as the "study of the role of genetics in drug response."[90] *Pharmacogenomics* is often used to refer to the broad spectrum of genetic variations that influence drug actions sometimes with comparisons between ethnically diverse populations (**Table 2**, discussed herein). A wide array of pharmacologic processes demonstrates inherited variations, ranging from drug receptors to transporters to enzymes involved in drug biotransformation. Although *pharmacogenetics* is usually used to describe inherited pharmacologic variations in individuals, the boundaries between pharmacogenomics and pharmacogenetics blurred until these terms have become interchangeable.[91]

The Human Genome Project (HGP) contributed many insights into pharmacogenetics/pharmacogenomics. Among the 20,000 to 25,000 genes discovered by the HGP, many related to pharmacologic processes that helped explain diseases and responses to drug therapy.[92] Comparison of genomes among individuals, revealed only a 0.1% difference among the DNA in their genes, but this variation can increase, decrease, or leave a pharmacologic process unchanged.

Single Nucleotide Polymorphisms

The HGP opened the door to discovery of many changes in DNA, termed single nucleotide polymorphisms (SNPs), in which a single nucleotide change in DNA causes a single nucleotide change in the message RNA (**Fig. 2**). Message RNA is translated into proteins by reading every 3 nucleotides as a codon, which identifies an amino acid or gives a signal to start or stop reading the RNA (see **Table 3**). A mutation in a single nucleotide in DNA (an SNP) can ultimately change the protein structure, change the

Table 2
Differences in the frequency of single nucleotide polymorphisms between races in the genes for the β1-adrenergic receptor (ADRB1) and the G receptor protein kinase 5 (GRK5) that change the proteins, and their activities

| | | | | Minor Allele Frequency (%) | |
| | | Nucleotide Position and | | | |
Gene Name	Common Name	Change	Amino Acid Changes	White	Black
ADRB1	β1AR	145 (A to G)	49 (Ser to Gly)	15	13
ADRB1	β1AR	1165 (C to G)	389 (Arg to Gly)	27	42
ADRB1	β1AR	1166 (G to T)	389 (Arg to Leu)	<0.1	0.9
GRK5	GRK5	122 (A to T)	41 (Gln to Leu)	1.3	23
GRK5	GRK5	840 (G to A)	304 (Arg to His)	<0.01	0
GRK5	GRK5	1274 (C to T)	425 (Thr to Met)	0	0.02
GRK5	GRK5	1624 (C to G)	542 (Pro to Ala)	<0.01	0

Amino acid abbreviations are shown in **Table 3**.
Data from Dorn GW, Liggett SB. Mechanisms of pharmacogenomic effects of genetic variation within the cardiac adrenergic network in heart failure. Mol Pharmacol 2009;76(3):466–80.

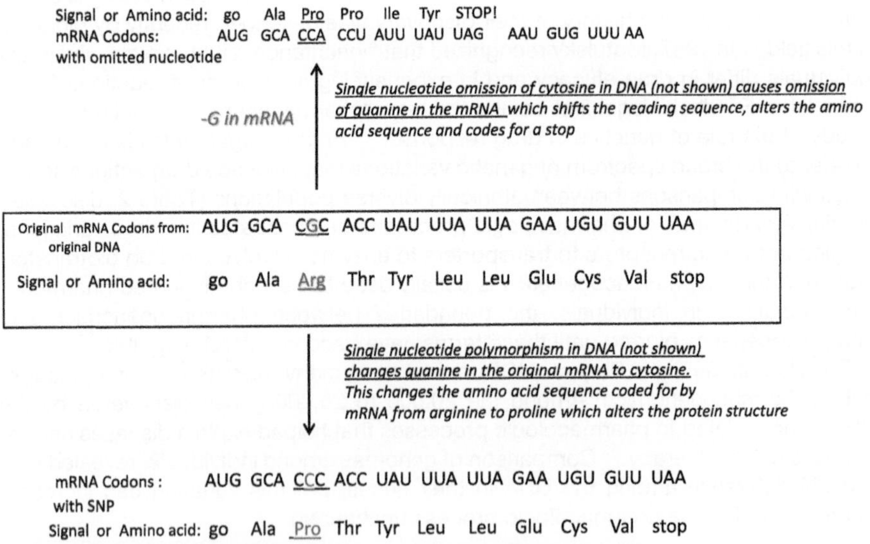

Fig. 2. Examples of single nucleotide polymorphisms (SNPs) in DNA (not shown) that have been transcribed into a different nucleotide sequence in message RNA, which in turn changes the nucleotide sequence of that change the amino sequence in a protein. The amino acid abbreviations are described in **Table 3**. The SNP at the top involves loss of guanine (*blue*) at position 8 in the message RNA, which shifts the reading sequence. The SNP at the bottom is a DNA substitution leading to a substitution cytosine (*blue*) for guanine (*blue*) in the original message RNA. This codes for a different amino acid, proline, rather than arginine. The key to the codons for specific amino acids is shown in **Table 3**.

Table 3
The sequences of 3 nucleotides in the message RNA (mRNA) comprise codons that code for each amino acid as well as some of the codes for starting and stopping translation of the amino acid into a protein

Amino Acid	Nucleotide Sequences	Amino Acid	Nucleotide Sequences
Alanine/A Ala	GCU, GCC, GCA, GCG	Leucine/L Leu	UUA, UUG, CUU, CUC, CUA, CUG
Arginine/R Arg	CGU, CGC, CGA, CGG, AGA, AGG	Lysine/K Lys	AAA, AAG
Asparagine/N Asn	AAU, AAC	Methionine/M Met	AUG
Aspartic acid/D Asp	GAU, GAC	Phenylalanine/F Phe	UUU, UUC
Cysteine/C Cys	UGU, UGC	Proline/P Pro	CCU, CCC, CCA, CCG
Glutamine/Q Gln	CAA, CAG	Serine/S Ser	UCU, UCC, UCA, UCG, AGU, AGC
Glutamic acid/E Glu	GAA, GAG	Threonine/T Thr	ACU, ACC, ACA, ACG
Glycine/G Gly	GGU, GGC, GGA, GGG	Tryptophan/W Trp	UGG
Histidine/H His	CAU, CAC	Tyrosine/Y Tyr	UAU, UAC
Isoleucine/I Ile	AUU, AUC, AUA	Valine/V Val	GUU, GUC, GUA, GUG
START	AUG	STOP	UAA, UGA, UAG

Data from Rodin AS, Szathmary E, Rodin SN. On origin of genetic code and tRNA before translation. Biology Direct 2011;6:1–24.

activity of an enzyme or a receptor, and even contribute to a disease, such as asthma or heart failure (see **Table 2**). Variations in the distribution of SNPs among populations can help to explain their increased or decreased frequencies of diseases and ethnically distributed changes in drug metabolism. For example, several SNPs in the β1-adrenergic receptor have been correlated with asthma and heart disease (see **Table 2**).

Another unexpected effect of SNPs was recently identified by Stockmann and colleagues.[93] They found that an SNP that inactivates CYP3A4, CYP3A4*22, identified pediatric patients with asthma whose symptoms were better controlled with inhaled fluticasone, a substrate for CYP3A4. Presumably the drug persists longer in the airway and creates more anti-inflammatory effects because of reduced metabolism.

Phenotypic Variations in Pharmacogenetics

Codeine is demethylated to form morphine by CYP2D6, which has undergone extensive genetic study.[94] Not only are there many different SNPs that can reduce its activity, some persons inherit multiple copies of genes for CYP2D6 producing supernormal activity.[95–97] In the perinatal period, mothers who are breastfeeding during treatment with codeine and who have supernormal activity of CYP2D6 can produce enough excess morphine to suppress respirations in their nursing newborn.[95–97] Warnings have been publicized about this potentially harmful or even lethal pharmacogenetic variation.

Developmental Expression of Drug-Metabolizing Enzymes

Pediatricians are used to developmental changes in growth and behavior. Developmental variations in the expression of genes related to pharmacologic processes affect therapeutic decisions.[98,99] CYP3A4 metabolizes more drugs in humans than any other enzyme. At birth, CYP3A4 activity to metabolize fentanyl varies 40% from the extremely premature newborn to the full-term newborn.[100] Some drug-metabolizing genes do not reach full adult levels of activity for several years, whereas others exceed adult activity for several years during childhood until adolescence, when they decrease to adult activities (**Fig. 3**). The maturation of drug metabolism in newborns and children does not follow a single pattern, and therefore requires knowledge of the individual patterns of clearance for specific drugs.

Personalized Medicine Reinterpreted

The HGP was expected to allow identification of single genetic changes (usually SNPs) that would identify causes of diseases as well as the best medical treatment for a disorder. This silver bullet for drug selection is unrealistic because of the multiple factors that can influence responses to drugs, including enzyme induction or inhibition and the effects of illness and maturation. Some health care systems are incorporating pharmacogenetic data within their electronic health records to assist prescribing physicians in avoiding drugs or for adjusting dosages in individuals with inactivating SNPs.[101]

Although more progress was expected after completion of the HGP in 2000, genetic variations are now beginning to explain some diseases and guide drug treatment in specific situations. Nebert and colleagues[90] caution, however, that personalized medicine will seldom provide unequivocal direction to optimal drug therapy. Rather, many pharmacogenomic discoveries provide guidance to optimal drug therapy that must be tempered by other conditions that influence drug metabolism and modulate responses to therapy. Within some health care organizations, however, pharmacogenetic data are associated with an individual's records to provide guidance to health

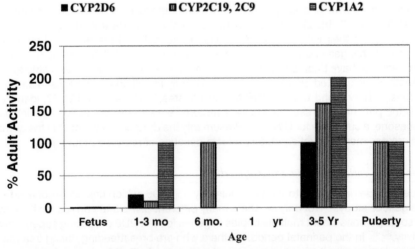

Fig. 3. Developmental changes in the activity of the cytochrome P450 (CYP) enzymes, CYP2D6 (*black columns*), CYP2C19 and CYP2C9 (*vertical stripes*), and CYP33A4 (*horizontal stripes*) with age after birth. (*Data from* Leeder JS, Kearns GL. Pharmacogenetics in pediatrics. Implications for practice. Pediatr Clin North Am 1997;44(1):55–77.)

care providers.[101] For example, a prescription for codeine to a female on the post partum floor may trigger an alert based on her previous pharmacogenetic testing that she lacks active CYP2D6 to activate codeine to morphine so it will be minimally effective or that she is an ultra-metabolizer with multiple CYP2D6 copies that will produce excessive amounts of morphine, placing her breastfeeding newborn at risk.

Summary

Pharmacogenomics can help to identify disease susceptibility and explain responses to drug therapy, but in neonatology it must be distinguished from the development of drug-metabolizing enzymes.

REFERENCES

1. Hudak ML, Tan RC. Neonatal drug withdrawal. Pediatrics 2012;129(2):e540–60.
2. Robinson S, Gregory GA. Fentanyl-air-oxygen anesthesia for ligation of patent ductus arteriosus in preterm infants. Anesth Analg 1981;60(5):331–4.
3. Oral R, Strang T. Neonatal illicit drug screening practices in Iowa: the impact of utilization of a structured screening protocol. J Perinatol 2006;26(11):660–6.
4. Hospital CCs. Universal drug testing for expectant mothers begins Sept. 1. 2013. Available at: http://www.cincinnatichildrens.org/professional/resources/ped-insights/2013/august/drug-testing/. Accessed January 3, 2015.
5. Montgomery D, Plate C, Alder SC, et al. Testing for fetal exposure to illicit drugs using umbilical cord tissue vs meconium. J Perinatol 2006;26(1):11–4.
6. Shah R, Diaz SD, Arria A, et al. Prenatal methamphetamine exposure and short-term maternal and infant medical outcomes. Am J Perinatol 2012;29(5):391–400.
7. Lester BM, Tronick EZ, LaGasse L, et al. The maternal lifestyle study: effects of substance exposure during pregnancy on neurodevelopmental outcome in 1-month-old infants. Pediatrics 2002;110(6):1182–92.
8. Rampono J, Simmer K, Ilett KF, et al. Placental transfer of SSRI and SNRI antidepressants and effects on the neonate. Pharmacopsychiatry 2009;42(3):95–100.
9. Moses-Kolko EL, Bogen D, Perel J, et al. Neonatal signs after late in utero exposure to serotonin reuptake inhibitors: literature review and implications for clinical applications. JAMA 2005;293(19):2372–83.
10. Jaques SC, Kingsbury A, Henshcke P, et al. Cannabis, the pregnant woman and her child: weeding out the myths. J Perinatol 2014;34(6):417–24.
11. Kellogg A, Rose CH, Harms RH, et al. Current trends in narcotic use in pregnancy and neonatal outcomes. Am J Obstet Gynecol 2011;204(3):259.e1–4.
12. Steg N. Narcotic withdrawal reactions in the newborn. AMA J Dis Child 1957;94(3):286–8.
13. Lipsitz PJ. A proposed narcotic withdrawal score for use with newborn infants. A pragmatic evaluation of its efficacy. Clin Pediatr (Phila) 1975;14(6):592–4.
14. Zahorodny W, Rom C, Whitney W, et al. The neonatal withdrawal inventory: a simplified score of newborn withdrawal. J Dev Behav Pediatr 1998;19(2):89–93.
15. Finnegan LP, Connaughton JF Jr, Kron RE, et al. Neonatal abstinence syndrome: assessment and management. Addict Dis 1975;2(1-2):141–58.
16. Smirk CL, Bowman E, Doyle LW, et al. How long should infants at risk of drug withdrawal be monitored after birth? J Paediatr Child Health 2014;50(5):352–5.
17. Velez M, Jansson LM. The Opioid dependent mother and newborn dyad: non-pharmacologic care. J Addict Med 2008;2(3):113–20.

18. McCarthy JJ, Posey BL. Methadone levels in human milk. J Hum Lact 2000; 16(2):115–20.
19. Isemann B, Meinzen-Derr J, Akinbi H. Maternal and neonatal factors impacting response to methadone therapy in infants treated for neonatal abstinence syndrome. J Perinatol 2011;31(1):25–9.
20. Hunseler C, Bruckle M, Roth B, et al. Neonatal opiate withdrawal and rooming-in: a retrospective analysis of a single center experience. Klin Padiatr 2013; 225(5):247–51.
21. Johnston A, Metayer J, Robinson E. Management of neonatal opioid withdrawal. Available at: http://www.pqcnc.org/documents/nas/nasresources/VCHIP_5NEONATAL_GUIDELINES.pdf. Accessed September 25, 2014.
22. Hufnagal-Miller C, Chuo J, Evans J, et al. Inpatient pathway for the evaluation/treatment of infants with neonatal abstinence syndrome. Available at: http://www.chop.edu/pathways/inpatient/neonatal-abstinence-syndrome/. Accessed September 25, 2014.
23. Leikin JB, Mackendrick WP, Maloney GE, et al. Use of clonidine in the prevention and management of neonatal abstinence syndrome. Clin Toxicol (Phila) 2009; 47(6):551–5.
24. Napolitano A, Theophilopoulos D, Seng SK, et al. Pharmacologic management of neonatal abstinence syndrome in a community hospital. Clin Obstet Gynecol 2013;56(1):193–201.
25. Coyle MG, Ferguson A, Lagasse L, et al. Diluted tincture of opium (DTO) and phenobarbital versus DTO alone for neonatal opiate withdrawal in term infants. J Pediatr 2002;140(5):561–4.
26. Backes CH, Backes CR, Gardner D, et al. Neonatal abstinence syndrome: transitioning methadone-treated infants from an inpatient to an outpatient setting. J Perinatol 2012;32(6):425–30.
27. Wallerstein E. Circumcision. The uniquely American medical enigma. Urol Clin North Am 1985;12(1):123–32.
28. Schechter NL. The undertreatment of pain in children: an overview. Pediatr Clin North Am 1989;36(4):781–94.
29. Humphrey T. Embryology of the central nervous system: with some correlations with functional development. Ala J Med Sci 1964;1:60–4.
30. Fitzgerald M, Beggs S. The neurobiology of pain: developmental aspects. Neuroscientist 2001;7(3):246–57.
31. Anand KJ, Hickey PR. Halothane-morphine compared with high-dose sufentanil for anesthesia and postoperative analgesia in neonatal cardiac surgery. N Engl J Med 1992;326(1):1–9.
32. Porter FL, Grunau RE, Anand KJ. Long-term effects of pain in infants. J Dev Behav Pediatr 1999;20(4):253–61.
33. Anand KJ, Scalzo FM. Can adverse neonatal experiences alter brain development and subsequent behavior? Biol Neonate 2000;77(2):69–82.
34. Bhutta AT, Anand KJ. Vulnerability of the developing brain. Neuronal mechanisms. Clin Perinatol 2002;29(3):357–72.
35. Taddio A, Katz J, Ilersich AL, et al. Effect of neonatal circumcision on pain response during subsequent routine vaccination. Lancet 1997;349(9052): 599–603.
36. Peters JW, Koot HM, de Boer JB, et al. Major surgery within the first 3 months of life and subsequent biobehavioral pain responses to immunization at later age: a case comparison study. Pediatrics 2003;111(1): 129–35.

37. Grunau RE, Oberlander TF, Whitfield MF, et al. Demographic and therapeutic determinants of pain reactivity in very low birth weight neonates at 32 Weeks' postconceptional Age. Pediatrics 2001;107(1):105–12.

38. Batton DG, Barrington KJ, Wallman C. Prevention and management of pain in the neonate: an update. Pediatrics 2006;118(5):2231–41.

39. Simons SH, van Dijk M, Anand KS, et al. Do we still hurt newborn babies? A prospective study of procedural pain and analgesia in neonates. Arch Pediatr Adolesc Med 2003;157(11):1058–64.

40. Porter FL, Wolf CM, Gold J, et al. Pain and pain management in newborn infants: a survey of physicians and nurses. Pediatrics 1997;100(4):626–32.

41. Gray L, Watt L, Blass EM. Skin-to-skin contact is analgesic in healthy newborns. Pediatrics 2000;105(1):e14.

42. Gray L, Miller LW, Philipp BL, et al. Breastfeeding is analgesic in healthy newborns. Pediatrics 2002;109(4):590–3.

43. Shah PS, Herbozo C, Aliwalas LL, et al. Breastfeeding or breast milk for procedural pain in neonates. Cochrane Database Syst Rev 2012;(12):CD004950.

44. Codipietro L, Ceccarelli M, Ponzone A. Breastfeeding or oral sucrose solution in term neonates receiving heel lance: a randomized, controlled trial. Pediatrics 2008;122(3):e716–21.

45. Iturriaga GS, Unceta-Barrenechea AA, Zarate KS, et al. Analgesic effect of breastfeeding when taking blood by heel-prick in newborns. An Pediatr (Barc) 2009;71(4):310–3 [in Spanish].

46. Marin Gabriel MA, del Rey Hurtado de Mendoza B, Jimenez Figueroa L, et al. Analgesia with breastfeeding in addition to skin-to-skin contact during heel prick. Arch Dis Child Fetal Neonatal Ed 2013;98(6):F499–503.

47. Curtis SJ, Jou H, Ali S, et al. A randomized controlled trial of sucrose and/or pacifier as analgesia for infants receiving venipuncture in a pediatric emergency department. BMC Pediatr 2007;7:27.

48. Ramenghi LA, Griffith GC, Wood CM, et al. Effect of non-sucrose sweet tasting solution on neonatal heel prick responses. Arch Dis Child Fetal Neonatal Ed 1996;74(2):F129–31.

49. Gibbins S, Stevens B, Hodnett E, et al. Efficacy and safety of sucrose for procedural pain relief in preterm and term neonates. Nurs Res 2002;51(6):375–82.

50. Harrison D, Johnston L, Loughnan P. Oral sucrose for procedural pain in sick hospitalized infants: a randomized-controlled trial. J Paediatr Child Health 2003;39(8):591–7.

51. Hatfield LA, Gusic ME, Dyer AM, et al. Analgesic properties of oral sucrose during routine immunizations at 2 and 4 months of age. Pediatrics 2008;121(2):e327–34.

52. Taddio A, Shah V, Hancock R, et al. Effectiveness of sucrose analgesia in newborns undergoing painful medical procedures. CMAJ 2008;179(1):37–43.

53. Stevens B, Yamada J, Lee GY, et al. Sucrose for analgesia in newborn infants undergoing painful procedures. Cochrane Database Syst Rev 2013;(1):CD001069.

54. Carbajal R, Lenclen R, Gajdos V, et al. Crossover trial of analgesic efficacy of glucose and pacifier in very preterm neonates during subcutaneous injections. Pediatrics 2002;110(2 Pt 1):389–93.

55. Okan F, Coban A, Ince Z, et al. Analgesia in preterm newborns: the comparative effects of sucrose and glucose. Eur J Pediatr 2007;166(10):1017–24.

56. Ramenghi LA, Webb AV, Shevlin PM, et al. Intra-oral administration of sweet-tasting substances and infants' crying response to immunization: a randomized, placebo-controlled trial. Biol Neonate 2002;81(3):163–9.

57. Lefrak L, Burch K, Caravantes R, et al. Sucrose analgesia: identifying potentially better practices. Pediatrics 2006;118(Suppl 2):S197–202.
58. Schechter NL, Zempsky WT, Cohen LL, et al. Pain reduction during pediatric immunizations: evidence-based review and recommendations. Pediatrics 2007; 119(5):e1184–98.
59. Ramenghi LA, Evans DJ, Levene MI. "Sucrose analgesia": absorptive mechanism or taste perception? Arch Dis Child Fetal Neonatal Ed 1999;80(2): F146–7.
60. Reboucas EC, Segato EN, Kishi R, et al. Effect of the blockade of mu1-opioid and 5HT2A-serotonergic/alpha1-noradrenergic receptors on sweet-substance-induced analgesia. Psychopharmacology 2005;179(2):349–55.
61. Colantuoni C, Rada P, McCarthy J, et al. Evidence that intermittent, excessive sugar intake causes endogenous opioid dependence. Obes Res 2002;10(6): 478–88.
62. Gradin M, Schollin J. The role of endogenous opioids in mediating pain reduction by orally administered glucose among newborns. Pediatrics 2005;115(4): 1004–7.
63. Johnston CC, Filion F, Snider L, et al. How much sucrose is too much sucrose? Pediatrics 2007;119(1):226.
64. Rushforth JA, Levene MI. Effect of sucrose on crying in response to heel stab. Arch Dis Child 1993;69(3):388–9.
65. Johnston CC, Filion F, Snider L, et al. Routine sucrose analgesia during the first week of life in neonates younger than 31 weeks' postconceptional age. Pediatrics 2002;110(3):523–8.
66. Abad F, Diaz-Gomez NM, Domenech E, et al. Oral sucrose compares favourably with lidocaine-prilocaine cream for pain relief during venepuncture in neonates. Acta Paediatr 2001;90(2):160–5.
67. Jain A, Rutter N. Does topical amethocaine gel reduce the pain of venepuncture in newborn infants? A randomised double blind controlled trial. Arch Dis Child Fetal Neonatal Ed 2000;83(3):F207–10.
68. Kaur G, Gupta P, Kumar A. A randomized trial of eutectic mixture of local anesthetics during lumbar puncture in newborns. Arch Pediatr Adolesc Med 2003; 157(11):1065–70.
69. Moore J. No more tears: a randomized controlled double-blind trial of Amethocaine gel vs. placebo in the management of procedural pain in neonates. J Adv Nurs 2001;34(4):475–82.
70. Stevens B, Johnston C, Taddio A, et al. Management of pain from heel lance with lidocaine-prilocaine (EMLA) cream: is it safe and efficacious in preterm infants? J Dev Behav Pediat 1999;20(4):216–21.
71. Taddio A, Ohlsson A, Einarson TR, et al. A systematic review of lidocaine-prilocaine cream (EMLA) in the treatment of acute pain in neonates. Pediatrics 1998;101(2):E1.
72. Taddio A, Stevens B, Craig K, et al. Efficacy and safety of lidocaine-prilocaine cream for pain during circumcision. N Engl J Med 1997;336(17): 1197–201.
73. Gradin M, Eriksson M, Holmqvist G, et al. Pain reduction at venipuncture in newborns: oral glucose compared with local anesthetic cream. Pediatrics 2002; 110(6):1053–7.
74. Lindh V, Wiklund U, Hakansson S. Heel lancing in term new-born infants: an evaluation of pain by frequency domain analysis of heart rate variability. Pain 1999;80(1–2):143–8.

75. Butler-O'Hara M, LeMoine C, Guillet R. Analgesia for neonatal circumcision: a randomized controlled trial of EMLA cream versus dorsal penile nerve block. Pediatrics 1998;101(4):E5.
76. Lehr VT, Cepeda E, Frattarelli DA, et al. Lidocaine 4% cream compared with lidocaine 2.5% and prilocaine 2.5% or dorsal penile block for circumcision. Am J Perinatol 2005;22(5):231–7.
77. Nioloux C, Floch-Tudal C, Jaby-Sergent MP, et al. Local anesthesia with Emla cream and risk of methemoglobinemia in a premature infant. Arch Pediatr 1995;2(3):291–2 [in French].
78. Couper RT. Methaemoglobinaemia secondary to topical lignocaine/prilocaine in a circumcised neonate. J Paediatr Child Health 2000;36(4):406–7.
79. Kumar AR, Dunn N, Naqvi M. Methemoglobinemia associated with a prilocaine-lidocaine cream. Clin Pediatr (Phila) 1997;36(4):239–40.
80. American Academy of Pediatrics Task Force on Circumcision. Male circumcision. Pediatrics 2012;130(3):e756–85.
81. Stang HJ, Snellman LW, Condon LM, et al. Beyond dorsal penile nerve block: a more humane circumcision. Pediatrics 1997;100(2):E3.
82. Kass FC, Holman JR. Oral glucose solution for analgesia in infant circumcision. J Fam Pract 2001;50(9):785–8.
83. Brady-Fryer B, Wiebe N, Lander JA. Pain relief for neonatal circumcision. Cochrane Database Syst Rev 2004;(4):CD004217.
84. Howard CR, Howard FM, Weitzman ML. Acetaminophen analgesia in neonatal circumcision: the effect on pain. Pediatrics 1994;93(4):641–6.
85. Lander J, Brady-Fryer B, Metcalfe JB, et al. Comparison of ring block, dorsal penile nerve block, and topical anesthesia for neonatal circumcision: a randomized controlled trial. JAMA 1997;278(24):2157–62.
86. Snellman LW, Stang HJ. Prospective evaluation of complications of dorsal penile nerve block for neonatal circumcision. Pediatrics 1995;95(5):705–8.
87. Maxwell LG, Yaster M, Wetzel RC, et al. Penile nerve block for newborn circumcision. Obstet Gynecol 1987;70(3 Pt 1):415–9.
88. Hardwick-Smith S, Mastrobattista JM, Wallace PA, et al. Ring block for neonatal circumcision. Obstet Gynecol 1998;91(6):930–4.
89. Machmouchi M, Alkhotani A. Is neonatal circumcision judicious? Eur J Pediatr Surg 2007;17(4):266–9.
90. Nebert DW, Zhang G, Vesell ES. From human genetics and genomics to pharmacogenetics and pharmacogenomics: past lessons, future directions. Drug Metab Rev 2008;40(2):187–224.
91. Evans WE, Relling MV. Pharmacogenomics: translating functional genomics into rational therapeutics. Science 1999;286(5439):487–91.
92. International Human Genome Sequencing Consortium. Finishing the euchromatic sequence of the human genome. Nature 2004;431:931–45.
93. Stockmann C, Fassl B, Gaedigk R, et al. Fluticasone propionate pharmacogenetics: CYP3A4*22 polymorphism and pediatric asthma control. J Pediatr 2013;162(6):1222–7, 1227.e1–2.
94. Ingelman-Sundberg M. Genetic polymorphisms of cytochrome P450 2D6 (CYP2D6): clinical consequences, evolutionary aspects and functional diversity. Pharmacogenomics J 2005;5(1):6–13.
95. Madadi P, Ciszkowski C, Gaedigk A, et al. Genetic transmission of cytochrome P450 2D6 (CYP2D6) ultrarapid metabolism: implications for breastfeeding women taking codeine. Curr Drug Saf 2011;6(1):36–9.

96. Madadi P, Amstutz U, Rieder M, et al. Clinical practice guideline: CYP2D6 genotyping for safe and efficacious codeine therapy. J Popul Ther Clin Pharmacol 2013;20(3):e369–96.

97. Koren G, Cairns J, Chitayat D, et al. Pharmacogenetics of morphine poisoning in a breastfed neonate of a codeine-prescribed mother. Lancet 2006;368(9536): 704.

98. Kearns GL, Abdel-Rahman SM, Alander SW, et al. Developmental pharmacology–drug disposition, action, and therapy in infants and children. N Engl J Med 2003;349(12):1157–67.

99. Leeder JS, Kearns GL. Pharmacogenetics in pediatrics. Implications for practice. Pediatr Clin North Am 1997;44(1):55–77.

100. Saarenmaa E, Neuvonen PJ, Fellman V. Gestational age and girth weight effects on plasma clearance of fentanyl in newborn infants. J Pediatr 2000;136:767–70.

101. Kullo IJ, Haddad R, Prows CA, et al. Return of results in the genomic medicine projects of the eMERGE network. Front Genet 2014;5:50.

Discharge Planning

Brian M. Barkemeyer, MD

KEYWORDS

- Neonatal intensive care unit • Discharge planning • Screening test • Circumcision
- Late preterm infant • High-risk infant

KEY POINTS

- Hospital discharge is a time of transition for infants and families that requires oversight of common postnatal adaptations, screening tests, and establishment of necessary follow-up care.
- Preterm infants face additional medical problems that vary in complexity by degree of prematurity, with infants born at lowest gestational age (<28 weeks) at highest risk for complicated neonatal course and adverse long-term outcomes.
- High-risk infants often have complex problems that require coordinated follow-up after discharge essential for improved outcomes.

INTRODUCTION

Initial hospital discharge of the infant is a time of great excitement and anxiety for the family. Health care provider and family anxiety may be heightened by any combination of actual or perceived medical and/or social risks. Preparation of the infant and family for discharge is an involved process that is best done through a consistent approach from all members of the health care team perceptive to the needs of the infant and family. Although most hospitals have routine patterns of newborn care, medical documentation, and discharge order sets, it is important that each relevant aspect of care is applied appropriately to each child at discharge. The optimal time for discharge of the apparently healthy newborn depends on several factors including the infant's condition, risk for evolving problems (eg, infection, poor feeding, jaundice, and drug withdrawal), the ability of the family to provide appropriate care for the infant, and the timely availability of appropriate follow-up.

Nursing, medical, and support staff should be attuned to the interaction of the infant and family throughout the initial hospital course to recognize concerns about the ability of the family to provide appropriate care. Additionally, variations from normal in an infant's health and behavior should be documented and communicated effectively by

Disclosure: None.
Neonatology, Louisiana State University Health Sciences Center, 200 Henry Clay Avenue, New Orleans, LA 70118, USA
E-mail address: bbarke@lsuhsc.edu

Pediatr Clin N Am 62 (2015) 545–556
http://dx.doi.org/10.1016/j.pcl.2014.11.013 **pediatric.theclinics.com**

all health care providers. Discharge examination of the newborn should be thorough with documentation of adequate transition from the intrauterine environment to include establishment of normal respirations, normal circulatory status, adequate feeding, normal voiding and stooling patterns, and adequate thermoregulation. Infants who fail to meet these criteria should not be discharged home and additional assessment may be needed. Before hospital discharge, physical examination should include assessment for the presence of a red reflex from the eyes bilaterally and for any evidence of developmental dysplasia of the hip. The red reflex should be bilateral, symmetric, and without dark spots or white opacity.[1] Female infants, infants born with breech presentation, and infants with a family history of this disorder are at highest risk for developmental dysplasia of the hip. When definite dislocation of the hip is noted, prompt referral to an orthopedist is warranted; when the examination is equivocal, serial follow-up examinations are warranted. If necessary, further assessment for developmental dysplasia of the hip can be performed with hip ultrasound.[2] The efficacy of these traditional recommendations for screening for developmental dysplasia of the hip and common interventions has more recently been questioned.[3]

SCREENING TESTS

Routine screening of mothers and infants for a variety of common and uncommon conditions has allowed for timely recognition and intervention resulting in ongoing significant improvements in perinatal outcomes. Many of these screening tools are discussed in greater detail elsewhere in this issue, and appropriate follow-up of abnormal results and pending studies is essential at hospital discharge. Follow-up of all relevant maternal screening tests requires effective communication between obstetric and newborn care providers. Timely identification of infants at risk for infection based on maternal screening tests (including gonorrhea, syphilis, HIV, hepatitis B, and group B streptococcus) should be accomplished in the immediate neonatal period, and follow-up on all such tests and their impact on the infant should be done at the time of discharge.

Although newborn metabolic screening results may not be available at the time of hospital discharge, it is important that specimens are obtained before discharge with proper follow-up mechanisms established. A hearing screen should be obtained before hospital discharge with awareness of ongoing factors, such as infection, ototoxic drug exposure, and severe jaundice, which may alter results. At-risk infants should be identified with appropriate follow-up testing in place at discharge.[4]

Screening for congenital heart disease should be performed with pulse oximetry after the first 24 hours of life in all infants, with infants with oxygen saturations less than 90% being evaluated immediately for potential cardiac malformation if there is no other obvious cause. Infants with oxygen saturations greater than or equal to 95% and less than 3% difference in saturation between right hand and either lower extremity are considered to have passed this screen.[5]

Because it is known that preterm and other infants may have apnea, bradycardia, and/or oxygen desaturation when placed semiupright in a car seat, it is recommended that infants of gestational age less than 37 weeks and other at-risk infants (eg, Down syndrome, hypotonia, congenital heart disease) undergo a period of observation in their car seat before discharge. This period of observation should be 90 to 120 minutes, or more if travel duration is longer. Infants who experience problems during this screen should be reassessed with changes in support or position to ensure safety. Family members should be educated in the importance of proper use of car restraints.[6]

Jaundice is a common problem in newborn infants during the first few days of life, which typically is self-limited or easily treated, but can put the infant at significant risk for adverse neurologic outcome if not monitored appropriately for timely intervention. Awareness of risk factors for excessive jaundice, such as hemolysis, excessive bruising, or poor feeding, is important along with visual screening and transcutaneous bilirubin determination. Transcutaneous bilirubin screening is noninvasive; relatively inexpensive; and avoids inadequacies of visual screening, such as poor lighting, poor color perception, or a newborn with darker skin tone. Comparison of screening bilirubin values with available time-dependent bilirubin nomograms helps identify higher-risk infants before hospital discharge. When transcutaneous bilirubin screening suggests a need for therapy, serum bilirubin should be promptly obtained to make appropriate clinical decisions. Infants who do not require intervention for hyperbilirubinemia and are otherwise ready for discharge may be safely discharged if timely follow-up of subsequent bilirubin levels is available.[7]

FEEDING

It is commonly accepted that exclusive breastfeeding is the optimal feeding method for infants for the first 6 months of life, and breastfeeding can continue beyond that up to 12 months or longer as mutually desired by the mother and infant. Achievement of higher sustained breastfeeding rates has significant medical benefits for infants and their mothers along with significant economic benefits for families and society. There are several barriers to effective breastfeeding including many within the birth hospital. Common hospital practices that have a negative influence on successful breastfeeding initiation include a lack of emotional and practical support for breastfeeding mothers, delays in initiation or limitations on duration of breastfeeding, and early introduction of supplemental formulas and pacifiers.[8] Pacifiers have been associated with a lower incidence of sudden infant death syndrome (SIDS), so if desired, their use should be restricted until after breastfeeding is well-established.[9]

Throughout the hospital stay and at the time of discharge, the adequacy of the mother's ability to breastfeed her infant should be assessed. Mothers with prior breast surgery, flat or inverted nipples, or difficult delivery are at greatest risk for problems in establishing adequate breastfeeding. Assessment of the mother's milk production, infant feeding practices, voiding and stooling patterns, and serial infant weight are needed. Because the establishment of breastfeeding is an ongoing process that typically continues after discharge, close monitoring of this evolution is necessary, especially for mother-infant pairs with suspicion or evidence of delays. Supplementation of breastfeeding should be limited in duration and for defined conditions (persistent hypoglycemia, dehydration as evidenced by inadequate voiding and stooling, and excessive weight loss >10% of birthweight). Breastfed infants should receive supplemental vitamin D, 400 IU per day.

Infants who are not breastfed need to have their intake, output, and weight monitored, although most infants quickly adapt to an ad lib intake. Mothers who decide against or are unable to breastfeed their child should be supported in this process. Formula-fed infants should receive an iron-fortified cow's milk–based formula unless there is a defined need for an alternative. There is no need for routine additional vitamin D supplementation of formula-fed infants.

CIRCUMCISION

Circumcision of newborn male infants has been a topic of great discussion and passion for several years. Although some medical benefits of circumcision are definite, opponents view any such benefits as limited given the risks and potential pain of the procedure. Proponents have argued that the procedure affords lifelong benefits with limited risk and can be safely done with appropriate anesthesia. In 2012, the American Academy of Pediatrics issued a Circumcision Policy Statement that stated, "preventive health benefits of elective circumcision of male newborns outweigh the risks of the procedure." Additionally, the policy states that circumcision lowers the risk of urinary tract infection (UTI) and acquisition of HIV and other sexually transmitted diseases, but these benefits are not so great to warrant routine circumcision for all male infants; if a family desires circumcision for medical and cultural reasons, the procedure should be safely done.

In addition to familiarity with the policy statements, such as that of the American Academy of Pediatrics, health care providers should be prepared to answer a family's questions about this procedure. The three primary benefits of circumcision are a reduced incidence of UTI, sexually transmitted diseases, and penile cancer. The number needed to treat for reduction of male UTI is 100, meaning that for every 100 circumcisions performed, one male UTI is prevented. Circumcision lowers transmission rates for HIV, herpes simplex virus type 2, and human papilloma virus. Penile cancer is rare, and current data to assess the impact of circumcision on risk are limited. Opponents to circumcision question the supportive data indicating reduction in sexually transmitted diseases and penile cancer are benefits of the procedure.

Circumcision done in the newborn period is generally safer and better-tolerated than in older males. Circumcision should be done by an appropriately trained provider using sterile technique. Appropriate anesthesia may include sucrose solution in addition to topical anesthetic or injectable local nerve block. There is no clear advantage to any of the three most commonly used techniques (Plastibell device, Gomco clamp, or Mogen clamp). Bleeding is the most frequent complication of circumcision, but it is usually limited. Significant complications are reported in 0.2% of all circumcisions. There is no evidence for diminished sexual pleasure or performance as a result of circumcision. Poor cosmetic outcome is a concern for some parents, but concerned parents should be advised that appearance will likely evolve to a more acceptable one over time.

Despite the available medical data, the decision for circumcision for most families is most strongly influenced by religious, cultural, and personal motives. At present, payment for the procedure by many third-party payors is limited.[10–13]

DISCHARGE OF THE LATE PRETERM INFANT

Lacking the physiologic maturity of the term infant, the late preterm infant is at higher risk of problems, such as feeding difficulty, hypoglycemia, hyperbilirubinemia, hypothermia, apnea, and respiratory distress. Because these infants lack some of the more obvious acute problems of infants born at earlier gestation and they are often managed in a regular nursery with full-term infants, a lack of awareness by caretakers and families of the potential for these problems may result in ever greater risks of morbidity and mortality. Additionally, there may be interplay between these problems, such as a late preterm infant with hypothermia with resulting tachypnea and further worsening of immature feeding processes, thus placing the infant at higher risk for hypoglycemia and hyperbilirubinemia.

The problems of the late preterm infant may not fully resolve at the time of discharge, and infants may regress in what initially seemed to be a normal feeding pattern. Sooner and more frequent outpatient follow-up may reduce the increased risk for readmission that these infants face. Ideally, the late preterm infant should be seen as an outpatient within 48 hours of discharge. At follow-up, close monitoring of feeding, voiding, and stooling is essential with serial weight measurements and observation of jaundice also necessary. Ultimately, the late preterm infant is at increased risk for developmental delays; close developmental follow-up is needed to provide timely allied health therapy interventions.[14,15]

DISCHARGE OF THE PRETERM INFANT AFTER NEONATAL INTENSIVE CARE UNIT STAY

Discharge of the preterm infant after neonatal intensive care unit (NICU) stay requires close attention to health care maintenance and follow-up for specific problems of prematurity that may require visits to several physicians and therapists. Timing of discharge for the complex infant is determined by the current stability and needs of the infant; the ability of caregivers to meet those needs in the home setting; and increasingly, outside pressures to limit duration of hospital stay. Thoughtful and thorough discharge planning may help reduce the high risks for morbidity, mortality, and hospital readmission these infants face.

In general, the preterm infant can be safely discharged from the NICU when the infant is able to feed adequately to allow for appropriate weight gain; is able to maintain appropriate body temperature without external heat sources; is able to receive any additional necessary medical care or therapy in the home setting; and is able to be cared for in a home with capable caretakers properly equipped with all necessary nutrition, medications, and equipment. Determining the readiness of a particular infant to meet each of these criteria depends on several variables in addition to gestational age and weight. Infants may meet one criteria (eg, adequate thermoregulation) but not another (eg, poor feeding); thus, it is not possible to routinely discharge a preterm infant at a given gestational age and weight. Although most infants are able to be safely discharged by 36 to 37 weeks postmenstrual age, some may be ready as early as 33 to 34 weeks, whereas others may require hospitalization well beyond these postmenstrual ages. Infants of lowest gestational age and birthweight are more likely to require discharge at a later gestational age.[16–18]

Oral feedings are typically introduced to preterm infants around 33 to 34 weeks postmenstrual age with appropriate maturation of the ability to coordinate sucking, swallowing, and breathing. Gaining proficiency at oral feedings varies by infant and depends on neurodevelopment and associated health problems; preterm infants with neurologic impairment or chronic lung disease may have significant delays in achieving proficiency at oral feeding. Gastroesophageal reflux is common in preterm infants; for most preterm infants without other comorbidities, gastroesophageal reflux is self-limited and typically does not require specific treatment. For preterm infants with comorbidities, such as neurologic impairment, chronic lung disease, or apnea, a variety of therapies for gastroesophageal reflux have been used including positional maneuvers, thickened feedings, acid-suppression medication, or prokinetic medication. There is no consensus among a variety of pediatric specialists for the optimal management of significant gastroesophageal reflux, but therapy should be provided in stepwise fashion with ongoing assessment for improvement.

A pattern of adequate growth on a specific feeding regimen that can be mimicked at home should be established before discharge. Breast milk is the optimal nutrition for preterm infants throughout the hospital stay and after discharge. Breast milk typically requires supplementation to augment calories, protein, sodium, and calcium intake in the preterm infant. In the hospital setting, this is often accomplished through the addition of commercial human milk fortifiers. Postdischarge, supplementation if necessary may be accomplished more economically by the addition of postdischarge formula to human milk intake. For the preterm infant not feeding breast milk, a fortified 22 calorie/

ounce preterm infant formula should be used after discharge. The duration of time postdischarge to use fortified human milk or 22 calorie/ounce preterm infant formula is variable and depends on degree of prematurity, growth, and associated medical problems, such as osteopenia. Infants born at less than 28 weeks gestation with ongoing medical problems may benefit for 12 months adjusted age, whereas infants of higher gestational age with few associated medical problems and steady growth may limit duration to 6 to 9 months adjusted age. Weight, length, and head circumference of the preterm infant after NICU discharge should be plotted regularly on growth curves designed for preterm infants.

Infants born at lower gestational ages (<28 weeks gestation) with prolonged total parenteral nutrition (TPN) use lack adequate bone mineralization at birth, which can develop into osteopenia of prematurity. Preterm infants who receive full or partial breast milk, or take in less than 1000 mL infant formula, should receive vitamin D, 400 IU daily.[19]

Despite advances in care for very low birthweight infants, nutritional care in the NICU is unable to match growth rates achieved in utero. Postdischarge, growth needs to be closely monitored with regular plotting of weight, length, and head circumference against standardized curves for the preterm infant. Because many preterm infants are at risk for developmental delay, it is essential that optimal nutrition for brain growth be provided in the first year of life.

Among very low birthweight infants who require TPN for more than 14 days, approximately 50% may develop TPN cholestasis with resultant elevation in direct bilirubin. Although TPN cholestasis is the most common cause for direct hyperbilirubinemia in the NICU population, there are a myriad of other potential causes for this problem that should not be overlooked. The extent of evaluation for any single infant to rule out other less common causes of elevated direct bilirubin is an individualized decision, but more common anatomic, infectious, and metabolic causes should be investigated. In most cases of TPN cholestasis, as feeds are resumed, a gradual resolution of the elevated direct bilirubin occurs. This resolution may continue after hospital discharge, necessitating serial laboratory observations to assess for return to normal of total and direct bilirubin levels. In some infants with more significant TPN cholestasis, therapy at hospital discharge may include specialty formulas with medium-chain triglycerides as the source of lipids, drugs that may increase bile acid flow (phenobarbital, ursodeoxycholic acid), and fat-soluble vitamin supplementation (vitamins A, D, E, K).[20]

A common hematologic problem in preterm infants is anemia of prematurity, which is an accentuation of the physiologic anemia that occurs in term infants, albeit sooner after birth and with resultant lower hemoglobin concentrations. Depending on the preterm infant's other problems of prematurity impacting oxygen delivery and oxygen needs, anemia of prematurity is more likely to be symptomatic than what occurs in term infants. During the acute stages of illness from prematurity, red blood cell transfusion may be necessary to replace ongoing losses from blood sampling for necessary laboratory tests. As the overall condition of the preterm infant improves closer to and beyond hospital discharge, the threshold for transfusion is unknown. Repeated transfusions late in the course of anemia of prematurity continue to delay recovery from this problem because the infant's own erythropoietin production is inhibited. In general, the preterm infant discharged from the hospital with anemia of prematurity should be monitored for adequate nutrition including sufficient iron in the diet, the absence of obvious symptoms related to anemia (persistent tachycardia, poor weight gain), and the gradual recovery of hemoglobin levels to normal. For infants with anemia of prematurity, evidence of spontaneous increase in hemoglobin concentration coupled with evidence of reticulocytosis is reassuring.

Apnea of prematurity is a common problem in preterm infants, especially those born at lower gestational ages. For most infants, resolution of apnea of prematurity occurs around the same time that other maturational events occur (oral feeding, thermoregulation). For some preterm infants, apnea of prematurity may continue after maturation in oral feeding and thermoregulation have occurred, thus delaying hospital discharge. Management of such infants varies, but in general, all infants should have a period of 3 to 7 days free of significant apnea or bradycardia before discharge. In some cases, methylxanthine therapy with caffeine or theophylline may be used to treat apnea of prematurity. Caffeine has a higher therapeutic index and once-daily dosing, thus it is the preferred drug for apnea of prematurity.

Apnea of prematurity typically resolves by 36 to 40 weeks postmenstrual age, but in infants born at less than 28 weeks gestation, it may persist to 44 weeks postmenstrual age. Management of infants otherwise ready for discharge who have ongoing minor cardiorespiratory events caused by apnea of prematurity varies. Caffeine therapy and/or home monitoring may be used to allow for earlier discharge of such infants. In most cases, caffeine therapy and/or home monitoring can be discontinued after 44 weeks postmenstrual age. Gastroesophageal reflux may coexist with apnea of prematurity in some infants, further complicating clinical assessment and decision making.

Although families may be concerned about potential links between apnea of prematurity and SIDS, the only link between these entities is that preterm infants are at increased risk for both. There is no evidence that preterm infants with apnea of prematurity are at a higher risk of SIDS than preterm infants without apnea of prematurity. Although acute management of preterm infants early in their hospital course may require prone positioning, most infants should be placed supine to sleep by 32 weeks postmenstrual age. The "Back to Sleep" campaign has reduced the rate of SIDS in term and preterm infants (**Box 1**).[21]

THE PRETERM INFANT WITH SPECIAL NEEDS AFTER DISCHARGE

A small subset of preterm infants may have special needs after discharge beyond their peers. Infants discharged on medications for ongoing medical problems, such as bronchopulmonary dysplasia, apnea of prematurity, or other complications related to prematurity, may require dosage adjustment for weight gain after discharge. Before hospital discharge, a plan of management for such complicated patients should be developed, including follow-up visits with pediatric specialists as needed to assist in management decisions.

Infants who continue to have feeding difficulties may require alternative means of feeding. In select instances, home gavage feedings may be used to allow for hospital discharge of an infant expected to progress to full oral feedings in a short period of time. Infants for whom home gavage feedings are used should be otherwise free of significant medical problems and have parents who are willing, capable, and trained to administer gavage feedings before discharge. Attempts at oral feedings should be continued with the family trained in the necessary skills to do so.

For infants unable to feed orally and unlikely to make progress to do so in a reasonable amount of time, placement of a feeding gastrostomy tube may be necessary. Parents should be educated in the administration of gastrostomy tube feedings, care of the gastrostomy site, and management when the gastrostomy tube is unexpectedly displaced. For any alternative feeding method, necessary supplies and replacements should be reliably provided.

Infants with severe bronchopulmonary dysplasia may require home oxygen therapy. Caretakers should be educated in the set-up and administration of supplemental

---

Box 1
Primary care checklist for the preterm NICU graduate

Nutrition

  Type, caloric density, volume, method of intake

  Use of growth chart (preterm specific)

Current medications

  Are they necessary?

  Are the doses appropriate for current weight?

Immunizations

  Are routine immunizations up to date?

  Is infant a palivizumab candidate?

Respiratory

  Any use of supplemental oxygen or aerosols?

  Any current issues with apnea of prematurity?

Anemia of prematurity

  Is there need for follow-up hemoglobin level?

Neurodevelopmental

  What are results of prior cranial imaging studies?

  Is there retinopathy of prematurity and is follow-up necessary?

  Is follow-up hearing assessment needed?

  Ongoing developmental screening

Car and home safety monitoring/guidance

Is family support appropriate for infant?

Other problems?

Other necessary follow-up?

---

home oxygen. Infants discharged on home oxygen therapy should be monitored with either continuous pulse oximetry or cardiorespiratory monitoring to recognize complications that may result from unexpected loss of supplemental oxygen. A plan for weaning home oxygen and appropriate follow-up should be established before discharge and modified based on the infant's condition.

Infants who require tracheostomy to establish an adequate airway are at risk for complications after discharge. Families should be instructed in tracheostomy care including suctioning, management of humidification and/or oxygen supplementation, and emergency tracheostomy replacement. Instruction should include assessment of independent skills in tracheostomy management. A care plan with outpatient subspecialty support should be established before discharge. As with all other specialty equipment, procurement of appropriate supplies before discharge is essential.

Intraventricular hemorrhage occurs inversely with gestational age, with significant intraventricular hemorrhage highest in infants of gestational age less than 28 weeks. Significant intraventricular hemorrhage (grades III or IV) is an important cause of adverse neurologic outcomes including mental retardation, cerebral palsy, or hydrocephalus. In most cases of posthemorrhagic hydrocephalus, the evolution of the problem and need for cerebrospinal fluid diversion (most often through ventriculoperitoneal shunt placement) occurs during the initial hospital stay. In some infants, evolution of hydrocephalus may continue after discharge necessitating serial evaluations of ventricular enlargement by head ultrasound or other neuroimaging studies. Assessment of head growth in all discharged preterm infants is an important part of ongoing follow-up to recognize inadequate or excessive head growth in a timely fashion.

Similar to other problems of prematurity, retinopathy of prematurity is most significant in infants born at lower gestational ages and full resolution of the problem may not occur until after hospital discharge. Most infants born at less than 28 weeks gestation develop retinopathy of prematurity, but most cases resolve without intervention and without visual loss. Timely recognition of retinopathy of prematurity is essential because current interventions with cryotherapy and/or intraocular bevacizumab if necessary can significantly improve visual outcomes when offered at optimal time. Unnecessary delays in referral, screening, or intervention can result in unnecessary blindness. It is essential that discharge plans for follow-up of infants at ongoing risk for retinopathy of prematurity be communicated effectively with parents and to the primary care physician; need for follow-up should be reinforced regularly with primary care follow-up visits.[22]

The most complicated preterm infant may remain medically fragile even after hospital discharge. Often these infants have illness involving multiple organ systems that may require various combinations of medications, oxygen therapy, respiratory support, specialty feedings, and multiple pediatric subspecialty follow-up visits. Although the complexity of illness involving any individual organ system may go beyond what is cared for by the general pediatrician, the general pediatrician as primary care provider is often placed in the role of gatekeeper or coordinator of care. It is essential that timely and thorough communication between the subspecialists and pediatrician be in place. In the role of primary care provider, the pediatrician must also assume the role of patient advocate for these complicated infants. Rehospitalization is much more common for the medically complicated infant because of exacerbations of existing problems or development of intercurrent illness, such as respiratory or gastrointestinal viral infections. Avoidance of sick contacts, frequent hand washing, and appropriate immunizations are essential to minimize the risk of intercurrent illness.

OUTCOME FOR THE PRETERM INFANT

Although the rate of preterm birth in the United States has declined slightly in recent years, births before 37 weeks gestation accounted for 11.6% of all births in 2012, with births of low birthweight infants (<2500 g) accounting for 8% of all births. Although all preterm infants have higher risks of short- and long-term complications compared with term infants, the greatest risk for mortality and long-term morbidity occurs in very low birthweight infants (<1500 g), which accounted for 1.4% of all United States deliveries in 2012 (**Table 1**).[23]

Improvements in neonatal care have allowed for progressive improvements in survival of preterm infants with survival rates for infants in the National Institute of Child Health and Human Development Neonatal Research Network ranging from 6% at 22 weeks gestation to 92% at 28 weeks gestation. Morbidity and mortality continue to be highest at the lower gestational ages. In general, lower gestational age and greater severity of short-term morbidities are associated with higher risks of long-term adverse neurodevelopmental outcome. Female gender, antenatal steroid use,

Table 1
Gestational age-specific outcome from National Institute of Child Health and Human Development network NICUs

Gestational Age	22 wk	23 wk	24 wk	25 wk	26 wk	27 wk	28 wk
Survival to discharge	6	26	55	72	84	88	92
Survival without major morbidity[a]	0	8	9	20	34	44	57

[a] Severe intraventricular hemorrhage, periventricular leukomalacia, bronchopulmonary dysplasia, necrotizing enterocolitis, infections, and retinopathy of prematurity stage $\geq$3.
Adapted from Stoll BJ, Hansen NI, Bell EF, et al. Neonatal outcomes of extremely preterm infants from the NICHD neonatal research network. Pediatrics 2010;126:443–56.

maternal education at or above high school, and the absence of major neonatal morbidities have been identified as independent predictors of unimpaired outcome at 30 months of age.[24]

Preterm infants born beyond 28 weeks are at limited risk for adverse medical and neurologic outcome when compared with infants born at lower gestational ages, with most infants born beyond 28 weeks gestation having normal outcomes. Despite the higher likelihood of normal outcome, because the risk of adverse outcome remains higher in this subgroup than that of term infants, close medical and developmental follow-up by the primary care physician is warranted.

Because of significantly higher risks of adverse medical and neurologic outcomes for infants born less than or equal to 28 weeks gestation, these infants require close follow-up for ongoing medical problems and neurodevelopmental impairment. High-risk follow-up clinics offer multidisciplinary resources that may be helpful in the ongoing evaluation and therapy for such infants. Most such high-risk clinics offer in depth neurodevelopmental follow-up, and some may also offer primary or specialty care for the NICU graduate. For infants who meet established inclusion criteria, referral to high-risk follow-up clinic should be done before hospital discharge.

Early intervention programs in the United States are federally funded programs administered by states to provide timely evaluation and intervention for infants from birth through 2 years of age who are experiencing developmental delays or at high risk for developmental delays based on established physical or mental conditions. Criteria for evaluation and services provided vary by state, but most high-risk NICU graduates meet these criteria.

THE HIGH-RISK FAMILY

For the family of any infant requiring NICU care, the hospital course and discharge planning process can be a stressful time. Even well-adjusted families need guidance and support through this difficult process. Families with independent risk factors for adverse outcomes, such as poverty, lack of education, lack of social support, domestic abuse, or substance abuse, may require extra resources and support leading up to and after discharge.

Families should be encouraged to visit their hospitalized child frequently, and they should be kept abreast of their child's problems and management plans. As the infant's condition stabilizes and especially as the time for discharge nears, the family should have progressive involvement in their child's care. Rooming-in opportunity should be provided for all parents, and mandated for at-risk parents or parents of infants with complex home care requirements. Postdischarge, resources that may aid in transition include early and frequent follow-up with the primary care provider, home health nursing, lactation specialist, and other available community support agencies.

In support of proper transition of care from the NICU to the home setting, effective communication of pertinent details from the hospital course to follow-up physicians and other care providers is important. Summarizing a lengthy NICU stay in a document that is understandable, is not too long, and provides relevant information for ongoing care is a skill that should be mastered by the neonatologist. In providing such a summary, the more practical details provided involve ongoing care rather than extensive details of resolved problems. Resolved problems are relevant, but should be mentioned in summary format. Electronic medical record access can be useful to identify more detailed information when necessary.

Care and support of the sick infant through a NICU stay requires an extensive amount of resources. For improved long-term outcomes to occur, successful transition of the high-risk infant from the hospital to home setting is necessary, including transition of care from the neonatologist to the primary care physician.

REFERENCES

1. American Academy of Pediatrics Section on Ophthalmology. Red reflex examination in neonates, infants, and children. Pediatrics 2008;122:1401–4.
2. Clinical practice guideline: early detection of developmental dysplasia of the hip. Subcommittee on Developmental Dysplasia of the Hip. American Academy of Pediatrics. Pediatrics 2000;105:896–905.
3. Shipman SA, Helfund M, Moyer VA, et al. Screening for developmental dysplasia of the hip: a systematic review for the US preventive services task force. Pediatrics 2006;117:e57–76.
4. American Academy of Pediatrics Joint Committee on Infant Hearing. Year 2007 position statement: principles and guidelines for early hearing detection and intervention programs. Pediatrics 2007;120:898–921.
5. Mahle WT, Newburger JW, Matherne GP, et al. Role of pulse oximetry in examining newborns congenital heart disease: a scientific statement from the AHA and AAP. Pediatrics 2009;124:123–36.
6. Bull MJ, Engle WA. Safe transportation of preterm and low birth weight infants at hospital discharge. Pediatrics 2009;123:1424–9.
7. American Academy of Pediatrics Subcommittee on Hyperbilirubinemia. Clinical practice guideline: management of hyperbilirubinemia in the newborn infant 35 or more weeks gestation. Pediatrics 2004;114:297–316.
8. Eidelman AI, Schanler RJ. American Academy of Pediatrics section on breastfeeding. Breastfeeding and the use of human milk. Pediatrics 2012;129:e827–41.
9. Hauck FR, Omojokun OO, Siadaty MS. Do pacifiers reduce the risk of sudden infant death syndrome? A meta-analysis. Pediatrics 2005;116:e716–23.
10. American Academy of Pediatrics Task Force on Circumcision. Circumcision policy statement. Pediatrics 2012;130:585–6.
11. American Academy of Pediatrics Task Force on Circumcision. Male circumcision. Pediatrics 2012;130:e756–85.
12. Frisch M, Aigrain Y, Barauskas V, et al. Cultural bias in the AAP's 2012 technical report and policy statement on male circumcision. Pediatrics 2013;131:796–800.
13. American Academy of Pediatrics Task Force on Circumcision. Cultural bias and circumcision: the AAP task force on circumcision responds. Pediatrics 2013;131:801–4.
14. Engle WA, Tomashek KM, Wallman C, Committee on Fetus and Newborn, American Academy of Pediatrics. Late-preterm infants: a population at risk. Pediatrics 2007;120:1390–401.

15. Kugelman A, Colin AA. Late preterm infants: near term but still in a critical developmental time period. Pediatrics 2013;132:741–51.
16. American Academy of Pediatrics Committee on Fetus and Newborn. Hospital discharge of the high-risk neonate: proposed guidelines. Pediatrics 1998;102:411–7.
17. American Academy of Pediatrics Committee on Fetus and Newborn. Hospital discharge of the high-risk neonate. Pediatrics 2008;122:1119–26.
18. Andrews B, Pellerite M, Myers P, et al. NICU follow-up: medical and developmental management age 0-3 years. Neoreviews 2014;15:e123–32.
19. Abrams SA, American Academy of Pediatrics Committee on Nutrition. Calcium and vitamin D requirements of enterally fed preterm infants. Pediatrics 2013;131:e1676–83.
20. Feldman AG, Sokol RJ. Neonatal cholestasis. Neoreviews 2013;14:e63–73.
21. American Academy of Pediatrics Task Force on Sudden Infant Death Syndrome Policy Statement. SIDS and other sleep-related infant deaths: expansion of recommendations for a safe sleeping environment. Pediatrics 2011;128:1030–9.
22. American Academy of Pediatrics Section on Ophthalmology Policy Statement. Screening examination of premature infants for retinopathy of prematurity. Pediatrics 2013;131:189–95.
23. Martin JA, Hamilton BE, Osterman MJ, et al. Births: final data for 2012. Natl Vital Stat Rep 2013;62:1–69, 72. Available at: http://www.cdc.gov/nchs/data/nvsr/nvsr62/nvsr62_09.pdf. Accessed September 23, 2014.
24. Stoll BJ, Hansen NI, Bell EF, et al. Neonatal outcomes of extremely preterm infants from the NICHD neonatal research network. Pediatrics 2010;126:443–56.

Index

Note: Page numbers of article titles are in **boldface** type.

Pediatr Clin N Am 62 (2015) 557–570
http://dx.doi.org/10.1016/S0031-3955(15)00034-6
0031-3955/15/$ – see front matter © 2015 Elsevier Inc. All rights reserved.

pediatric.theclinics.com

Moving?

Make sure your subscription moves with you!

To notify us of your new address, find your **Clinics Account Number** (located on your mailing label above your name), and contact customer service at:

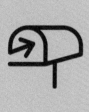

Email: journalscustomerservice-usa@elsevier.com

800-654-2452 (subscribers in the U.S. & Canada)
314-447-8871 (subscribers outside of the U.S. & Canada)

Fax number: 314-447-8029

Elsevier Health Sciences Division
Subscription Customer Service
3251 Riverport Lane
Maryland Heights, MO 63043

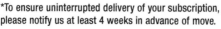

*To ensure uninterrupted delivery of your subscription, please notify us at least 4 weeks in advance of move.

ELSEVIER

Printed and bound by CPI Group (UK) Ltd, Croydon, CR0 4YY

08/06/2025

01896875-0001